Thieme

Neurosurgery Primary Examination Review

Questions and Answers

Syed I. Khalid, MD
Resident Physician
Department of Neurosurgery
University of Illinois
Chicago, Illinois, USA

Jonathan Citow, MD
Chief of Neurosurgery
Advocate Condell Medical Center
Libertyville, Illinois, USA

196 Illustrations

Thieme
New York • Stuttgart • Delhi • Rio de Janeiro

Library of Congress Cataloging-in-Publication Data
is available from the publisher.

Thieme Publishers New York
333 Seventh Avenue, 18th Floor,
New York, NY 10001, USA
www.thieme.com
+1 800 782 3488,
customerservice@thieme.com

Cover design: ©Thieme
Cover Image source: © Thieme
Typesetting by Thomson Digital, Noida, India

Printed in India by Replika Press Pvt. Ltd. 5 4 3 2 1

DOI: 10.1055/b000000958
ISBN: 978-1-68420-614-8

Also available as an e-book:
eISBN (PDF): 978-1-68420-615-5
eISBN (epub): 978-1-68420-616-2

To Dr. Brittany Hunter, my wife and unwavering foundation, whose love, strength, and patience have made every step of this journey possible. To Dr. Jonathan Citow, whose mentorship ignited my passion for neurosurgical education and the development of meaningful board review resources; to Dr. John H. Shin, whose guidance continues to shape my surgical vision and drive for innovation; to Dr. Sandi Lam, whose example has shaped my understanding of compassionate care and inspired my commitment to organizational excellence; to Dr. Ankit I. Mehta, who believed in me, brought me to the University of Illinois at Chicago, and opened the door to a career in neurosurgery; to Dr. Alan R. Cohen, who saw potential in me early on and supported my path; and to Dr. Fady T. Charbel, whose visionary leadership has been a guiding light in my pursuit of surgical excellence. This book is dedicated to each of you—and to all the mentors whose wisdom and generosity continue to shape my work at the intersection of surgery, education, and innovation.

Syed I. Khalid, MD

I would like to dedicate this book to my mother, Phyllis, who loved reading, learning, teaching, and challenging her brilliant mind every way she could.

Jonathan Citow, MD

Contents

Preface

Preparing for the neurosurgery primary examination is a pivotal milestone in a neurosurgical resident's training. This examination assesses a foundation of core neurosurgical knowledge and serves as a benchmark for residents as they progress through their clinical and operative training. Recognizing the challenges of mastering the breadth and depth of neurosurgical topics, we developed *Neurosurgery Primary Examination Review: Questions and Answers* to provide a structured and high-yield resource for residents at every stage of their preparation.

This book is designed to serve as both a comprehensive question bank and an active learning tool, offering carefully curated multiple-choice questions that mirror the style and content of the examination. Each question is accompanied by detailed explanations, emphasizing key concepts, relevant clinical pearls, and essential board-tested facts. We have structured the content to align with the primary examination's core topics, ensuring coverage of neuropathology, neuroanatomy, neurophysiology, neuro-oncology, spine, vascular, trauma, and critical care.

Our goal was to create a resource that goes beyond rote memorization. By focusing on the clinical application of concepts and the reasoning behind correct and incorrect answer choices, we hope to foster deeper learning and reinforce test-taking strategies. The explanations in this book provide insights that will aid in passing the examination and enhancing clinical decision-making and operative preparedness.

This work would not have been possible without the mentorship and guidance of countless educators whose dedication to neurosurgical training has shaped our approach to learning and teaching. We are particularly grateful to our colleagues who reviewed the content, provided invaluable feedback, and shared their expertise refining this question bank.

We hope this book will be a trusted companion throughout your examination preparation and beyond. Whether you are tackling the primary examination for the first time or reviewing high-yield concepts for continued learning, we trust that this resource will solidify your knowledge and help you to succeed in your neurosurgical training.

Best of luck in your studies and your journey through neurosurgery.

Syed I. Khalid, MD
Jonathan Citow, MD

Contributors

Ali Alaraj, MD
Professor and Section Chief,
Endovascular Neurosurgery
Department of Neurology
University of Illinois Hospital and Health Sciences System
Chicago, Illinois, USA

Gursant Atwal, MD
Assistant Professor, Neuroendovascular/
Neurovascular
Department of Neurosurgery
University of Illinois Hospital and Health Sciences System
Chicago, Illinois, USA

Fady T. Charbel, MD
Head and Residency Program Director
Richard L. and Gertrude W. Fruin Professor
Department of Neurosurgery
University of Illinois
Chicago, Illinois, USA

Mark Dapash, MD
Resident
Department of Neurological Surgery
Northwestern University
Feinberg School of Medicine
Chicago, Illinois, USA

Jared M. Davis, MD
Assistant Professor
Program Director, Neurology Residency
Neurocritical Care
Department of Neurology and Rehabilitation
Department of Neurosurgery
University of Illinois
Chicago, Illinois, USA

Faten El Ammar, MD
Assistant Professor, Neurocritical Care
Department of Neurology and Rehabilitation
University of Illinois
Chicago, Illinois, USA

Aladine Elsamadicy, MD
Resident
Department of Neurological Surgery
Yale-New Haven Hospital
New Haven, Connecticut, USA

Hamad Farhat, MD
Chairman
Department of Neurosurgery
Advocate Christ Medical Center
Oak Lawn, Illinois, USA

Sean Hogan, PhD
Vice President
Research and Evaluation at ACGME
Visiting Professor
Department of Medical Education
University of Illinois at Chicago
Chicago, Illinois, USA

Mariyam Humayun, MD
Assistant Professor
Department of Neurology and Rehabilitation
University of Illinois
Chicago, Illinois, USA

Syed I. Khalid, MD
Resident Physician
Department of Neurosurgery
University of Illinois
Chicago, Illinois, USA

Sandi Lam, MD, MBA
Division Chief Pediatric Neurosurgery and
Fellowship Director
Ann & Robert H. Lurie Children's Hospital of Chicago
Chicago, Illinois, USA

Maciej S. Lesniak, MD, MHCM
Professor of Neurosurgery
Chair
Department of Neurological Surgery
Northwestern University
Feinberg School of Medicine
Chicago, Illinois, USA

Lei Liu, MD, PhD
Resident
Department of Neurological Surgery
Northwestern University
Feinberg School of Medicine
Chicago, Illinois, USA

Laura McGuire, MD
Assistant Professor
Department of Neurological Surgery
University of Wisconsin
School of Medicine and Public Health
Madison, Wisconsin, USA

Yoon Soo Park, PhD
Professor
Head of Department of Medical Education
University of Illinois
Chicago, Illinois, USA

Zachary A. Pennington, MD
Resident
Department of Neurological Surgery
Mayo Clinic
College of Medicine and Science
Rochester, Minnesota, USA

Nate Pertsch, MD
Resident
Department of Neurosurgery
Rush University Medical Center
Chicago, Illinois, USA

Francesco Pucci, MD
Assistant Professor
Department of Neurosurgery
University of Illinois Hospital and Health Sciences System
Chicago, Illinois, USA

Ciro Ramos-Estebanez, MD, PhD, MBA
Associate Professor
Neurocritical Care Division Chief
Department of Neurology and Rehabilitation
Chicago, Illinois, USA

Sepehr Sani, MD
Professor
Department of Neurosurgery
Rush University Medical Center
Chicago, Illinois, USA

Jonathan Scoville, MD
Physician
Department of Neurosurgery
Anne & Robert H. Lurie Children's Hospital of Chicago
Chicago, Illinois, USA

John H. Shin, MD, MBA
Neurosurgeon
Director, Penn Spine Center
Division Head, Spine and Peripheral Nerve
Penn Spine Center Pennsylvania
Penn Neurosurgery Pennsylvania
Philadelphia, Pennsylvania, USA

Konstantin Slavin, MD
Professor and Head of Section of Stereotactic and Functional Neurosurgery
University of Illinois Hospital and Health Sciences System
Chicago, Illinois, USA

Robert J. Spinner, MD
Neurosurgeon
Orthopedic Surgeon
Chair, Neurosurgery
Mayo Clinic
Rochester, Minnesota, USA

1 Vascular and Endovascular Neurosurgery

Syed I. Khalid, Laura McGuire, Hamad Farhat, Gursant Atwal, Ali Alaraj, Fady T. Charbel

▸▸ Question 1

A 52-year-old female with a history of hypertension presents with a Hunt and Hess Grade II subarachnoid hemorrhage. Angiography reveals a 7-mm anterior communicating artery aneurysm with a wide neck. Which of the following treatment options should be considered first for this patient?

- A. Conservative management with serial imaging
- B. Endovascular coiling
- C. Microsurgical clipping
- D. Stereotactic radiosurgery
- E. Pharmacological therapy with antifibrinolytics

Correct answer is B

The decision between endovascular coiling and microsurgical clipping is influenced by several factors, including the aneurysm's size, location, morphology, and patient-specific factors. The International Subarachnoid Aneurysm Trial (ISAT) showed that in patients with ruptured intracranial aneurysms suitable for both coiling and clipping, endovascular coiling was associated with better outcomes in terms of survival free of disability at 1 year (▸ Table 1.1).

(A) Conservative management with serial imaging is generally not recommended for ruptured aneurysms due to the high risk of rebleeding, which can be catastrophic. **(C) Microsurgical clipping** involves craniotomy and the placement of a clip at the aneurysm's neck to isolate it from blood flow. While effective, this method is more invasive and may pose a higher risk of complications for aneurysms that are difficult to access surgically or have complex anatomy. **(D) Stereotactic radiosurgery** does not play a role in the current management paradigm for cerebral aneurysms. **(E) Pharmacological therapy with antifibrinolytics** can be used temporarily to reduce the risk of early rebleeding before definitive treatment, but it is not a standalone treatment option for ruptured aneurysms.[1]

Table 1.1 Outcomes of endovascular coiling versus microsurgical clipping

Outcome	Endovascular coiling	Microsurgical clipping
Dead or dependent at 1 year	23.5%	30.9%
Rebleeding after initial treatment	Slightly higher risk	Lower risk
Epilepsy	Lower risk	Higher risk

▸▸ Question 2

A 45-year-old man presents with a 1-year history of progressive lower extremity weakness and urinary incontinence. A spinal MRI shows a thoracic spinal dural arteriovenous fistula. Which of the following symptoms is most directly attributable to this condition?

- A. Cervical radiculopathy
- B. Lumbar disk herniation
- C. Myelopathic symptoms due to venous congestion
- D. Neurogenic claudication
- E. Peripheral neuropathy

Correct answer is C

Spinal dural arteriovenous fistulas (SDAVFs) are the most common type of spinal arteriovenous malformations (AVMs) and are a significant cause of adult myelopathy. They are characterized by an abnormal connection between a radicular artery and the radicular vein or the venous plexus of the spinal cord, leading to venous hypertension and congestion. This venous congestion can impair spinal cord function due to decreased perfusion and hypoxia, leading to progressive neurological symptoms such as weakness and sensory changes. The classification of spinal AVMs is summarized in ▸ Table 1.2.

The myelopathic symptoms due to venous congestion in SDAVFs are a direct result of venous hypertension that impairs spinal cord perfusion. This leads to a classic presentation of progressive lower extremity weakness, sensory changes, and bladder or bowel dysfunction. The symptoms typically worsen over time and can be exacerbated by activities that increase venous pressure, such as standing or exercise.

Table 1.2 Classification of spinal AVMs

Type	Location	Characteristics	Clinical presentation
Type I—SDAVFs	Often thoracolumbar spine	Abnormal connection between a dural branch of a spinal artery and a radicular vein	Venous congestion and myelopathy
Type II—Intramedullary spinal cord AVMs (glomus AVMs)	Within the spinal cord, parenchyma	Compact nidus with direct arteriovenous shunting	Hemorrhage or myelopathy
Type III—Juvenile or giant AVMs	Extensive, involving much of the spinal cord and surrounding structures	High-flow lesions with multiple feeding arteries and dilated draining veins	Hemorrhage or severe neurological deficits
Type IV—Perimedullary AVMs	On the surface of the spinal cord	Direct fistulas between the feeding arteries and draining veins without a nidus	Subarachnoid hemorrhage or myelopathy

Abbreviations: AVMs, arteriovenous malformations; SDAVFs, spinal dural arteriovenous fistulas.

The diagnosis of SDAVFs typically involves spinal MRI to identify the signal changes associated with venous congestion and spinal angiography to identify the fistula definitively. Treatment usually involves endovascular embolization or surgical ligation of the fistula to prevent further venous congestion and potentially reverse some neurological deficits.[2]

▸▸ Question 3

A 75-year-old man with a history of smoking and hypercholesterolemia presents with a transient ischemic attack characterized by right-sided weakness and aphasia. Carotid duplex ultrasound reveals 80% stenosis of the left internal carotid artery, confirmed on digital subtraction angiography (▸ Fig. 1.1). What is the most appropriate next step in management?

- A. Antiplatelet therapy
- B. Carotid endarterectomy
- C. Carotid stenting
- D. High-intensity statin therapy
- E. Lifestyle modifications

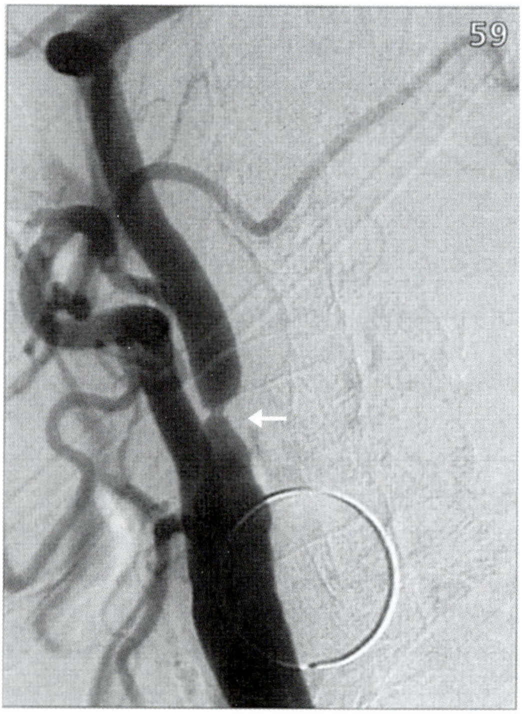

Fig. 1.1 (Source: Reproduced from Ischemic Stroke. In: Borsody M, ed. Comprehensive Board Review in Neurology. 2nd Edition. New York: Thieme; 2012.)

Correct answer is B

The decision for carotid endarterectomy (CEA) over other management strategies is supported by several key trials, which have demonstrated its effectiveness in reducing the risk of future strokes in patients with significant symptomatic carotid artery stenosis.

For a 75-year-old man with a history of smoking, hypercholesterolemia, and a recent transient ischemic attack, along with 80% stenosis of the left internal carotid artery, CEA is the most appropriate next step. This is based on evidence showing that CEA significantly reduces the risk of stroke in patients with symptomatic carotid stenosis by 70% or more. The key trials and their findings have been summarized in the table below. Additionally, studies such as the CREST trial demonstrated improved outcomes in patients older than 70 years with CEA compared to carotid stenting.

Patient selection is key, and (C) **Carotid stenting** may be preferred for the treatment of carotid stenosis in patients younger than 70 years and with significant cardiac medical history.

(A) **Antiplatelet therapy**, (D) **High-intensity statin therapy**, and (E) **Lifestyle modifications** are essential components of the management strategy for patients with carotid artery disease but, in this case, do not address the immediate risk of stroke as effectively as CEA for symptomatic high-grade stenosis (▶ Table 1.3).[3,4,5,6,7]

▸▸ Question 4

A 32-year-old woman on oral contraceptives presents with headache, papilledema, and seizures. MRV shows thrombosis in the superior sagittal sinus. Which of the following is the initial treatment of choice?

- A. Acetazolamide
- B. Anticoagulation with heparin
- C. Decompressive craniectomy
- D. Endovascular thrombectomy
- E. High-dose corticosteroids

Correct answer is B

Dural venous sinus thrombosis (DVST) can be precipitated by several factors, including oral

Table 1.3 Key findings of carotid endarterectomy and stenting trials

Trial name	Year	Comparison	Key findings	Citations
NASCET	1991	CEA vs. medical therapy	CEA significantly reduced the risk of ipsilateral stroke in patients with symptomatic carotid stenosis of 70–99%	Barnett HJM, Taylor DW, Haynes RB, et al. N Engl J Med 1991;325(7):445–453
ECST	1998	CEA vs. medical therapy	CEA offered significant stroke prevention benefits over medical treatment in patients with symptomatic high-grade carotid artery stenosis	European Carotid Surgery Trialists' Collaborative Group. Lancet 1998;351 (9113):1379–1387
ACST	2004	CEA vs. medical therapy (asymptomatic)	CEA reduces the risk of stroke in asymptomatic patients, especially in men and those over 75 years	Halliday A, Mansfield A, Marro J, et al. Lancet 2004;363(9420):1491–1502
SAPPHIRE	2004	CAS vs. CEA (high-risk patients)	CAS was noninferior to CEA in patients at high risk for surgical complications	Yadav JS, Wholey MH, Kuntz RE, et al. N Engl J Med 2004;351(15):1493–1501
CREST	2010	CEA vs. CAS	CEA and CAS were effective for carotid revascularization in symptomatic and asymptomatic patients with different risk profiles. Patients older than 70 fared better with CEA. The risk of stroke was higher in CAS. The risk of MI was higher in CEA	Brott TG, Hobson RW II, Howard G, et al. N Engl J Med 2010;363(1):11–23

contraceptive use, which is likely relevant in the case of the 32-year-old woman described. (B) **Anticoagulation with heparin** is the initial treatment of choice for DVST, regardless of intracranial hemorrhage. This approach aims to stop the clot from growing and prevent new clots from forming, allowing the body's natural fibrinolytic mechanisms to dissolve the existing clot. Anticoagulation therapy typically starts with intravenous heparin, followed by transition to oral anticoagulants.

(A) **Acetazolamide** reduces cerebrospinal fluid production and can help relieve symptoms associated with increased intracranial pressure, but it does not address the underlying cause of DVST. (C) **Decompressive craniectomy** may be considered in cases where there is evidence of significant brain edema or venous infarct leading to a risk of herniation or when medical therapy fails to control increased intracranial pressure. It is a more invasive option and not the first line of treatment. (D) **Endovascular thrombectomy** may be an option in some instances where there is a large or extensive thrombus causing significant venous obstruction, mainly if there is a poor response to medical therapy. However, it is not typically the initial treatment choice. (E) **High-dose corticosteroids** have been used to reduce cerebral edema in CVST, but their efficacy is controversial, and they are not considered a first-line treatment.[8,9]

▸▸ Question 5

A 39-year-old female, 3 days post-ruptured middle cerebral artery aneurysm repair, develops a worsening headache and confusion. Transcranial Doppler shows increased flow velocities. Which of the following should be the next step in the treatment for suspected cerebral vasospasm?

- A. Calcium channel blockers
- B. Corticosteroids
- C. Hyperbaric oxygen therapy
- D. Increased fluid administration and induction of hypertension
- E. Intravenous magnesium sulfate

Correct answer is D

Upon detection of cerebral vasospasm following aneurysmal subarachnoid hemorrhage (SAH), as evidenced by clinical symptoms and increased flow velocities on transcranial Doppler, the active intervention aims to alleviate the vasospasm and improve cerebral perfusion. The traditional triple H therapy (hypervolemia, hypertension, hemodilution) seeks to enhance blood flow to ischemic brain regions affected by the vasospasm. The central component of this therapy, particularly for symptomatic vasospasm, is induced hypertension, facilitated by vasopressors to elevate systemic blood pressure and drive blood flow through the narrowed vessels.

While there has been a move toward more nuanced management strategies in recent years, induced hypertension remains a cornerstone for treating symptomatic cerebral vasospasm, supported by clinical experience and expert consensus. The American Heart Association/American Stroke Association (AHA/ASA) guidelines for the management of aneurysmal subarachnoid hemorrhage recommend the use of hemodynamic augmentation, including induced hypertension, for patients with symptomatic vasospasm, despite the specific mention of triple H therapy being less emphasized in recent guidelines due to potential complications associated with hypervolemia and hemodilution.

(A) **Calcium channel blockers (nimodipine)**, while not directly reversing established vasospasm, play a crucial prophylactic role in reducing the risk of delayed cerebral ischemia (DCI) by preventing calcium influx into smooth muscle cells of the vessel wall. (E) **Intravenous magnesium sulfate** and (B) **Corticosteroids** have been explored for their potential benefits in vasospasm management; however, clinical trials and current evidence do not support their effectiveness in this specific context, with magnesium sulfate showing no significant benefit, and corticosteroids not being recommended due to a lack of efficacy in treating vasospasm. (C) **Hyperbaric oxygen therapy**, aiming to increase oxygen delivery to ischemic brain tissue, presents an interesting approach, yet it remains a nonstandard treatment with limited evidence supporting its use in cerebral vasospasm.[10,11,12,13,14,15]

▸▸ Question 6

A 60-year-old man presents with a sudden onset of headache, nausea, and left-sided weakness. Noncontrast CT of the head reveals a right basal ganglia hemorrhage with intraventricular extension and no clinical signs of hydrocephalus

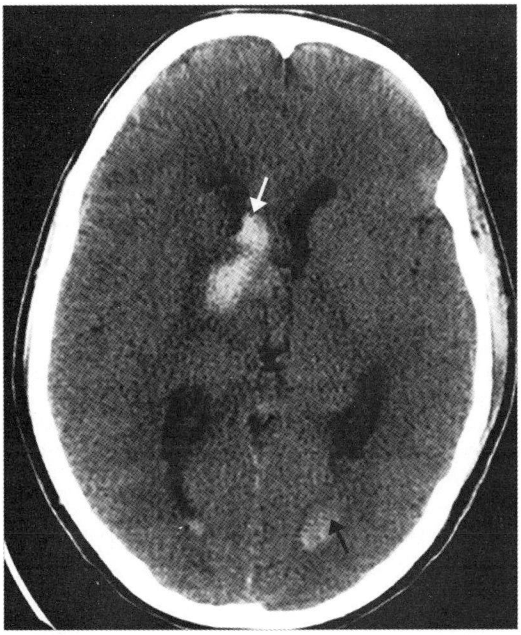

Fig. 1.2 (Source: Reproduced from Clinical presentation. In: Riascos R, Bonfante E, Calle S, eds. RadCases Plus Q 2018.)

(▶ Fig. 1.2). Which of the following is the most appropriate initial management?
- A. Immediate anticoagulation
- B. Surgical evacuation of the hematoma
- C. Conservative management with blood pressure control
- D. Intraventricular fibrinolysis
- E. Ventriculostomy

Correct answer is C

In the scenario of a 60-year-old man presenting with sudden-onset headache, nausea, and left-sided weakness, where noncontrast CT of the head reveals a right basal ganglia hemorrhage with intraventricular extension and no evidence of ventriculomegaly or clinical hydrocephalus, the most appropriate initial management is conservative treatment focusing on blood pressure control. This approach aims to stabilize the patient's condition, mitigate the risk of hematoma expansion, and manage symptoms while minimizing potential complications.

(B) Surgical evacuation of the hematoma might be considered in specific circumstances, such as when the hematoma is accessible and causing significant mass effect. Specifically, the size and location of the hematoma governs surgical evacuation. Larger hematomas, especially those greater than 30 cm^3 in volume, located superficially within 1 cm of the cortical surface, may benefit from surgical evacuation, particularly if the patient's neurological status is deteriorating due to mass effect from the hematoma. **(D) Intraventricular fibrinolysis** may be utilized in cases where there is significant intraventricular hemorrhage leading to hydrocephalus. While this approach can help alleviate hydrocephalus by breaking down blood clots in the ventricles, it is not typically the first line of management for basal ganglia hemorrhage without significant ventricular involvement. In the setting of hydrocephalus, **(E) Ventriculostomy** should be performed for cerebrospinal fluid diversion and intracranial pressure management.[16,17]

▸▸ Question 7

A 7-year-old child presents with recurrent transient ischemic attacks affecting the right side. Angiography shows stenosis of the bilateral internal carotid arteries with a "puff-of-smoke" appearance (▶ Fig. 1.3). Which of the following surgical treatments is most appropriate?
- A. Carotid endarterectomy
- B. Direct superficial temporal artery to middle cerebral artery bypass

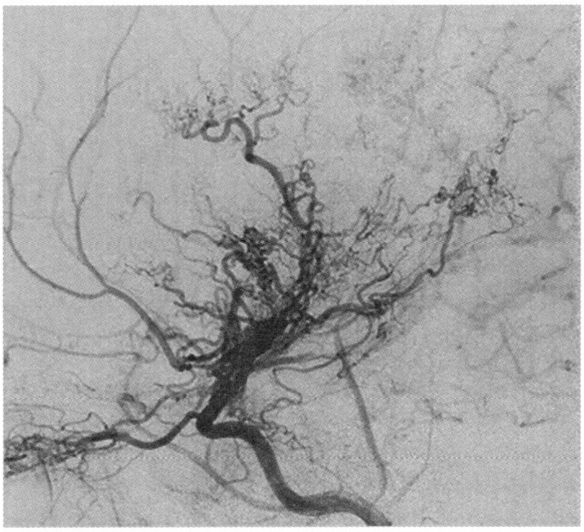

Fig. 1.3 (Source: Reproduced from Moyamoya syndrome and disease. In: Theodore N, Lonser R, eds. The Brain, Spine and Nerves in Sports. 1st ed. New York: Thieme; 2024.)

- C. Endovascular stenting of the internal carotid arteries
- D. Encephaloduroarteriosynangiosis (EDAS)
- E. Vertebral artery angioplasty

Correct answer is B

A 7-year-old child presenting with recurrent transient ischemic attacks affecting the right side and showing angiographic evidence of bilateral internal carotid artery stenosis with a "puff-of-smoke" appearance is indicative of Moyamoya disease. This condition is characterized by progressive stenosis of the intracranial internal carotid arteries and their main branches, with the development of an abnormal vascular network at the base of the brain compensating for the stenosis.

Grading of Moyamoya disease:

Moyamoya disease is staged based on angiographic findings and according to the Suzuki stages, ranging from Grade I (incipient stage with narrowing of the carotid fork) to Grade VI (most severe stage with disappearance of the Moyamoya network and reliance on external carotid artery for blood supply). They are summarized in ▸ Table 1.4.

(B) Direct superficial temporal artery to middle cerebral artery bypass involves the anastomosis between the harvested donor vessel (superficial temporal artery) and the cortical recipient vessel (middle cerebral artery, M4), and it offers an immediate boost in collateral blood flow. Studies have shown that direct bypass can offer more immediate symptomatic relief and a lower risk of perioperative stroke in Moyamoya patients with significant ischemic symptoms. **(D) Encephaloduroarteriosynangiosis (EDAS)**: Indirect revascularization techniques, such as EDAs, involve laying a donor artery on the surface of the brain to encourage new blood vessel growth over time. While these procedures are less invasive and can be effective, they typically take longer to establish improved blood flow and may not be sufficient for patients with severe or rapidly progressing symptoms. The choice between direct and indirect bypass in Moyamoya disease is informed by several factors, including the patient's age, severity of symptoms, specific characteristics of cerebral blood flow compromise, and size and quality of the potential recipient and donor vessels. **(A) Carotid endarterectomy**, **(C) Endovascular stenting of the internal carotid arteries**, and **(E) Vertebral artery angioplasty** do not play a role in the management of Moyamoya disease.[18,19]

▸▸ Question 8

A 55-year-old male with a known glioblastoma multiforme presents with acute onset of hemiparesis. MRI brain shows a new area of restricted diffusion adjacent to the tumor site. Which of the following is the most likely cause of this finding?

- A. Radiation necrosis
- B. Tumor progression
- C. Postsurgical changes
- D. Tumor-associated stroke
- E. Chemotherapy-induced leukoencephalopathy

Table 1.4 Grading of Moyamoya disease

Grade	Description
I	Narrowing of the carotid bifurcation
II	Initiation of the Moyamoya network at the base of the brain (initial Moyamoya blush)
III	Intensification of the Moyamoya network (increased blush), loss of proximal ACA and MCA, leptomeningeal collaterals from PCA
IV	Minimization of the Moyamoya network (reduced blush), progressive ICA occlusion, with the development of ECA collateral routes
V	Reduction of the Moyamoya network (reduced blush) and increased prominence of ECA collaterals
VI	Disappearance of the Moyamoya network and full reliance on ECA for blood supply

Abbreviations: ACA, anterior cerebral artery; ECA, external carotid artery; ICA, internal carotid artery; MCA, middle cerebral artery; PCA, posterior cerebral artery.

Correct answer is D

This type of stroke can occur in patients with high-grade gliomas due to several tumor-related factors, including vascular endothelial proliferation, increased intracranial pressure leading to compromised blood flow, and the propensity of these tumors to invade or compress adjacent blood vessels.

(A) **Radiation necrosis** is a delayed complication of radiation therapy that typically occurs months to years after treatment. While it can mimic tumor progression on imaging, its onset is generally not associated with acute neurological deficits like hemiparesis without preceding signs. (B) **Tumor progression** could explain new neurological symptoms and imaging changes, but the specific finding of restricted diffusion on MRI is more indicative of acute ischemia than of tumor growth alone. (C) **Postsurgical changes** can include a variety of findings on MRI, depending on the extent and location of surgery. While surgery can lead to changes in brain structure and function, an acute onset of hemiparesis and restricted diffusion on MRI are more suggestive of an acute vascular event. (E) **Chemotherapy-induced leukoencephalopathy** typically presents with more diffuse changes on MRI and a more gradual onset of neurological symptoms, rather than acute hemiparesis and localized restricted diffusion.[20,21]

▸▸ Question 9

A 70-year-old man develops a sudden onset of paraplegia following thoracoabdominal aneurysm repair. Which of the following is the most likely cause?

- A. Acute herniated lumbar disk
- B. Spinal cord ischemia due to artery of Adamkiewicz occlusion
- C. Postoperative hematoma compressing the spinal cord
- D. Acute epidural abscess
- E. Neurogenic shock

Correct answer is B

The artery of Adamkiewicz is a critical blood vessel that supplies blood to the lower two-thirds of the spinal cord, including the lumbar and sacral regions. During thoracoabdominal aneurysm repair, inadvertent damage or occlusion of this artery can lead to a significant reduction in blood flow to the spinal cord, resulting in ischemia and subsequent paraplegia.

(A) **Acute herniated lumbar disk** typically presents with radicular pain and possible weakness in the lower extremities, but sudden paraplegia immediately following surgery suggests a vascular rather than mechanical cause. (C) **Postoperative hematoma compressing the spinal cord** is a possible cause of acute neurological deterioration postsurgery, but this condition would likely be identifiable on imaging studies and might not present as abruptly as ischemia. (D) **Acute epidural abscess** generally develops over a longer period and is associated with infection signs, making it less likely in the immediate postoperative period without preceding infection. (E) **Neurogenic shock** can occur after spinal cord injury but is characterized by hypotension and bradycardia, alongside potential motor and sensory deficits, not isolated acute paraplegia.[22,23]

▸ Fig. 1.4 shows a diagram illustrating the spinal cord's blood supply, highlighting the artery of Adamkiewicz.

▸▸ Question 10

A 10-year-old child presents with sudden severe headache and loss of consciousness. Imaging reveals a ruptured cerebral aneurysm. Which of the following factors is most commonly associated with pediatric cerebral aneurysms?

- A. Atherosclerosis
- B. Connective tissue disorders
- C. Hypertension
- D. Smoking
- E. Diabetes mellitus

Correct answer is B

In pediatric patients, cerebral aneurysms are relatively rare compared to the adult population and often have different underlying causes. Among these, **connective tissue disorders** are the most commonly associated factor with the development of cerebral aneurysms in children. These disorders, which include conditions like Marfan syndrome, Ehlers-Danlos syndrome, and others, can lead to weaknesses in the blood vessel walls, making them more prone to bulging and aneurysm formation.

(A) **Atherosclerosis** is uncommon in children due to the shorter exposure time to risk factors that contribute to atherosclerotic changes, and while it may contribute to cerebral aneurysm formation, it is not a leading cause. (C) **Hypertension** is a significant risk factor for aneurysm development, particularly in adulthood, and can

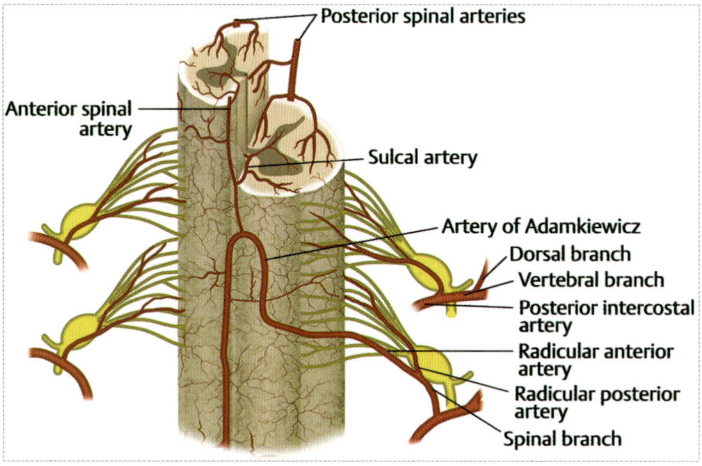

Fig. 1.4 (Source: Reproduced from 5.4 Muscular anatomy. In: Singh K, ed. Spine Essentials Handbook: A Bulleted Review of Anatomy, Evaluation, Imaging, Tests, and Procedures. 1st ed. New York: Thieme; 2019.)

contribute to aneurysm formation by increasing the stress on blood vessel walls. However, it is less commonly the primary factor in pediatric cases compared to connective tissue disorders. **(D) Smoking** is a well-established risk factor for the development of aneurysms in adults but is unlikely to be a significant factor in pediatric populations due to less exposure. **(E) Diabetes mellitus** is associated with vascular complications over time but is not directly linked to the formation of cerebral aneurysms, especially in pediatric cases.[24,25]

▸▸ Question 11

For a patient with a saccular middle cerebral artery aneurysm measuring 6 mm in diameter and a 3-mm neck, which of the following endovascular treatments is most appropriate?

- A. Flow diversion
- B. Coiling
- C. Stenting
- D. Balloon angioplasty
- E. Conservative management with observation

Correct answer is B

Endovascular coiling is a preferred treatment for small saccular middle cerebral artery aneurysms with favorable aspect ratios, providing a safe and effective means of preventing rupture. The decision-making process involves careful consideration of aneurysm morphology, including size, neck width, and aspect ratio, to determine the most appropriate treatment approach and the potential need for adjunctive techniques. Of note, recent endovascular innovations, such as intrasaccular flow diverting devices (the WEB), have emerged as a possible treatment option for cerebral aneurysms with favorable configurations.

Aspect Ratios of Aneurysms:

The aspect ratio, which is the height of the aneurysm dome divided by the neck width, is a crucial morphological feature in determining the suitability of an aneurysm for coiling and the likelihood of requiring adjunctive techniques. A higher aspect ratio indicates a more favorable geometry for coiling. An aspect ratio of < 1.6 often predicts the need for adjunctive techniques such as balloon or stent assistance to secure the coils within the aneurysm. Aneurysms with an aspect ratio of < 1.2 almost always require these adjunctive techniques for successful coiling.

Wide-Neck Cerebral Aneurysm:

A wide-neck cerebral aneurysm is most commonly defined by a neck diameter of ≥ 4 mm or a dome-to-neck ratio of < 2. These morphologic features make endovascular treatment more challenging due to the increased risk of coil herniation into the parent vessel. In such cases, adjunctive techniques or alternative treatments may be considered.

(A) Flow diversion and **(C) Stenting** are typically reserved for aneurysms that are not suitable for coiling due to their size, shape, or neck width. Flow diverters are particularly useful for larger aneurysms with wide necks. **(D) Balloon angioplasty** is not a primary treatment for aneurysms but may be used adjunctively to remodel the vessel or assist in coiling. (E) **Conservative management with observation** is generally considered for small aneurysms (<7 mm) that are incidentally found and have a low risk of rupture, depending on the patient's overall risk profile and aneurysm characteristics (▶ Fig. 1.5).[26,27]

▸▸ Question 12

A patient presents with vertigo, dysphagia, hoarseness, and hiccups. MRI shows a stroke in the lateral medulla. Which artery is most likely occluded?

- A. Anterior inferior cerebellar artery
- B. Posterior inferior cerebellar artery (PICA)
- C. Superior cerebellar artery
- D. Basilar artery
- E. Vertebral artery

Correct answer is B

A patient presenting with vertigo, dysphagia, hoarseness, and hiccups, coupled with an MRI showing a stroke in the lateral medulla, is highly indicative of occlusion of the **posterior inferior cerebellar artery (PICA)**. These symptoms are classic for lateral medullary syndrome (also known as Wallenberg's syndrome), which is most commonly caused by the occlusion of PICA.

(A) **Anterior inferior cerebellar artery (AICA)** typically presents with symptoms that can include hearing loss and facial weakness, due to its supply area involving the inner ear and facial nerve. (C) **Superior cerebellar artery** occlusion would more likely affect coordination and movement, given its supply to the upper part of the cerebellum. (D) **Basilar artery** involvement often leads to more widespread brainstem symptoms due to its larger territory, potentially including severe motor and consciousness disturbances. (E) **Vertebral artery** could be a broader answer that might encompass PICA since PICA branches off the vertebral artery. However, the specificity of the symptoms and the area of the brain affected as shown on MRI directly point to PICA as the most precise answer.[28,29]

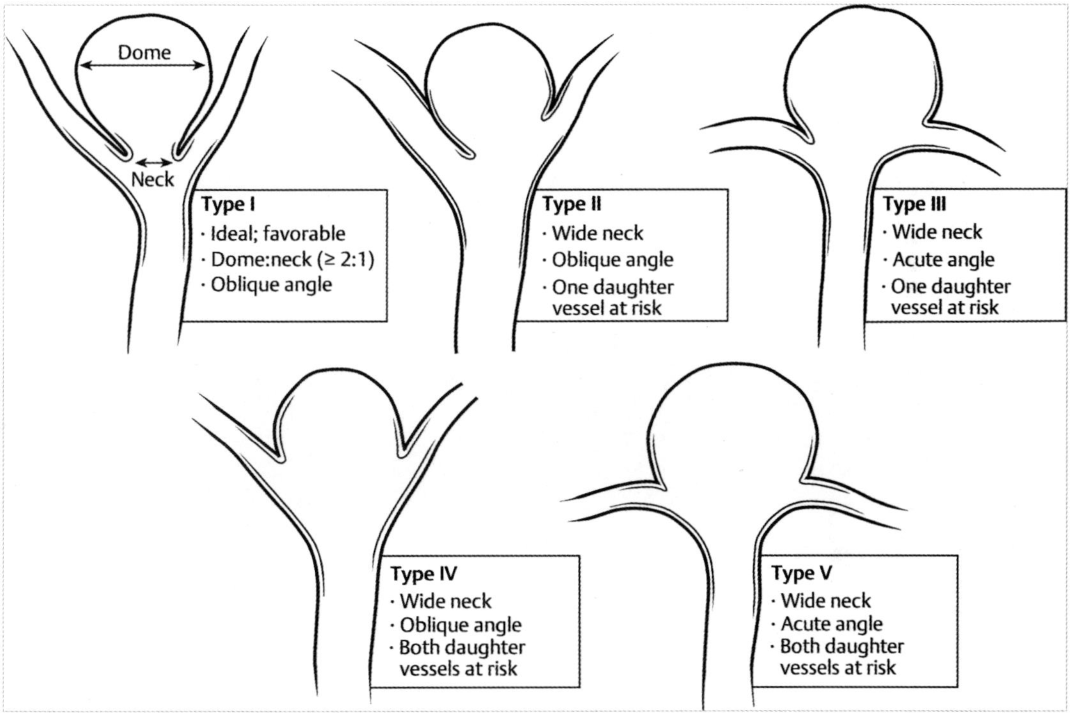

Fig. 1.5 (Source: Reproduced from Type I: Favorable dome-to-neck ratio (≥ 2:1). In: Spetzler R, Kalani M, Nakaji P, ed. Neurovascular Surgery. 2nd ed. New York: Thieme; 2015.)

▸▸ Question 13

A 45-year-old male presents with headache, cognitive decline, and multifocal neurologic deficits. Brain biopsy confirms primary CNS vasculitis. What is the mainstay of treatment?

- A. Anticoagulation
- B. Corticosteroids and cyclophosphamide
- C. Surgical resection of lesions
- D. Endovascular angioplasty
- E. High-dose aspirin

Correct answer is B

The treatment of primary CNS vasculitis focuses on rapidly controlling inflammation and modulating the immune response to prevent further vessel damage and neurological compromise.

(A) **Anticoagulation** is not typically used as the primary treatment for primary CNS vasculitis because the core problem is inflammation of the vessel wall rather than blood clotting. However, it may be considered in certain situations if there is a specific risk of thrombosis. (C) **Surgical resection of lesions** is not applicable in this context because primary CNS vasculitis is a diffuse process affecting multiple blood vessels rather than a single, resectable lesion. (D) **Endovascular angioplasty** is not a standard treatment for primary CNS vasculitis, as the disease involves inflammation and potential damage to the vessel walls rather than blockages that can be opened with angioplasty. (E) **High-dose aspirin** is used in various vasculitides for its anti-inflammatory properties, but it is not sufficient as the mainstay therapy for primary CNS vasculitis, where more potent immunosuppressive therapy is required.[30,31]

▸▸ Question 14

A 55-year-old man presents with progressive myelopathy. MRI and spinal angiography confirm a spinal dural arteriovenous fistula (DAVF) at the L2 level (▸ Fig. 1.6). Of the following, what is the most appropriate treatment?

- A. Observation and physical therapy
- B. High-dose corticosteroids
- C. Laminectomy and fistula ligation
- D. Systemic anticoagulation
- E. Radiation therapy

Correct answer is C

Surgical treatment, specifically laminectomy and fistula ligation, is the most effective approach for managing spinal dural arteriovenous fistulas,

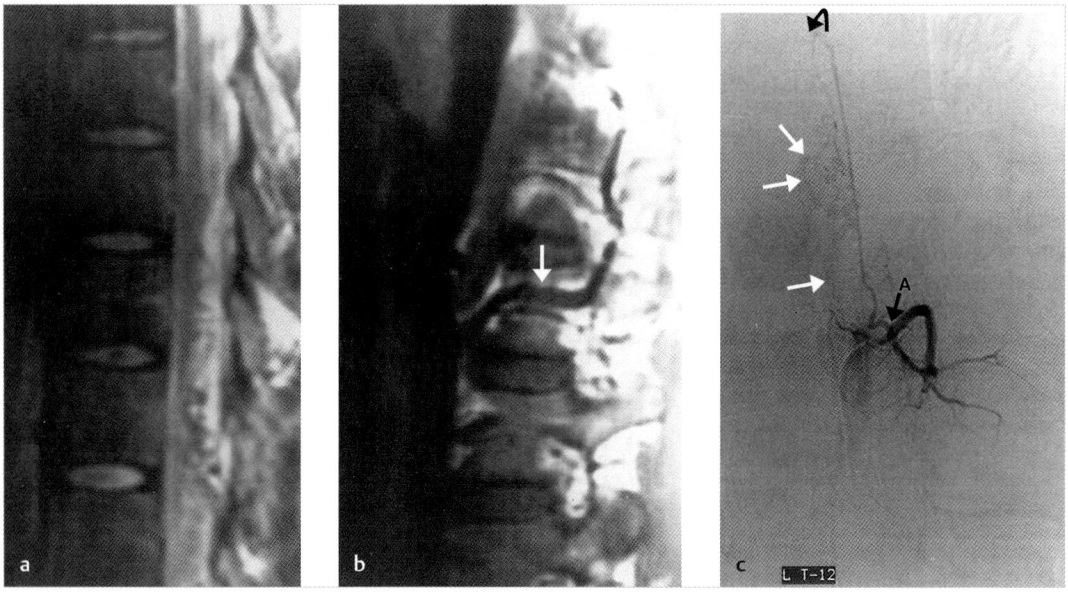

Fig. 1.6 (Source: Reproduced from XXV. Spinal vascular diseases. In: Citow J, Macdonald R, Puffer R, Khalid S, Carter B, Cohen A, Spinner R, Refai D, eds. Comprehensive Neurosurgery Board Review. 3rd ed. New York: Thieme; 2019.)

directly addressing the cause of myelopathy by eliminating the arteriovenous shunting. Endovascular treatment can sometimes be an option on a case-by-case assessment, based on the accessibility of the feeder vessel and fistulous point of the DAVF.

(A) **Observation and physical therapy** are not adequate for treating the underlying vascular abnormality and can lead to further neurological deterioration. (B) **High-dose corticosteroids** may temporarily alleviate symptoms by reducing edema but do not address the root cause of the DAVF and its hemodynamic effects. (D) **Systemic anticoagulation** is not indicated as a treatment for spinal DAVFs. While it might prevent thrombosis in the aberrant vessels, it does not eliminate the fistula or the risk of bleeding. (E) **Radiation therapy** can be considered for certain intracranial arteriovenous malformations but is less commonly used for spinal DAVFs due to the risk of radiation myelopathy and the effectiveness of surgical options.

▸▸ Question 15

A patient develops new hemiparesis and aphasia 3 days following clipping of an anterior communicating artery aneurysm. Which complication is most likely responsible for these new deficits?

- A. Hydrocephalus
- B. Vasospasm
- C. Rebleeding of the aneurysm
- D. Seizure
- E. Embolic stroke

Correct answer is B

Vasospasm is a critical and common complication following subarachnoid hemorrhage due to aneurysmal rupture. Recognizing the signs of cerebral ischemia due to vasospasm is crucial for timely intervention to mitigate the risk of permanent neurological injury. If the patient developed symptoms immediately following surgical intervention, a major concern would be procedure-related stroke, which can occur due to temporary clipping of the afferent vessel, flow-limiting stenosis of the parent vessel secondary to the aneurysm clip, or perforator stroke.

(A) **Hydrocephalus** generally causes global symptoms, such as alteration of level of consciousness, worsening headache, or nausea and vomiting. (C) **Rebleeding**, while possible, would be less likely following aneurysm clipping, and the development of focal deficits also points against this differential diagnosis. (D) **Seizure** can occur following aneurysm rupture, and patients with subarachnoid hemorrhage are treated with prophylactic antiepileptic medication. While atypical, this clinical presentation could possibly be attributed to seizure, but evaluating and ruling out ischemia secondary to vasospasm would be imperative. (E) **Embolic stroke** can cause focal deficits, such as these, but in the absence of known risk factors, it would be less likely in this clinical case.[34,35]

▸▸ Question 16

A patient presents with a 2.5-cm partially thrombosed aneurysm of the ophthalmic artery, causing optic nerve compression (▸ Fig. 1.7). What is the most appropriate management strategy?

- A. Microsurgical clipping
- B. Endovascular coiling
- C. Flow diversion with a pipeline embolization device
- D. Conservative management with serial imaging
- E. Stereotactic radiosurgery

Correct answer is C

The most appropriate management for a large (2.5 cm), partially thrombosed aneurysm of the ophthalmic segment causing optic nerve compression, is flow diversion with a pipeline embolization device (PED). Flow diverters are endoluminal devices that redirect blood flow away from the aneurysm sac, promoting thrombosis within the aneurysm and allowing for reconstruction of the parent artery. This technique is particularly effective for large or giant, wide-necked aneurysms that are difficult to treat with traditional methods like clipping or coiling.

(A) Microsurgical clipping with optic nerve decompression involves a high risk due to the complex anatomy and the need for extensive skull base exposure. The proximity to critical neurovascular structures increases the potential for morbidity, including worsening visual deficits. (B) Endovascular coiling may not be effective for large, partially thrombosed aneurysms because it often fails to achieve complete occlusion and has a higher risk of recurrence. (D) Conservative management is inappropriate in this case due to

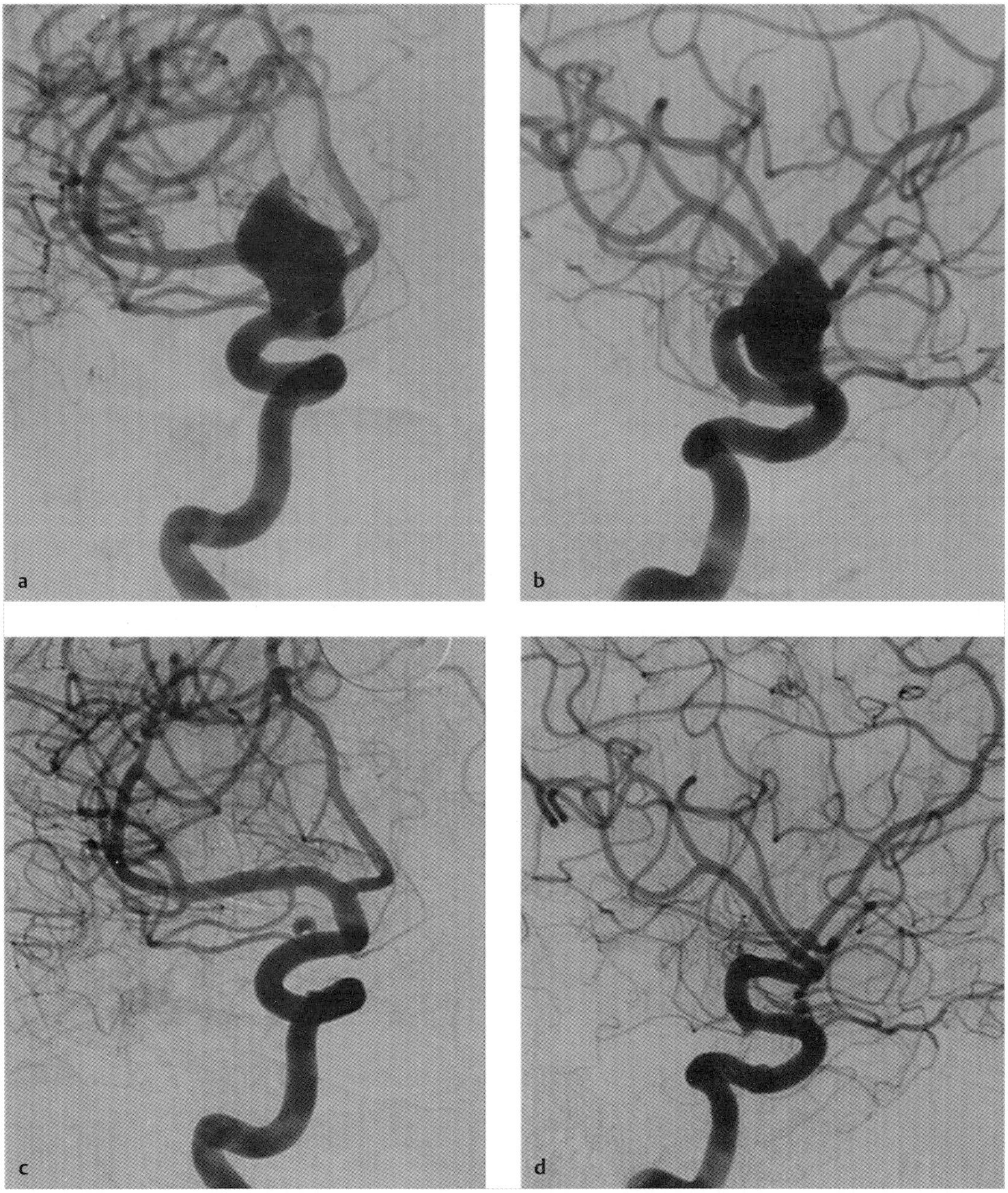

Fig. 1.7 (Source: Reproduced from Necessary aneurysm residual. In: Park M, Taussky P, Albuquerque F, McDougall C, eds. Flow Diversion of Cerebral Aneurysms. 1st ed. New York: Thieme; 2017.)

the progressive visual loss and the risk of aneurysm rupture or further growth causing irreversible damage. (E) **Stereotactic radiosurgery** does not play a role in the management of cerebral aneurysms.

Flow diversion has emerged as a preferred treatment for large or complex intracranial aneurysms that are unsuitable for traditional surgical or endovascular techniques. It not only reduces the risk of aneurysm rupture but can also alleviate mass effect symptoms by promoting aneurysm thrombosis and subsequent shrinkage.[36,37]

▸▸ Question 17

A Spetzler-Martin Grade III cerebral AVM is identified in a 25-year-old patient presenting with a seizure. Which definitive treatment option is most appropriate?

- A. Observation and medical management of seizures
- B. Embolization followed by surgical resection
- C. Stereotactic radiosurgery alone
- D. Immediate antiepileptic drug therapy
- E. Intravenous thrombolysis

Correct answer is B

Embolization followed by surgical resection offers a balanced approach for treating Grade III cerebral AVMs, aiming to reduce the risks associated with surgery by minimizing the AVM's flow and complexity. The Spetzler-Martin grading system assesses AVMs based on size, eloquence of adjacent brain tissue, and pattern of venous drainage, with higher grades indicating more complex AVMs that are traditionally considered challenging for surgical resection alone (▸ Fig. 1.8). The SM grading system is summarized in ▸ Table 1.5. Additionally, Grade and recommended treatment are further summarized in ▸ Table 1.6.

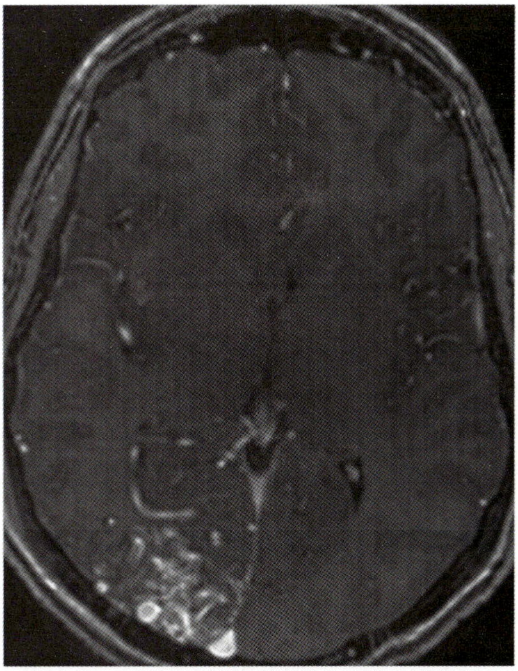

Fig. 1.8 (Source: Reproduced from Case overview: CASE 40.10 vertebral artery dissection/occlusion rescued with flow diversion stenting using the floss technique. In: Rangel-Castilla L, Siddiqui A, Levy E, Lanzino G, Hopkins L, Davies J, ed. Video Atlas of Neuroendovascular Procedures. 1st ed. New York: Thieme; 2020.)

Table 1.5 SM grading system

Feature	Details
Size of AVM	Small (< 3 cm): 1 point Medium (3–6 cm): 2 points Large (> 6 cm): 3 points
Eloquence of adjacent brain tissue	Non-eloquent area: 0 points Eloquent area: 1 point
Pattern of venous drainage	Superficial only: 0 points Deep venous drainage: 1 point

(A) **Observation and medical management of seizures** might be considered for asymptomatic AVMs or those with a high surgical risk, but it does not address the risk of hemorrhage or the potential for future seizures directly related to the AVM. (C) **Stereotactic radiosurgery alone** is typically reserved for smaller AVMs or those in eloquent areas where surgery poses too high a risk. It may not be as effective for a Grade III AVM due to size and complexity. (D) **Immediate antiepileptic drug therapy** is essential for managing seizures in this patient but does not address the underlying AVM or offer definitive treatment,

Table 1.6 Grade and recommended treatment

Grade	Recommended treatment
1	Surgical resection or radiosurgery, lower risk of neurological deficit
2	Multidisciplinary approach, individual risk–benefit assessment
3	Embolization followed by surgical resection or radiosurgery, higher risk requires careful consideration
4	Generally high risk, conservative management or embolization, consider surgery in selected cases
5	Conservative management preferred, intervention generally not recommended due to high risk

which continues to pose a risk for hemorrhage, seizure in this case, and further neurological damage. (E) **Intravenous thrombolysis** is not a treatment option for AVMs; it is used in the acute management of ischemic stroke.[38,39,40,41]

▸▸ Question 18

A 45-year-old woman presents with the worst headache of her life. CT scan shows diffuse subarachnoid hemorrhage (SAH). Cerebral angiography does not reveal an aneurysm. What is the most likely diagnosis, and what is the next best step in management?

- A. Arteriovenous malformation, proceed with MRI brain
- B. Traumatic SAH, observe and manage conservatively
- C. Aneurysmal SAH, repeat angiography in 1 week
- D. Venous sinus thrombosis, start anticoagulation
- E. Migraine, treat symptomatically

Correct answer is C

In cases where the initial angiography does not reveal an aneurysm, it is possible that vasospasm, thrombosis, or the technical limitations of the study have obscured the aneurysm. With this clinical and radiographic presentation, suspicion remains high for the vascular source of the hemorrhage, and thus, repeat angiography would be indicated. Repeating angiography in 1 week allows time for potential vasospasms or thrombosis to resolve and provides a second opportunity to identify the aneurysm.

(A) **Arteriovenous malformation** is unlikely to be the diagnosis with a fully negative diagnostic cerebral angiogram. (B) **Traumatic subarachnoid hemorrhage** does not match the patient's clinical presentation in the absence of stated trauma. (D) **Venous sinus thrombosis** can present with intracerebral hemorrhage due to venous congestion and hypertension, but it usually presents with hemorrhage localized near the thrombosed venous structure and not diffuse SAH. (E) **Migraine** would not be an appropriate diagnosis in this case due to the presence of accompanying hemorrhage on the imaging with the symptom of headache.[42,43]

▸▸ Question 19

A patient on warfarin therapy presents with an intracerebral hemorrhage. What is the most appropriate initial management?

- A. Continue warfarin with close INR monitoring
- B. Administer vitamin K and fresh frozen plasma
- C. Immediate reversal with protamine sulfate
- D. Surgical evacuation of the hematoma
- E. Initiate low molecular weight heparin

Correct answer is B

In a patient on warfarin therapy who presents with an intracerebral hemorrhage (ICH), the most appropriate initial management is to **administer vitamin K and fresh frozen plasma**. Other agents, such as prothrombin complex concentrate (PCC), can be used as well to reverse warfarin and have less fluid volume than plasma, which may be more suitable for some patients, although this was not an option above.

(A) **Continue warfarin with close INR monitoring** is not appropriate in the context of an ICH due to the ongoing risk of hemorrhage. (C) **Immediate reversal with protamine sulfate** is used for heparin reversal and is not effective against the anticoagulation effects of warfarin. (D) **Surgical evacuation of the hematoma** may be necessary in cases where there is significant mass effect or risk of herniation, but the immediate priority is to reverse the anticoagulation to prevent further bleeding. (E) **Initiate low-molecular-weight heparin** is not indicated in the setting of an acute

Table 1.7 Anticoagulants and their reversal agents

Anticoagulant	Reversal agent
Warfarin	Vitamin K and fresh frozen plasma or prothrombin complex concentrate
Unfractionated heparin	Protamine sulfate
Low-molecular-weight heparin	Protamine sulfate (partial reversal)
Direct oral anticoagulants (DOACs) —thrombin inhibitor (dabigatran)	Idarucizumab
DOACs—Factor Xa inhibitors (e.g., rivaroxaban, apixaban)	Andexanet alfa or prothrombin complex concentrate

hemorrhage and ongoing anticoagulation; indeed, it would exacerbate the risk of further bleeding.[44,45]

Anticoagulants and their reversal agents are provided in ▶ Table 1.7.

▸▸ Question 20

What is the preferred management strategy for acute ischemic stroke due to large vessel occlusion in a pregnant woman who presents 6 hours after symptom onset?

- A. Intravenous thrombolysis with alteplase
- B. Mechanical thrombectomy
- C. Antiplatelet therapy
- D. Conservative management with antihypertensives
- E. Anticoagulation with heparin

Correct answer is B

In the context of a pregnant woman experiencing an acute ischemic stroke due to large vessel occlusion 6 hours after symptom onset, mechanical thrombectomy represents the most appropriate and effective treatment option. The decision to proceed with mechanical thrombectomy should be made in a timely manner to optimize outcomes for both the mother and the developing fetus.

(A) **Intravenous thrombolysis** with tissue plasminogen activator (tPA) is listed as a relative contraindication in pregnancy but may be considered when anticipated benefits of treating moderate or severe stroke outweigh anticipated increased risks of uterine bleeding, according to the 2018 Guidelines, but it has been noted that tPA is not known to be teratogenic and is a large molecule that does not cross the placenta. (C) **Antiplatelet therapy** is not an appropriate treatment in the setting of acute ischemic stroke; however, depending on the source of the stroke, antiplatelet therapy may be recommended. While the U.S. Food and Drug Administration (FDA) generally recommends avoiding the use of nonsteroidal anti-inflammatory drugs, including aspirin, after 19th week of pregnancy due to concern for rare but serious renal issues in fetal development, low-dose aspirin has not been found to be harmful during pregnancy and is used in conditions such as preeclampsia. (D) **Conservative management** would not be appropriate given that the patient is presenting with a suspected large vessel occlusion within the time window for intervention. (E) **Anticoagulation with heparin** does not represent a treatment option for acute ischemic stroke (▶ Table 1.8).[46,47]

▸▸ Question 21

Which imaging modality is most sensitive in the early detection of cerebral vasospasm following subarachnoid hemorrhage?

- A. CT angiography
- B. Transcranial Doppler ultrasound
- C. MRI with diffusion-weighted imaging
- D. Digital subtraction angiography
- E. PET scan

Correct answer is B

Transcranial Doppler (TCD) ultrasound is the most sensitive imaging modality for the early detection of cerebral vasospasm following subarachnoid hemorrhage (SAH). TCD ultrasound measures the velocity of blood flow through the cerebral arteries, which increases in the presence of vasospasm due to the narrowed lumen of the affected vessels. This noninvasive, bedside modality allows for daily monitoring, making it an invaluable tool in the early detection and management of vasospasm, a common and severe complication of SAH.

Table 1.8 Absolute and relative contraindications to thrombolytics

Absolute contraindications to thrombolytics	Relative contraindications to thrombolytics
• Significant head trauma or prior stroke in the previous 3 mo • Symptoms suggest subarachnoid hemorrhage • Arterial puncture at a noncompressible site in previous 7 d • History of previous intracranial hemorrhage • Intracranial neoplasm, AVM, or an aneurysm • Recent intracranial or intraspinal surgery • Elevated blood pressure (systolic > 185 mm Hg or diastolic > 110 mm Hg) • Active internal bleeding • Acute bleeding diathesis, including but not limited to: ○ Platelet count less than 100,000/mm^3 ○ Heparin received within 48 h resulting in abnormally elevated aPTT above the upper limit of normal ○ Current use of anticoagulant with INR > 1.7 or PT > 15 s ○ Current use of direct thrombin inhibitors or direct factor Xa inhibitors with elevated sensitive laboratory tests (e.g., aPTT, INR, platelet count, ECT, TT, or appropriate factor Xa activity assays) ○ Blood glucose concentration < 50 mg/dL (2.7 mmol/L) ○ CT demonstrates multilobar infarction (hypodensity greater than one-third cerebral hemisphere)	• Only minor or quickly improving stroke symptoms (clearing automatically) • Pregnancy • Seizure at the onset with postictal residual neurological impairments • Major surgery or serious trauma within prior 14 d • Recent GI or urinary tract hemorrhage (within previous 21 d) • Recent acute myocardial infarction (within preceding 3 mo)

Abbreviations: aPTT, activated partial thromboplastin time; INR, international normalized ratio; ECT, ecarin clotting time; TT, thrombin time.

(D) Digital subtraction angiography (DSA) is considered the gold standard for visualizing cerebral vasculature and can definitively diagnose vasospasm and also treat it, through the administration of intra-arterial calcium channel blockers or balloon angioplasty. However, DSA is invasive, requiring arterial catheterization, and unsuitable for routine or daily monitoring. **(A) CT angiography**, **(C) MRI with diffusion-weighted imaging**, and **(E) PET scan** would not represent the best tests for detecting cerebral vasospasm following aneurysmal subarachnoid hemorrhage.[48,49]

▸▸ Question 22

During routine follow-up imaging 1 year after endovascular coiling of a posterior communicating artery aneurysm, a patient is found to have a recurrent aneurysm at the same site. Which factor is most predictive of recurrence in this scenario?

- A. Patient's age
- B. Initial aneurysm size
- C. Coil density
- D. Hypertension control
- E. Use of antiplatelet therapy

Correct answer is C

In the scenario where a patient has a recurrent aneurysm 1 year after endovascular coiling of a posterior communicating artery aneurysm, the factor most predictive of recurrence is **coil density**. Coil density, or packing density, refers to the percentage of the aneurysm volume that is filled with coils. A higher coil density is associated with a lower risk of coil compaction and thus aneurysm recurrence, as it implies less space within the aneurysm sac for blood to enter and potentially cause regrowth or rebleeding.

(A) Patient's age: While age may influence the overall risk profile for aneurysms and vascular diseases, it is not directly predictive of aneurysm recurrence after coiling. **(B) Initial aneurysm size**: Although larger aneurysms have a higher risk of recurrence after treatment due to their complex geometry and the potential for incomplete occlusion, the specific factor of coil density within the aneurysm plays a more direct role in determining the likelihood of recurrence. **(D) Hypertension control**: While poorly controlled hypertension is a risk factor for the formation and rupture of aneurysms, its role as a predictive factor for recurrence after coiling is less direct compared to coil density.

Effective hypertension control is essential for overall vascular health and may impact long-term outcomes, but it does not explicitly predict recurrence in the same way as coil packing density. (E) **Use of antiplatelet therapy**: Antiplatelet therapy is often used in the context of endovascular treatment to prevent thromboembolic complications, particularly when stents have been deployed. While necessary for patient management, its use does not directly predict aneurysm recurrence post-coiling.[50,51,52,53]

▸▸ Question 23

Which of the following features of a cerebral arteriovenous malformation (AVM) most significantly increases the risk of hemorrhagic stroke?

- A. Size of AVM > 3 cm
- B. Location in the frontal lobe
- C. Presence of deep venous drainage
- D. Presence of an associated aneurysm
- E. AVM located superficially

Correct answer is C

The risk of hemorrhagic stroke in patients with cerebral AVMs is influenced by several factors related to the characteristics of the AVM itself. Among these factors, the **presence of deep venous drainage** is significantly associated with an increased risk of bleeding. This is because AVMs draining into deep venous systems are more likely associated with higher venous pressures, contributing to the risk of rupture and hemorrhage.

(A) Size of AVM > 3 cm: While larger AVMs might seem intuitively at a higher risk of hemorrhage, the literature suggests that smaller AVMs are more prone to bleeding. This counterintuitive finding is thought to be related to the higher flow velocities and pressures found in smaller AVMs. **(B) Location in the frontal lobe**: The location of an AVM within the brain (e.g., frontal lobe vs. basal ganglia or brainstem) does not consistently predict hemorrhage risk. Hemorrhagic risk is more closely related to the venous drainage pattern and the presence of associated aneurysms rather than the specific cerebral location. **(D) Presence of an associated aneurysm**: While the presence of an associated aneurysm with an AVM can increase the risk of hemorrhage, it is not as universally predictive of hemorrhagic stroke as the venous drainage pattern. Aneurysms related to AVMs can increase the risk due to the increased flow and pressure exerted on the arterial feeders and the nidus itself. **(E) AVM located superficially**: Superficial versus deep location of an AVM does not inherently increase the risk of hemorrhage. Instead, the risk is more closely related to the characteristics of the AVM's vascular architecture, such as the presence of deep venous drainage and associated aneurysms.[54,55,56]

▸▸ Question 24

A 45-year-old man presents with a history of pulsatile tinnitus and was found to have a dural arteriovenous fistula (DAVF) on imaging. Which feature, if present, is the most critical determinant in assessing the patient's risk of intracranial hemorrhage?

- A. The size of the fistula
- B. The presence of cortical venous drainage
- C. The location of the fistula within the dural layers
- D. The presence of arterial aneurysms within the fistula
- E. The flow rate through the fistula

Correct answer is B

In evaluating and classifying DAVFs, the presence of **cortical venous drainage** stands out as the most critical determinant in assessing the risk of intracranial hemorrhage. This is highlighted in both the Borden and Cognard classification systems, which categorize DAVFs based on their drainage patterns and the associated risks of aggressive neurological symptoms, including hemorrhage. The Borden and Cognard classification systems are summarized below (▸ Table 1.9, ▸ Table 1.10, and ▸ Fig. 1.9).[57,58]

Table 1.9 Borden classification

Type	Drainage pattern	Hemorrhage risk
I	Drainage into dural venous sinuses or meningeal veins without cortical venous drainage	Low
II	Drainage into dural venous sinuses with retrograde flow into cortical veins	Intermediate
III	Direct cortical venous drainage without sinus involvement	High

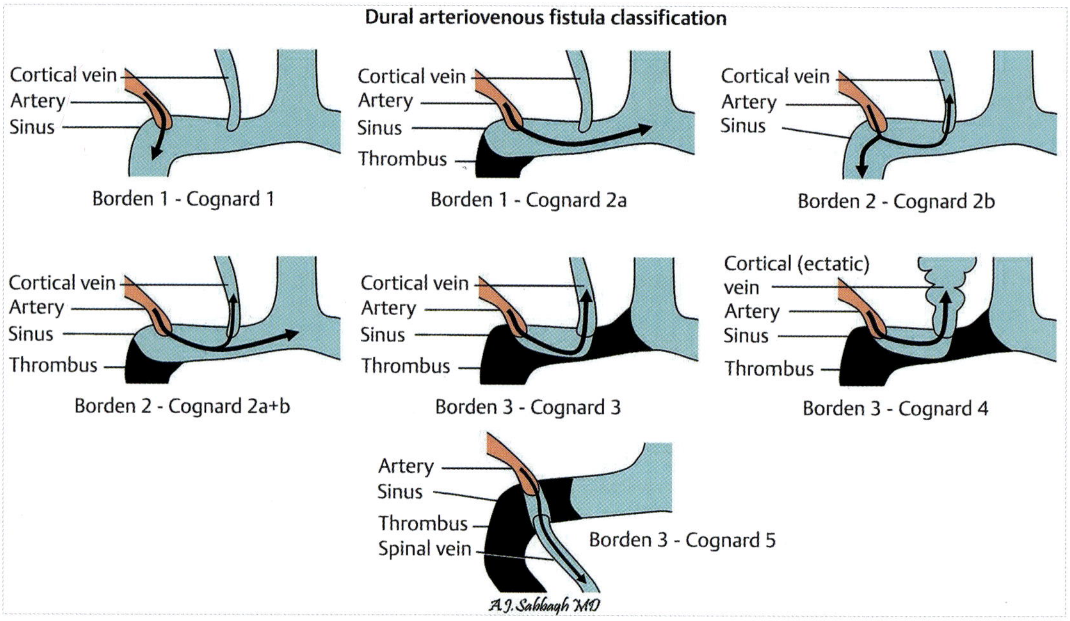

Fig. 1.9 (Source: Reproduced from Case 31 Dural arteriovenous fistula. In: Nader R, Sabbagh A, Elbabaa S, Al-Jehani H, Gasco J, Gragnaniello C, ed. Neurosurgery Case Review: Questions and Answers. 2nd ed. New York: Thieme; 2020.)

Table 1.10 Cognard classification

Type	Drainage pattern	Hemorrhage risk
I	Antegrade drainage into the dural sinus without cortical venous drainage	Low
IIa	Antegrade drainage into the dural sinus with reflux into the sinus	Low
IIb	Antegrade drainage into cortical vein without reflux into sinus or ectasia	Intermediate
IIa + b	Antegrade drainage into the dural sinus with reflux into both the sinus and cortical veins	High
III	Direct cortical venous drainage without venous ectasia	High
IV	Direct cortical venous drainage with venous ectasia	Very high
V	Spinal perimedullary venous drainage	Variable

▸▸ Question 25

During a carotid endarterectomy, blood pressure decreases from 170/90 to 70/40 mm Hg following plaque removal but before arteriotomy closure; pulse remains 60/min. Which of the following is the most appropriate next step in management?

- A. Administer intravenous fluids
- B. Perform a carotid sinus massage
- C. Administer atropine
- D. Administer phenylephrine
- E. Increase anesthetic depth

Correct answer is D

Hypotension, bradycardia, or both are relatively common phenomenon during or after carotid surgery, occurring in more than half of all procedures, due to direct autonomic stimulation in the carotid sinus. Phenylephrine is a vasopressor that can increase blood pressure by stimulating alpha-adrenergic receptors, which is necessary in this hypotensive situation. Phenylephrine helps counteract the drop in blood pressure and maintain cerebral perfusion during carotid endarterectomy.[59,60,61]

►► Question 26

Division of the ansa hypoglossi during carotid endarterectomy can result in which of the following adverse effects?

- A. Loss of taste on the anterior two-thirds of the tongue
- B. Difficulty swallowing
- C. Vocal cord paralysis
- D. Loss of sensation on the face
- E. Difficulty shrugging the shoulder

Correct answer is B

Dividing the ansa hypoglossi (ansa cervicalis) is routine in carotid endarterectomy surgery. The ansa hypoglossi gives muscular branches to the geniohyoid muscle of the suprahyoid group and most of the infrahyoid muscles (excluding the thyrohyoid muscle). These muscles play a role in swallowing through movement of the larynx. Injury to the ansa cervicalis can potentially impair motor function, affecting the swallowing mechanism. However, dysphagia following carotid endarterectomy can also be caused by injury to the vagus nerve, pharyngeal manipulation, soft tissue swelling in the neck, and pre- or perioperative stroke.[62]

►► Question 27

Which of the following factors is associated with increased procedural risk of cerebral ischemia after carotid artery stenting (CAS), but not after carotid endarterectomy (CEA)?

- A. Age over 70 years
- B. History of stroke
- C. Severe contralateral carotid stenosis
- D. Recent myocardial infarction
- E. Presence of carotid artery ulceration

Correct answer is A

Several trials have compared CAS to CEA. In two meta-analyses of multiple randomized controlled trials, CEA was shown to be superior to CAS in patients aged 70 years and older due to increased periprocedural stroke risk in patients within this age group treated with CAS.

The presence of (C) **Severe contralateral carotid stenosis** raises the risk of stroke due to lack of collaterals; however, this has not been shown to increase the risk in carotid stenting over CEA. (E) **Presence of carotid artery ulceration** raises the risk of stroke in general, but it has not been shown to increase the risk of stroke in one procedure over the other. (D) **Recent myocardial infarction** (MI) does not inherently increase the risk of stroke; however, CAS has demonstrated lower risk of periprocedural MI compared to CEA.[63,64]

►► Question 28

Which of the following is likely to provide the most conclusive evidence of the anatomic integrity of the facial nerve in a patient with facial paralysis following a basilar skull fracture?

- A. CT scan of the temporal bone
- B. MRI with contrast of the facial nerve
- C. Electromyography
- D. Nerve conduction study
- E. Facial nerve decompression surgery

Correct answer is B

MRI with contrast can provide detailed imaging of the facial nerve and surrounding structures, helping to determine the cause and extent of paralysis. It is the preferred imaging modality for assessing facial nerve integrity following trauma (► Fig. 1.10).[65,66] ► Table 1.11 summarizes the major functional components of the facial nerve.

►► Question 29

A 67-year-old man with type 2 diabetes mellitus, hyperlipidemia, and hypertension presents with transient aphasia and right-sided weakness. MR imaging demonstrates a watershed infarct in the left hemisphere. CT angiography shows focal 70% left M1 stenosis (► Fig. 1.11). Which of the following is the most appropriate treatment?

- A. Intravenous heparin
- B. Carotid endarterectomy
- C. Carotid artery stenting
- D. Medical management with antiplatelet therapy
- E. Surgical bypass

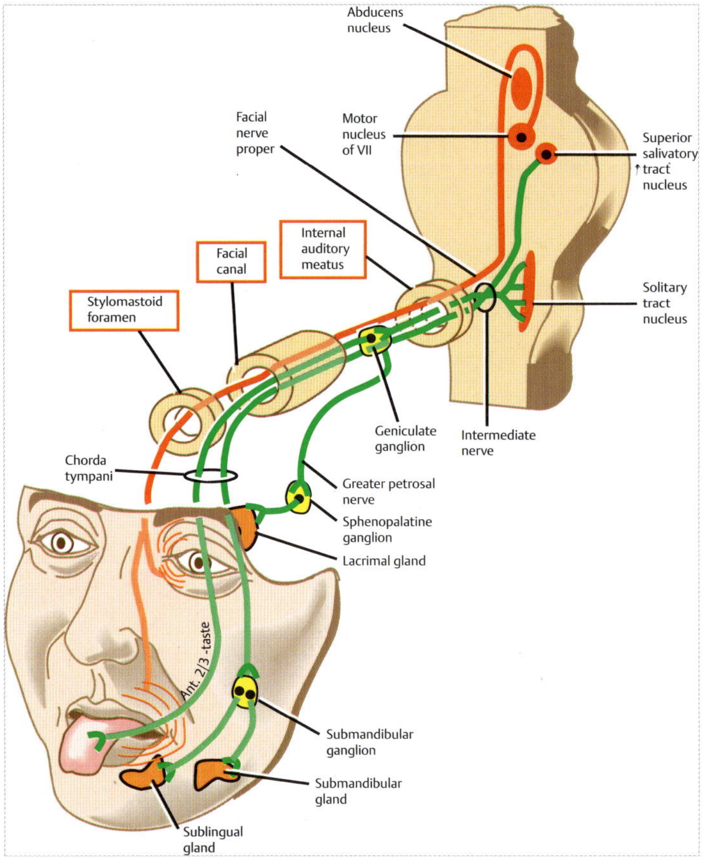

Fig. 1.10 (Source: The Intermediate Nerve. In: Alberstone C, Benzel E, Jones S, Wang Z, Steinmetz M, ed. Anatomic Basis of Neurologic Diagnosis. 2nd Edition. New York: Thieme; 2023.)

Table 1.11 Functional components of the facial nerve (VII)

Components	Ganglia	Nuclei	Exit through skull	Target organ	Function
Somatic motor		Facial motor	Internal auditory meatus	Muscles of facial expression; stylohyoid, posterior digastric muscles; platysma	Multiple actions in the face and neck
Visceral motor	Pterygopalatine	Superior salivatory		Lacrimal gland	Gland secretion
	Submandibular			Submandibular and sublingual glands	
Special sense	Geniculate	Solitary tract		Taste buds in the anterior two-thirds of the tongue	Taste

Correct answer is D

D. Medical management with antiplatelet therapy is typically the first-line treatment for patients with symptomatic intracranial atherosclerosis. This approach includes optimizing medical therapy for risk factors such as diabetes, hypertension, and hyperlipidemia.

In this case, **(A) Intravenous heparin** is generally not considered in the management of intracranial atherosclerotic disease. **(B) Carotid**

endarterectomy and (C) **Carotid stenting** would be inappropriate for disease that was intracranial, as these procedures treat the extracranial carotid artery. However, in the case of a tandem lesion, treating the cervical carotid artery would be indicated. (E) **Surgical bypass** is controversial for intracranial atherosclerotic disease, but it is typically considered only after failure of medical management.[67,68,69]

▸▸ Question 30

Which of the following is the most appropriate treatment for a symptomatic carotid-cavernous fistula (CCF) in the digital subtraction angiogram shown (▸ Fig. 1.12)?

- A. Observation
- B. Intravenous corticosteroids
- C. Endovascular embolization
- D. Open surgical repair
- E. Radiation therapy

Correct answer is C

Symptomatic CCFs, including both direct and indirect fistulas, are often treated with endovascular embolization. This minimally invasive approach can effectively close the fistula and alleviate symptoms such as pulsatile tinnitus, headache, and vision changes.

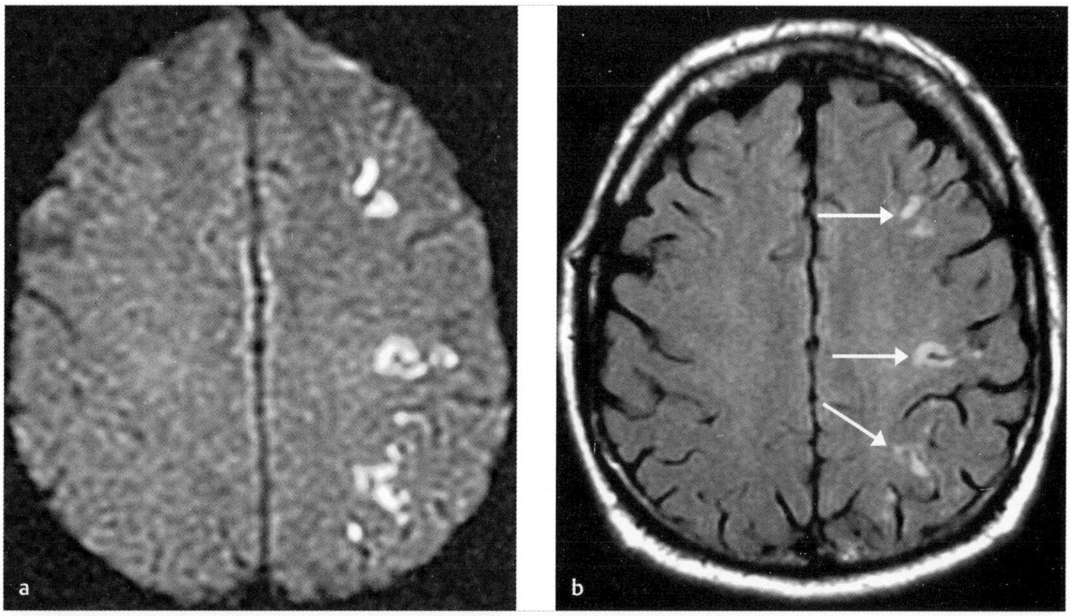

Fig. 1.11 (Source: Reproduced from Table 1.4 Multiple intra-axial lesions in the brain. In: Meyers S, ed. Differential Diagnosis in Neuroimaging: Brain and Meninges. 1st ed. New York: Thieme; 2016.)

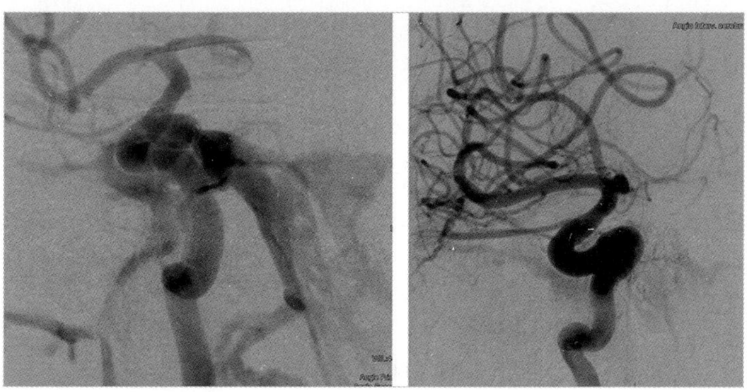

Fig. 1.12 (Source: Reproduced from Direct CCFs (Type A). In: Spetzler R, Kalani M, Nakaji P, ed. Neurovascular Surgery. 2nd ed. New York: Thieme; 2015.)

(A) **Observation** would not be an appropriate course of action in the setting of a symptomatic fistula. (B) **Intravenous corticosteroids** may play a role in symptom management following treatment; they do offer an appropriate management strategy and will not resolve the CCF. (D) **Open surgical repair** may be a potential treatment approach in some dural arteriovenous fistulas, particularly in those with failed endovascular embolization and/or lack of endovascular access; however, this is generally not considered a first-line approach. (E) **Radiation therapy** has been described in the treatment of some CCFs, in particular indirect CCF, but due to this case representing a symptomatic CCF and the long obliteration process required with radiation, endovascular embolization would be preferred as a first-line treatment.[70,71,72,73]

▸▸ Question 31

A 35-year-old woman is evaluated because of persistent, severe, right-sided retro-orbital pain that came on suddenly 2 days ago. Three hours ago, she had an episode of transient right eye blindness that lasted 2 minutes. The patient has no history of serious illness and takes no medication. Examination shows a miotic pupil and ptosis on the right. Which of the following is the most likely diagnosis?

- A. Cluster headache
- B. Carotid artery dissection
- C. Trigeminal neuralgia
- D. Migraine with aura
- E. Glaucoma

Correct answer is B

Carotid artery dissection can present with severe unilateral pain, Horner's syndrome (miotic pupil and ptosis), and transient vision loss due to retinal ischemia. This condition requires prompt diagnosis and treatment to prevent further ischemic events (▸ Fig. 1.13 and ▸ Fig. 1.14).[74,75]

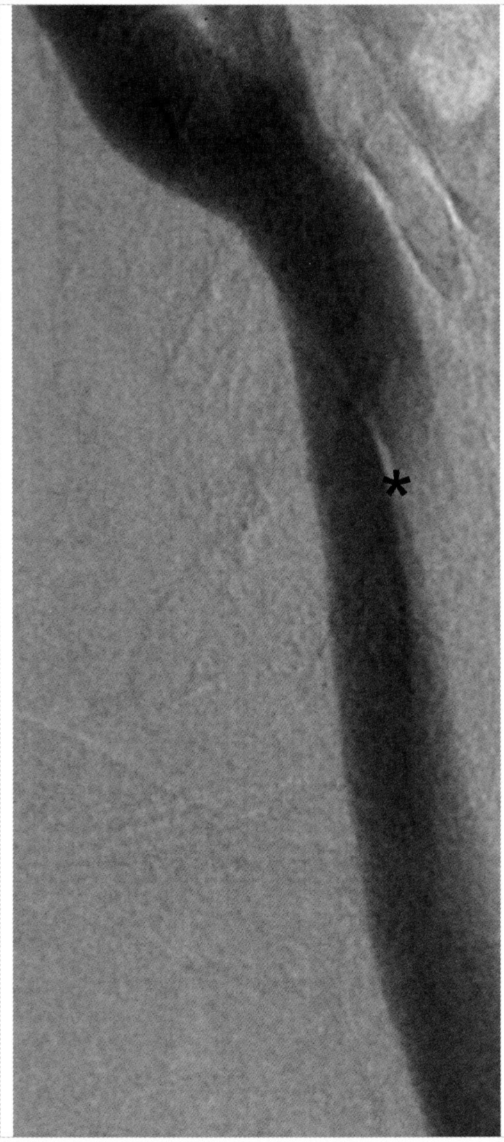

Fig. 1.13 (Source: Reproduced from Spontaneous cerebrovascular injuries. In: Spetzler R, Kalani M, Nakaji P, ed. Neurovascular Surgery. 2nd ed. New York: Thieme; 2015.)

▸▸ Question 32

A 79-year-old woman is evaluated because of a Hunt and Hess grade 4 and Fisher's grade 4 subarachnoid hemorrhage with left hemiplegia. CT scan of the head shows a subarachnoid hemorrhage isolated to the cervicomedullary junction and posterior fossa. CT angiography shows an 8-mm right posterior inferior cerebral artery (PICA) aneurysm with a 2-mm neck in addition to a 2-mm left middle cerebral artery (MCA) aneurysm. Which of the following is the most appropriate treatment for this patient (▶ Fig. 1.15)?

- A. Observation
- B. Medical management with antihypertensive therapy
- C. Surgical clipping of the PICA aneurysm
- D. Endovascular coiling of the PICA aneurysm
- E. Stereotactic radiosurgery

Correct answer is D

Endovascular coiling is often preferred for aneurysms located in difficult surgical locations such as the PICA. This minimally invasive approach can reduce the risk of rebleeding and manage the aneurysm effectively. In this case, the aneurysm is described as having a narrow neck and a dome-to-neck ratio of 4, which makes it favorable for endovascular intervention (▶ Fig. 1.16).

(A) Observation is not appropriate in the setting of a ruptured aneurysm, especially one amenable to treatment, due to the high risk of rerupture. **(B) Medical management with antihypertensive therapy** might be necessary in the setting of vasospasm, once the ruptured aneurysm has been secured. **(C) Surgical clipping of the PICA aneurysm** is an option if endovascular therapy fails. **(E) Stereotactic radiosurgery** does not play a role in the management of cerebral aneurysms.[76]

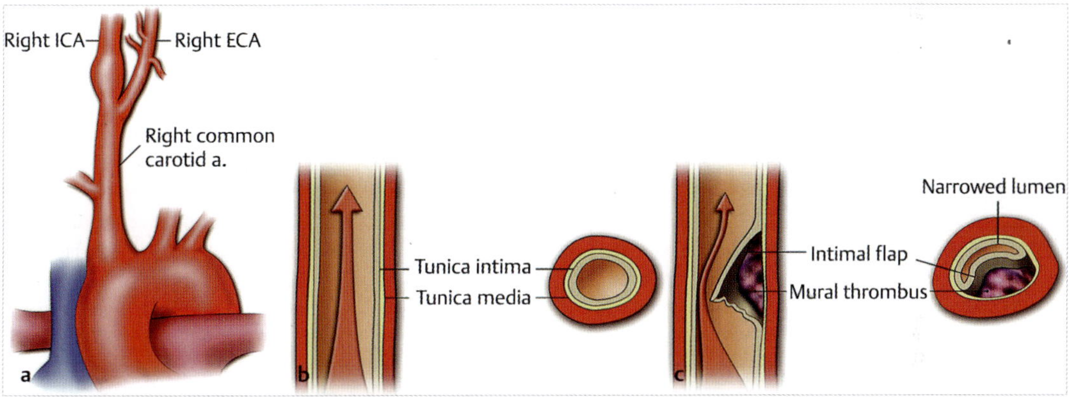

Fig. 1.14 (Source: Reproduced from Pathophysiology and natural history. In: Bendok B, Batjer H, ed. Hemorrhagic and Ischemic Stroke: Medical, Imaging, Surgical, and Interventional Approaches. 2nd ed. New York: Thieme; 2024.)

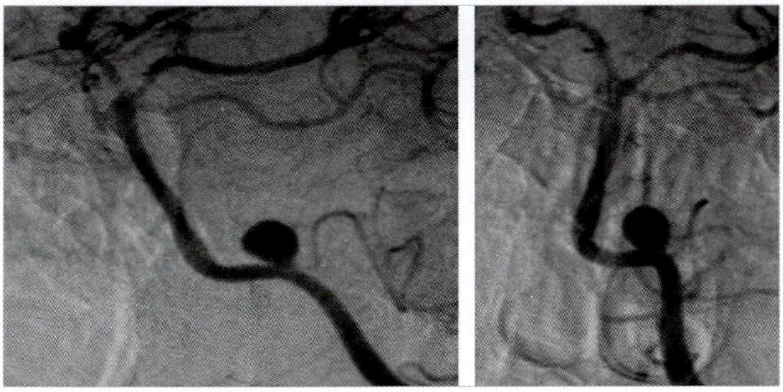

Fig. 1.15 (Source: Reproduced from Case Overview: CASE 23.8 Large Posterior Inferior Cerebellar Artery Aneurysm. In: Rangel-Castilla L, Siddiqui A, Levy E, Lanzino G, Hopkins L, Davies J, eds. Video Atlas of Neuroendovascular Procedures. 1st ed. New York: Thieme; 2020.)

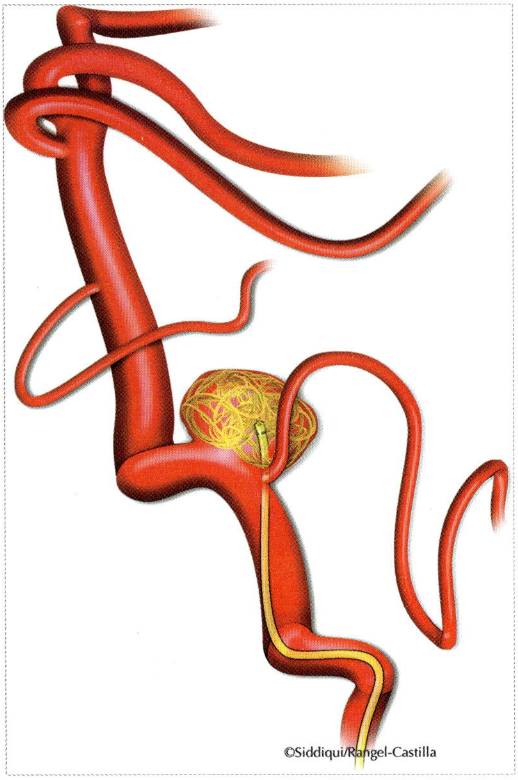

Fig. 1.16 (Source: Reproduced from Case Overview: CASE 23.8 Large Posterior Inferior Cerebellar Artery Aneurysm. In: Rangel-Castilla L, Siddiqui A, Levy E, Lanzino G, Hopkins L, Davies J, eds. Video Atlas of Neuroendovascular Procedures. 1st ed. New York: Thieme; 2020.)

▸▸ Question 33

A 45-year-old man is evaluated because of a 2-week history of headaches. MR angiography shows a 13-mm smooth left middle cerebral artery aneurysm. Which of the following factors would put this patient at increased risk for future hemorrhage?

- A. Aneurysm size
- B. Patient age
- C. Presence of diabetes
- D. Location of aneurysm in the anterior circulation
- E. History of smoking

Correct answer is A

In this case, **(A) Aneurysm size** would be the answer choice that brings the highest risk of rupture. The size of the aneurysm is a critical factor in determining the risk of future hemorrhage. Aneurysms larger than 10 mm are associated with a significantly higher risk of rupture. The question prompt does not state whether it was confirmed that the aneurysm might have ruptured in a sentinel event; however, prior rupture would place the patient at high risk for future hemorrhage. According to the International Study of Unruptured Intracranial Aneurysms (ISUIA) study, an unruptured middle cerebral artery aneurysm measuring between 7 and 12 mm has a 2.5% 5-year rupture risk (▸ Table 1.12). **(D) Location of the aneurysm in the anterior circulation** carries a lower risk of rupture when compared to posterior circulation aneurysms.[77,78,79]

Table 1.12 Five-year cumulative rupture rates according to size and location of unruptured aneurysm and according to patient group in the ISUIA study

	<7 mm Group 1	<7 mm Group 2	7–12 mm	13–24 mm	≥25 mm
Cavernous	0%	0%	0%	3.0%	6.4%
AComm/MCA/ICA	0%	1.5%	2.6%	14.5%	40%
Posterior/PComm	2.5%	3.4%	14.5%	18.4%	50%

Abbreviations: AComm, anterior communicating artery; ICA, internal carotid artery; MCA, middle cerebral artery; PComm, posterior communicating artery.
Group 1: no history of subarachnoid hemorrhage (SAH).
Group 2: history of SAH from a separate aneurysm.

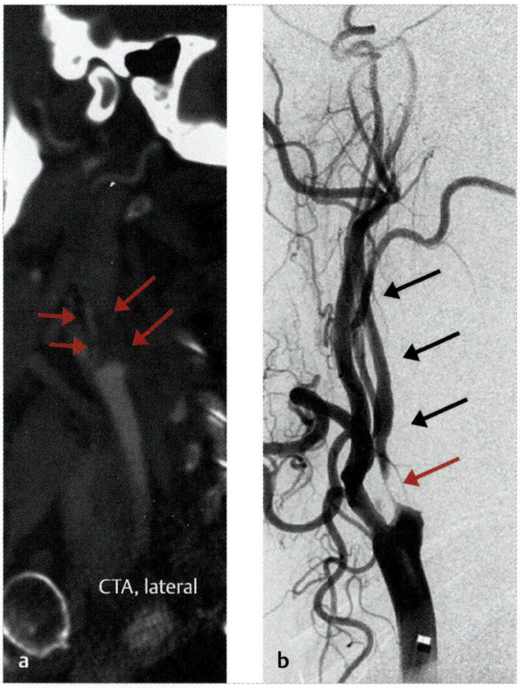

Fig. 1.17 (Source: Reproduced from Anatomical and imaging aspects. In: Mokin M, Levy E, Siddiqui A, eds. Video Atlas of Acute Ischemic Stroke Intervention. 1st ed. New York: Thieme; 2022.)

▸▸ Question 34

A 70-year-old woman with severe congestive heart failure is evaluated because of several episodes of word-finding difficulty and right-arm weakness. CT angiography shows 90% stenosis of the left internal carotid artery at the level of C2 according to North American Symptomatic Carotid Endarterectomy Trial (NASCET) criteria. The right internal carotid artery demonstrates 40% stenosis. Left ventricular ejection fraction is 25% (▸ Fig. 1.17). Which of the following is the most appropriate treatment option for this patient's carotid stenosis?

- A. Medical management with antiplatelet therapy
- B. Carotid endarterectomy
- C. Carotid artery stenting
- D. Carotid artery bypass surgery
- E. Observation and follow-up imaging in 6 months

Correct answer is C

For patients with severe cardiac disease (congestive heart failure in this case) and significant carotid artery stenosis, carotid artery stenting (CAS) is often preferred over endarterectomy due to the lower perioperative risk associated with the procedure, as CAS can be performed under monitored anesthetic care or moderate sedation rather than general anesthesia. CAS has been shown to have less risk of myocardial infarction when compared to **(B) Carotid endarterectomy** (CEA), and thus, CAS is preferred in patients with cardiac history. Patients who are 70 years old or older may be better suited for CEA, in the absence of significant medical comorbidities. The key trials and their findings have been summarized in ▸ Table 1.13.

(A) Medical management with antiplatelet therapy is an option but not preferred in the setting of symptomatic carotid stenosis > 50%. **(D) Carotid artery bypass** is not a first-line option. **(E) Observation and follow-up imaging** would not be appropriate in either symptomatic or asymptomatic high-grade carotid artery stenosis (▸ Table 1.12).[80,81,82,83,84]

▸▸ Question 35

Which of the following best describes cranial nerves that are contained within the superior orbital fissure?

- A. Cranial nerves III, IV, V1, and VI
- B. Cranial nerves II, III, IV, and V2
- C. Cranial nerves III, V1, V2, and VI
- D. Cranial nerves II, III, IV, and VI
- E. Cranial nerves III, IV, V1, V2, and VI

Correct answer is A

This question ensures a clear understanding of the anatomical structures related to the cranial nerves passing through the superior orbital fissure (SOF). CN III has two divisions, the inferior and superior, both of which pass through the SOF, and both of which are contained within the annulus of Zinn. CN IV passes through the SOF but remains outside of the annulus of Zinn. CN V1 has multiple branches, some of which go through the SOF and some go through the inferior orbital fissure. Of the branches of CN V1, the lacrimal nerve, frontal nerve, and nasociliary nerve go through the SOF, and of these branches, only the nasociliary nerve passes in the annulus of Zinn. Lastly, CN VI goes

Table 1.13 Key findings of carotid endarterectomy and stenting trials

Trial name	Year	Comparison	Key findings	Citations
NASCET	1991	CEA vs. medical therapy	CEA significantly reduced the risk of ipsilateral stroke in patients with symptomatic carotid stenosis of 70–99%	Barnett HJM, Taylor DW, Haynes RB, et al. N Engl J Med 1991;325(7):445–453
ECST	1998	CEA vs. medical therapy	CEA offered significant stroke prevention benefits over medical treatment in patients with symptomatic high-grade carotid artery stenosis	European Carotid Surgery Trialists' Collaborative Group. Lancet 1998;351 (9113):1379–1387
ACST	2004	CEA vs. medical therapy (asymptomatic)	CEA reduces the risk of stroke in asymptomatic patients, especially in men and those over 75 y	Halliday A, Mansfield A, Marro J, et al. Lancet 2004;363(9420):1491–1502
SAPPHIRE	2004	CAS vs. CEA (high-risk patients)	CAS was noninferior to CEA in patients at high risk for surgical complications	Yadav JS, Wholey MH, Kuntz RE, et al. N Engl J Med 2004;351(15):1493–1501
CREST	2010	CEA vs. CAS	CEA and CAS were effective for carotid revascularization in symptomatic and asymptomatic patients with different risk profiles. Patients older than 70 fared better with CEA. Risk of stroke was higher in CAS. Risk of MI was higher in CEA	Brott TG, Hobson RW 2nd, Howard G, et al. N Engl J Med 2010;363(1):11–23

through the SOF and also through the annulus of Zinn. In addition to the nerves passing in the SOF, the superior ophthalmic vein travels through the SOF and often a branch of the inferior ophthalmic vein (▶ Fig. 1.18).

▸▸ Question 36

A 45-year-old woman is evaluated for carotid artery stenosis. Doppler ultrasound reveals 70% stenosis by NASCET criteria in the cervical right internal carotid artery. She has no symptoms of stroke or transient ischemic attack. Which of the following is the most appropriate management?

- A. Carotid endarterectomy or carotid artery stenting
- B. Repeat Doppler ultrasound now
- C. Medical management with antiplatelet therapy and statins
- D. Observation and follow-up imaging in 6 months
- E. Lifestyle and diet modification

Correct answer is A

In asymptomatic patients with carotid artery stenosis 70% or higher, intervention should be recommended according to the joint guidelines in order to prevent future stroke. In a patient with low anesthetic risk, carotid endarterectomy could be entertained over carotid artery stenting, although both are viable options. In a recent systematic review and meta-analysis comparing CAS to CEA in asymptomatic carotid artery stenosis, CAS has comparable perioperative and long-term composite outcomes compared with CEA. However, CAS may have a higher risk of any stroke and nondisabling stroke in the perioperative period.

(B) **Repeat Doppler ultrasound now** would not be necessary unless there was some question of technique or poor image acquisition. One might consider additional imaging for surgical planning, such as CTA or digital subtraction angiography. (C) **Medical management with antiplatelet therapy and statins** would be the treatment recommendation in patients with lower grade stenosis and no

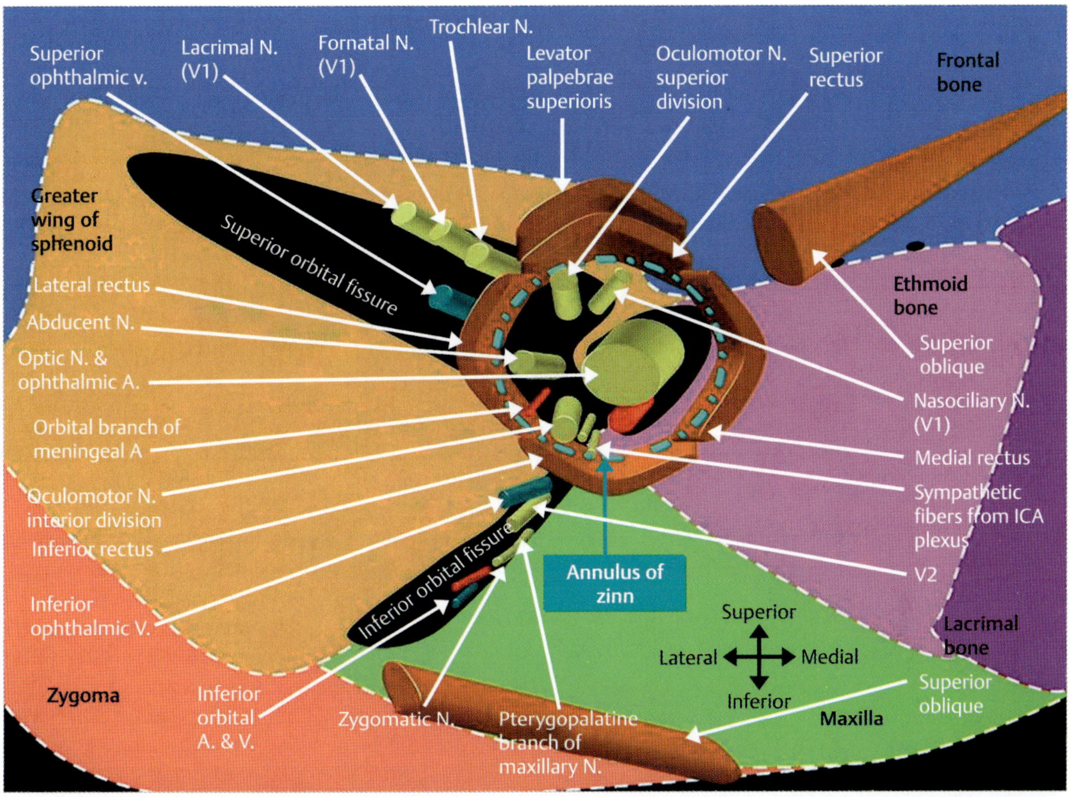

Fig. 1.18 (Source: Reproduced from Case 23 Orbital tumor. In: Nader R, Sabbagh A, Elbabaa S, Al-Jehani H, Gasco J, Gragnaniello C, eds. Neurosurgery Case Review: Questions and Answers. 2nd ed. New York: Thieme; 2020.)

symptomatology, and while antiplatelet and statin therapy play a role in this case, it would not appropriate to recommend as the only management option. (**D**) **Observation and follow-up imaging** would not be the right course of action, as the stenosis appears to be high grade, even though asymptomatic. (**E**) **Lifestyle and diet modification** would be useful to prevent further development of vascular disease, but in the setting of high-grade stenosis, it would not be enough to protect the patient from future stroke.[85,86,87]

▸▸ Question 37

Which of the following factors is associated with increased procedural risk of cerebral ischemia after carotid artery stenting, but not after carotid endarterectomy?

- A. Advanced age
- B. Hypertension
- C. Diabetes mellitus
- D. Presence of aortic arch atheroma
- E. Contralateral carotid occlusion

Correct answer is D

The presence of aortic arch atheroma increases the risk of cerebral ischemia during carotid artery stenting due to the potential for embolization, but it does not similarly affect carotid endarterectomy. Having vascular disease of the aorta is thought to contribute to the increased risk of periprocedural stroke following carotid artery stenting in patients older than 70 years when compared to carotid endarterectomy.[88,89]

▸▸ Question 38

Which of the following characteristics confers the highest risk of hemorrhage for patients harboring dural arteriovenous fistulas (DAVFs)?

- A. Location in the anterior cranial fossa
- B. Presence of cortical venous reflux

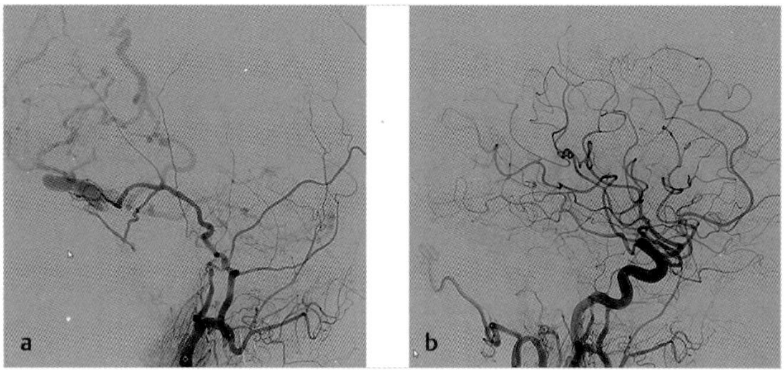

Fig. 1.19 (Source: Reproduced from Classification, presentation, and natural history. In: Macdonald R, ed. Neurosurgical Operative Atlas: Vascular Neurosurgery. 3rd ed. New York: Thieme; 2018.)

- C. High flow rate through the fistula
- D. Multiple feeding arteries
- E. Young patient age

Correct answer is B

DAVFs are acquired lesions and represent complex vascular malformations that involve an abnormal connection between the arterial and venous systems surrounding the nervous system. The fistulous point resides within the dura. Typically, they are supplied by multiple feeders from arteries that supply the relevant part of the meninges but can also recruit regional scalp vessels and intracranial feeders. The presence of cortical venous reflux is the most significant risk factor for hemorrhage in patients with DAVFs. The significance of cortical venous reflux is reflected in both the Borden and Cognard classification systems, which assign higher grades to DAVFs exhibiting cortical venous reflux (▶ Fig. 1.19).[90,91]

▸▸ Question 39

A 62-year-old woman presents with a sudden severe headache and is found to have a Hunt and Hess grade 3 subarachnoid hemorrhage. Angiography reveals a 9-mm saccular aneurysm at the bifurcation of the anterior communicating artery. Which of the following factors in this case was most predictive of this aneurysm's rupture risk?

- A. Location of the aneurysm
- B. Size of the aneurysm
- C. Patient's age
- D. Presence of multiple aneurysms
- E. Aneurysm shape (irregular or multilobulated)

Correct answer is B

The risk of aneurysm rupture increases with the size of the aneurysm. Aneurysms larger than 7 mm are at a significantly higher risk of rupture compared to smaller aneurysms. Other factors, such as (A) **Aneurysm location** (posterior circulation aneurysms have higher rupture risks), (**C**) **Patient age**, and (**D**) **Presence of multiple aneurysms**, also contribute to the risk. The shape of the aneurysm, particularly irregular or multilobulated shapes, can further increase the likelihood of rupture, and the presence of a bleb or daughter sac on an aneurysm can often represent the site of rupture. Management strategies are guided by these risk factors to prevent catastrophic outcomes. In this case, the patient had an aneurysm of the anterior circulation without any irregularity but over 7 mm in size. Thus, the size of the aneurysm was the factor most related to rupture in this patient. According to the International Study of Unruptured Intracranial Aneurysms (ISUIA) study, an unruptured middle cerebral artery aneurysm measuring between 7 and 12 mm has a 2.5% 5-year rupture risk (▶ Table 1.14).[92,93]

▸▸ Question 40

A 50-year-old woman with a 5-mm ruptured anterior communicating artery aneurysm undergoes endovascular coiling. During the procedure, the patient develops new neurological deficits. Which of the following complications is most likely responsible for these deficits?

- A. Coil migration
- B. Aneurysm rerupture
- C. Thromboembolic event
- D. Vasospasm
- E. Coil compaction

Table 1.14 Five-year cumulative rupture rates according to size and location of unruptured aneurysm and according to patient group in the ISUIA study

	<7 mm Group 1	<7 mm Group 2	7–12 mm	13–24 mm	≥25 mm
Cavernous	0%	0%	0%	3.0%	6.4%
AComm/MCA/ICA	0%	1.5%	2.6%	14.5%	40%
Posterior/PComm	2.5%	3.4%	14.5%	18.4%	50%

Abbreviations: AComm, anterior communicating artery; ICA, internal carotid artery; MCA, middle cerebral artery; PComm, posterior communicating artery.
Group 1: no history of subarachnoid hemorrhage (SAH).
Group 2: history of SAH from a separate aneurysm.

Correct answer is C

(C) **Thromboembolic events** are a common complication during and after endovascular coiling procedures. These events can lead to ischemic strokes, resulting in new neurological deficits. About one in every two patients undergoing endovascular treatment of an aneurysm will have DWI-positive lesion on MRI following the procedure, with the highest rates found in flow diversion placement. Preventive measures, including heparinization during the procedure, can reduce the risk of thromboembolic complications. Other potential complications include (A) **Coil migration**, (B) **Aneurysm rerupture**, (D) **Vasospasm**, and (E) **Coil compaction**. Coil migration, aneurysm rerupture, and vasospasm could all lead to the development of neurological deficit; however, these would also be observed during the procedure and were not noted in the question stem. Each of these complications requires prompt identification and management to minimize patient morbidity and mortality. Coil compaction is a later sequelae that can occur following this treatment modality but does not cause neurological deficit.[94,95,96,97]

▸▸ Question 41

A 58-year-old woman develops a new onset of aphasia and right hemiparesis immediately after surgical clipping of a left middle cerebral artery aneurysm. Which of the following is the most likely cause of these new deficits?

- A. Cerebral vasospasm
- B. Aneurysm rerupture
- C. Intraoperative thrombosis
- D. Clip slippage
- E. Ischemic stroke due to clip occlusion of perforating arteries

Correct answer is E

Ischemic stroke resulting from the occlusion of perforating arteries by the aneurysm clip is a recognized complication of surgical clipping of intracranial aneurysms. The middle cerebral artery bifurcation is particularly prone to this complication due to the presence of numerous small perforating vessels supplying critical areas of the brain. Ischemic stroke may also occur due to flow-limiting stenosis of the parent vessels secondary to clip placement. Intraoperative assessment, including neuromonitoring, meticulous clip placement, visual inspection with indocyanine green angiography, and possible intraoperative blood flow measurement of the inflow and outflow vessels, is essential to minimize this risk. Postoperative imaging and prompt intervention are necessary if complications arise.

Other answer choices are plausible but less likely given the scenario. (A) **Cerebral vasospasm** can occur due to subarachnoid hemorrhage but usually occurs a few days after ictus and the risk remains present until up to 21 days after rupture. (B) **Aneurysm rerupture** could certainly lead to new deficits, but this event would be noted intraoperatively and less likely to occur postoperatively if the clip ligation were complete. (C) **Intraoperative thrombosis** might occur during temporary clipping of the inlet and outlet vessels of the aneurysm, which could potentially cause new neurologic deficit, but can be minimized with short temporary clipping times. (D) **Clip slippage** is an unlikely occurrence and, in itself, would not cause new neurological deficits.[98,99]

▸▸ Question 42

A 58-year-old man with aneurysmal subarachnoid hemorrhage is at risk for vasospasm. Which of the following is the standard pharmacologic intervention to prevent delayed cerebral ischemia due to vasospasm?

- A. Intravenous mannitol
- B. Oral nimodipine
- C. Intravenous heparin
- D. Oral corticosteroids
- E. Intravenous tissue plasminogen activator

Correct answer is B

Nimodipine, a calcium channel blocker, is the standard pharmacologic agent used to prevent delayed cerebral ischemia due to vasospasm in patients with aneurysmal subarachnoid hemorrhage. It has been shown to improve clinical outcomes in this patient population, although it is not necessarily correlated with a reduction in the radiographic incidence and appearance of vasospasm. The recommended regimen is 60 mg orally every 4 hours for 21 days. Early intervention and continuous monitoring are critical for optimizing patient outcomes.[100,101]

▸▸ Question 43

A 70-year-old woman with a history of smoking and hypertension presents with sudden onset of a severe headache. She is diagnosed with a subarachnoid hemorrhage and treated with endovascular coiling of the ruptured aneurysm. On postprocedure day 5, she develops new neurological deficits, including left-sided weakness and aphasia. What is the most likely cause of her new symptoms?

- A. Rerupture of the aneurysm
- B. Cerebral vasospasm
- C. Hydrocephalus
- D. Electrolyte imbalance
- E. Coil migration

Correct answer is B

Cerebral vasospasm is a common and serious complication of subarachnoid hemorrhage, typically occurring between days 4 and 14 posthemorrhage. It can lead to delayed cerebral ischemia and new neurological deficits, which may be transient or permanent. Early detection and aggressive management, including maintaining euvolemia, induced hypertension, and administration of nimodipine, are essential for reducing the risk of permanent deficits and improving patient outcomes (▸ Fig. 1.20).

(A) **Rerupture of the aneurysm** in the acute setting is possible but unlikely after a successfully

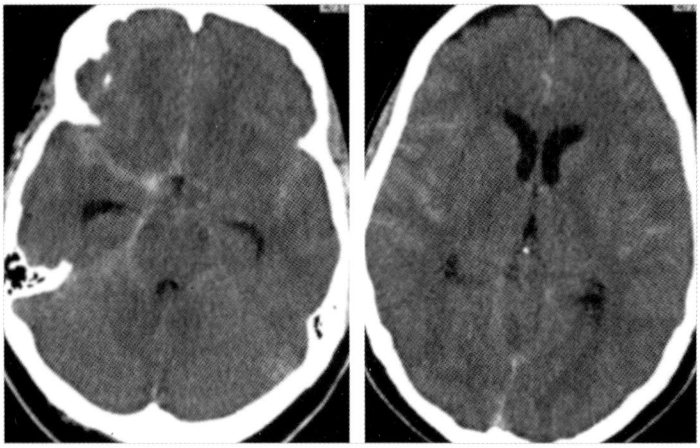

Fig. 1.20 (Source: Reproduced from Case Overview: CASE 23.3 Very Small Ruptured Anterior Cerebral Artery Aneurysm: Primary Coiling. In: Rangel-Castilla L, Siddiqui A, Levy E, Lanzino G, Hopkins L, Davies J, eds. Video Atlas of Neuroendovascular Procedures. 1st ed. New York: Thieme; 2020.)

treated aneurysm. (**C**) **Hydrocephalus** can occur after subarachnoid hemorrhage but usually does not cause focal deficits; rather, it tends to produce global neurological signs, such as decreased mentation. (**D**) **Electrolyte imbalance** can also cause altered mental status, but it would be unusual to produce focal deficits. (**E**) **Coil migration** is a rare complication following endovascular treatment of cerebral aneurysms and, if it occurs, typically happens intraprocedurally; thus, cerebral vasospasm would be the more likely culprit. Although not an answer choice, seizures are worth mentioning as a possible cause of focal but transient deficits following aneurysmal subarachnoid hemorrhage, and patients are usually treated prophylactically with antiepileptic medications.[102,103]

▸▸ Question 44

A 35-year-old man presents with seizures and is diagnosed with an arteriovenous malformation (AVM) on MRI (▶ Fig. 1.21). The AVM is located in the right parietal lobe, measures 4 cm, and has superficial venous drainage. According to the Spetzler-Martin grading system, what is the grade of this AVM?

- A. Grade 1
- B. Grade 2
- C. Grade 3
- D. Grade 4
- E. Grade 5

Correct answer is C

The Spetzler-Martin grading system is used to predict the surgical risk of AVMs. It assigns points based on the size of the AVM, the pattern of venous drainage, and the location of the AVM in eloquent brain areas (▶ Table 1.15).

This patient's AVM is 4 cm (2 points), has superficial venous drainage (0 points), and is in the parietal lobe (eloquent brain, 1 point), resulting in a total of 3 points, which corresponds to Grade 3.[104,105]

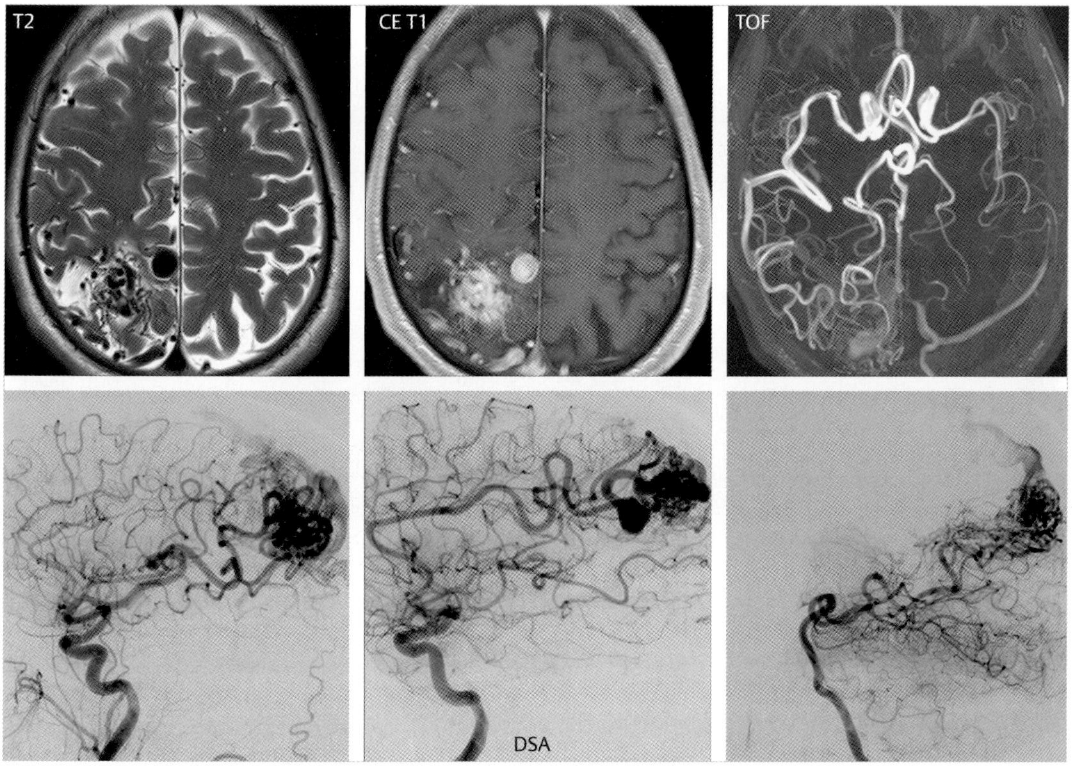

Fig. 1.21 (Source: Reproduced from Arteriovenous malformation. In: Runge V, ed. Imaging of Cerebrovascular Disease. 1st ed. New York: Thieme; 2016.)

Table 1.15 Spetzler–Martin grading system

Feature	Points
Size	
Small (< 3 cm) Medium (3–6 cm) Large (> 6 cm)	1 point 2 points 3 points
Venous drainage	
Superficial only Deep	0 points 1 point
Location	
Noneloquent Eloquent	0 points 1 point

▸▸ Question 45

A 28-year-old woman is diagnosed with an incidentally found unruptured arteriovenous malformation (AVM) located in the left frontal lobe. The AVM measures 2 cm and has superficial venous drainage. She is asymptomatic. Which of the following treatment options is most appropriate for this patient?

- A. Observation with serial imaging
- B. Microsurgical resection
- C. Stereotactic radiosurgery
- D. Embolization
- E. Combined modality treatment

Correct answer is A

Management of unruptured AVMs is controversial and depends on factors such as AVM size, location, patient age, and symptomatology. In asymptomatic patients with small AVMs and no high-risk features for rupture, studies, such as ARUBA, support the recommendation of conservative management with observation and serial imaging. This approach minimizes the risk of treatment-related complications, but the risks and benefits of treatment must be carefully weighed with the patient on a case-by-case basis.

It is important to note, however, that AVMs in general carry a rupture risk of 2 to 4% per year, and assuming a life expectancy of 70 years, a young patient may benefit from treatment, even in the setting of unruptured and asymptomatic presentation. In this patient of 28 years of age, her lifetime rupture risk would be 77%. Any high-risk features, such as a feeder artery aneurysm or draining vein stenosis, may further point toward active treatment.[106,107,108]

▸▸ Question 46

A 50-year-old woman undergoes microsurgical resection of a left occipital arteriovenous malformation (AVM). Postoperatively, she develops right homonymous hemianopia. Which of the following best describes the cause of this complication?

- A. Damage to the optic nerve
- B. Ischemic injury to the occipital lobe
- C. Edema around the surgical site
- D. Vasospasm
- E. Hemorrhagic transformation

Correct answer is B

Postoperative complications following AVM resection can include neurological deficits due to ischemic injury to brain regions adjacent to the AVM. In this case, the right homonymous hemianopia is likely due to ischemic damage to the left occipital lobe during surgery. It is also possibly the result of resection of eloquent brain matter surrounding the AVM, although this is not an option in the question above. Understanding potential complications and their management is crucial for optimizing patient outcomes.[109,110]

▸▸ Question 47

A 55-year-old man undergoes surgical clipping of a ruptured anterior communicating artery aneurysm. Postoperatively, he is noted to have difficulty with short-term memory and exhibits confabulatory behavior. Which of the following is the most likely cause of his symptoms (▸ Fig. 1.22)?

- A. Anterior cerebral artery ischemia
- B. Basal forebrain damage
- C. Vasospasm
- D. Hydrocephalus
- E. Posterior cerebral artery infarction

Correct answer is B

Damage to the basal forebrain, particularly structures such as the septal nuclei and the nucleus basalis of Meynert, can result in short-term memory deficits and confabulation. This region is

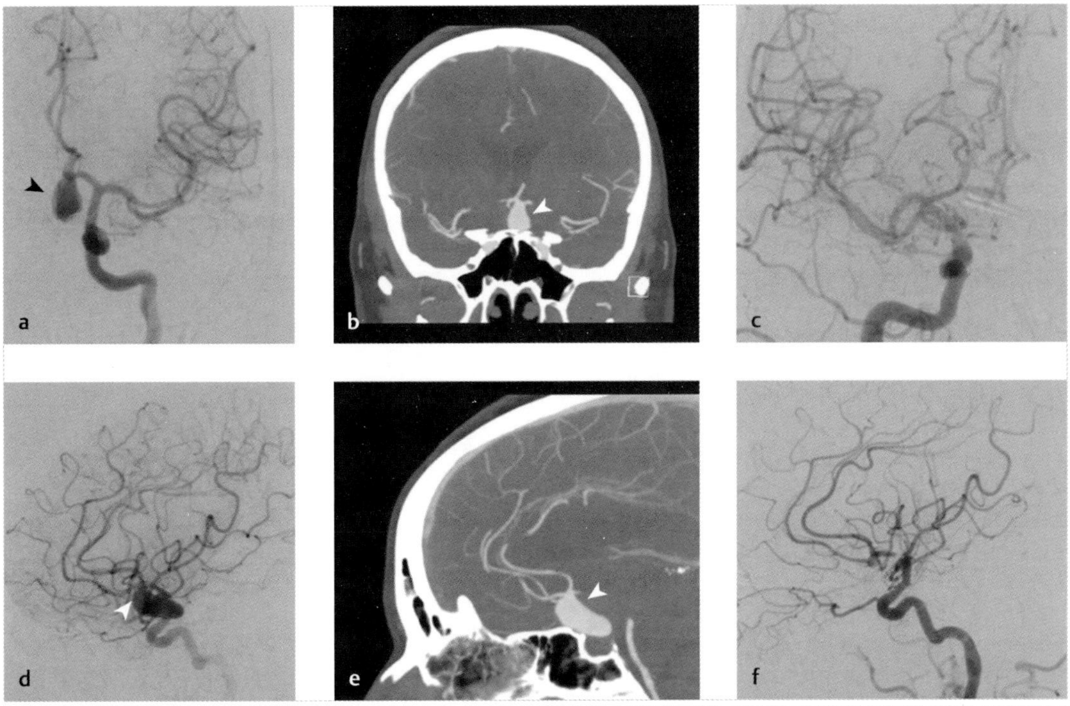

Fig. 1.22 (Source: Reproduced from Authors' recommendations. In: Lai L, Gragnaniello C, eds. Neurosurgical Diseases: An Evidence-Based Approach to Guide Practice. 1st ed. New York: Thieme; 2021.)

susceptible during anterior communicating artery aneurysm surgery due to its proximity to the aneurysm and manipulation of the structures during dissection and retraction.

The septal nuclei—located medially in the cerebral hemispheres inferior to the rostrum of the corpus callosum, anterior to the third ventricle, and into the base of the septum pellucidum—appear to play a role in emotional behaviors, sexual behavior, aggressive behavior, modulation of autonomic functions, and attention and memory functions (from the cholinergic neurons). The nucleus basalis of Meynert is a structure in the basal forebrain, located inferior to the globus pallidus interna, which provides the major source of cholinergic innervation to the cortex. Prevention of this injury with technique is key, but recognizing and managing such complications is critical for optimal postoperative care, including appropriate rehabilitation.[111]

▸▸ Question 48

A 60-year-old woman presents with a subarachnoid hemorrhage due to a ruptured anterior communicating artery aneurysm. She is classified as Hunt and Hess grade 2. Which of the following is the most appropriate method for monitoring and detecting vasospasm during the critical period after aneurysm rupture?

- A. Serial CT angiography
- B. Digital subtraction angiography
- C. Transcranial Doppler ultrasound
- D. MRI with perfusion sequences
- E. Clinical examination only

Correct answer is C

Transcranial Doppler ultrasound is a noninvasive method that is frequently used to monitor for vasospasm in patients with subarachnoid hemorrhage. It allows for the detection of changes

Table 1.16 Transcranial Doppler criteria for vasospasm of middle cerebral artery and basilar artery

Severity of vasospasm of MCA	MFV (cm/s)	MFV-MCA: MFV-EICA ratio (Lindegaard ratio)
Hyperemia	< 120	< 3
Mild	120–149	3–6
Moderate	150–200	3–6
Severe	> 200	> 6
Severity of vasospasm of BA	**MFV (cm/s)**	**MFV-BA:MFV-EVA ratio (modified Lindegaard ratio)**
Hyperemia	< 70	< 2
Mild	70–85	> 2
Moderate	> 85	> 2.5
Severe	> 85	> 3

Abbreviations: MCA, middle cerebral artery; MFV, mean flow velocity; EICA, extracranial internal carotid artery; BA, basilar artery; EVA, extracranial vertebral artery.

in cerebral blood flow velocities, which can indicate the development of vasospasm. Early detection and management of vasospasm are crucial to prevent ischemic complications (▸ Table 1.16).[112]

▸▸ Question 49

A 40-year-old woman with an unruptured arteriovenous malformation (AVM) is being considered for treatment. Which of the following factors would most strongly favor a conservative management approach over surgical intervention?

- A. AVM located in an eloquent brain area
- B. AVM smaller than 3 cm
- C. Presence of associated aneurysms
- D. Patient's age below 50 years
- E. Presence of deep venous drainage

Correct answer is A

Management of AVMs involves weighing the risks of intervention against the natural history of the lesion. AVMs located in eloquent brain areas (regions responsible for critical functions such as language, motor control, and sensory processing) are associated with a higher risk of neurological deficits following surgery. Therefore, conservative management is often favored in these cases unless there are compelling reasons for intervention, such as recurrent hemorrhage or progressive neurological deficits.[113,114]

▸▸ Question 50

A 55-year-old man undergoes stereotactic radiosurgery for a cerebral arteriovenous malformation (AVM). Which of the following is the most likely long-term complication associated with this treatment modality?

- A. Immediate hemorrhage
- B. Radiation necrosis
- C. Infection
- D. Hydrocephalus
- E. Venous thrombosis

Correct answer is B

Stereotactic radiosurgery is a noninvasive treatment option for AVMs, particularly those that are small and located in eloquent brain areas. However, a potential long-term complication unique to this treatment is radiation necrosis, which can occur months to years after the procedure. This results from the delayed effects of radiation on the surrounding brain tissue and can lead to edema, neurological deficits, and sometimes necessitate further treatment.[115]

▸▸ Question 51

A 38-year-old man with an arteriovenous malformation (AVM) presents with an acute headache and loss of consciousness. CT scan shows an intracerebral hemorrhage. Which of the following characteristics of AVMs is most strongly associated with an increased risk of hemorrhage?

- A. Small AVM size
- B. Superficial venous drainage
- C. Associated feeder aneurysms
- D. History of prior hemorrhage
- E. Age over 30 years

Correct answer is D

(D) **History of prior hemorrhage** is a risk factor that has consistently been identified across studies as a risk factor for future hemorrhage. Studies have demonstrated that deep AVM location and deep venous drainage, as opposed to (B) **Superficial venous drainage**, potentially increase the risk of hemorrhage. Additional newer studies have suggested (A) **Smaller AVM size** may impart a higher risk of rupture compared to larger AVMs, although this risk is not as high as that conveyed by previous hemorrhage. The presence of (C) **Associated feeder aneurysms** may also increase the risk of rupture. Other vascular anomalies, such as intranidal aneurysms and venous varices, also represent high-risk features for rupture. (E) **Age over 30 years** does not inherently increase the risk of rupture of cerebral AVM; however, the lifetime risk of a rupture event increases as patients get older.[116]

▸▸ **Question 52**

A 65-year-old man with a history of poorly controlled hypertension presents with a sudden onset of headache, nausea, and right-sided weakness. CT scan of the head shows this hemorrhage. Which of the following is the most likely underlying cause of this patient's hemorrhage?

- A. Cerebral amyloid angiopathy
- B. Hypertensive vasculopathy
- C. Arteriovenous malformation
- D. Ruptured aneurysm
- E. Coagulopathy

Correct answer is B

▸ Fig. 1.23 shows an intraparenchymal hemorrhage in the basal ganglia. Hypertensive vasculopathy is the most common cause of spontaneous intracerebral hemorrhage in the basal ganglia. Chronic hypertension leads to small vessel lipohyalinosis and Charcot-Bouchard microaneurysms, which can rupture and cause hemorrhage. Prompt blood pressure control is essential in managing these patients to prevent further bleeding and reduce morbidity.[117,118]

▸▸ **Question 53**

A 75-year-old woman on warfarin therapy for atrial fibrillation presents with a sudden onset of left-sided weakness and a headache. CT scan reveals a right parietal intracerebral hemorrhage. Her INR is 3.2. What is the most appropriate initial step in the management of her anticoagulant-associated intracerebral hemorrhage?

- A. Administer vitamin K
- B. Administer fresh frozen plasma (FFP)
- C. Administer prothrombin complex concentrate (PCC)
- D. Discontinue warfarin
- E. Perform immediate surgical evacuation

Correct answer is C

In patients with warfarin-associated intracerebral hemorrhage (ICH), the most urgent priority is to rapidly reverse anticoagulation to limit hematoma expansion and reduce morbidity and mortality. PCC is the preferred first-line treatment, as

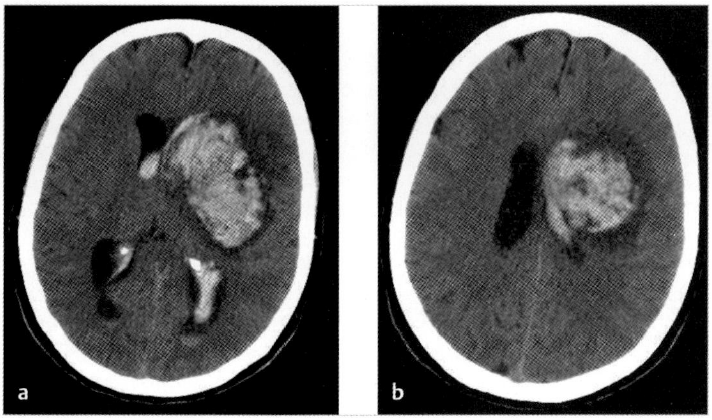

Fig. 1.23 (Source: Reproduced from Postprocedure care. In: Mendes Pereira V, Dmytriw A, Slater L, Power S, Krings T, ed. Endovascular Management of Ischemic Stroke: A Case-Based Approach. 1st ed. New York: Thieme; 2021.)

it provides rapid normalization of the INR and has been shown to be more effective and faster-acting than FFP. PCC contains clotting factors II, VII, IX, and X and can reverse warfarin coagulopathy within minutes.

Vitamin K should also be administered concurrently, as it promotes endogenous clotting factor synthesis, but its onset of action is delayed (typically several hours), so it is not sufficient as a standalone initial intervention. FFP is less favored due to its slower onset, requirement for blood type matching, larger infusion volume, and increased risk of volume overload—especially problematic in elderly or heart failure patients.

Discontinuation of warfarin is necessary as part of the broader management plan but does not address the immediate need to reverse coagulopathy. Surgical evacuation may be indicated in select patients (e.g., large hemorrhages with mass effect or clinical deterioration), but it is not the first step—anticoagulation reversal is the immediate priority before considering surgical intervention. Thus, PCC is the most appropriate initial step in the acute management of this patient.[119,120]

▸▸ Question 54

A 70-year-old woman presents with a spontaneous intracerebral hemorrhage while on rivaroxaban for atrial fibrillation. What is the most appropriate agent for reversing the anticoagulant effect of rivaroxaban in this patient?

- A. Vitamin K
- B. Fresh frozen plasma (FFP)
- C. Prothrombin complex concentrate (PCC)
- D. Andexanet alfa
- E. Desmopressin (DDAVP)

Correct answer is D

Andexanet alfa is a specific reversal agent for direct factor Xa inhibitors, such as rivaroxaban and apixaban. It rapidly reverses the anticoagulant effects and is used in cases of life-threatening bleeding, such as intracerebral hemorrhage. **(C) Prothrombin complex concentrate (PCC)** can also be used, but it is not as specific or effective as andexanet alfa for reversing factor Xa inhibitors.[121]

▸▸ Question 55

A 62-year-old man presents with a large lobar intracerebral hemorrhage causing significant midline shift and deteriorating consciousness. What is the most appropriate next step in management?

- A. Continue conservative medical management
- B. Initiate hyperosmolar therapy
- C. Immediate surgical evacuation
- D. Begin intravenous antihypertensive therapy
- E. Transfer to a stroke unit for observation

Correct answer is C

Surgical evacuation is indicated in select patients with large lobar intracerebral hemorrhages (ICH), particularly when there is evidence of significant mass effect and neurological deterioration. Early surgical intervention can be life-saving and may improve functional outcomes in appropriately selected cases.

Several key factors guide the decision to proceed with surgery. Hematoma volume is one of the most important—bleeds greater than 30 mL are generally considered for surgical evacuation. Location also matters: lobar hemorrhages are more accessible and more likely to benefit from surgery than deep-seated hemorrhages (such as those in the basal ganglia or thalamus), where surgery may pose greater risk and offer less benefit.

The neurological status of the patient is critical; worsening level of consciousness, signs of herniation, or evidence of increased intracranial pressure—particularly midline shift greater than 5 mm—are strong indications for surgical intervention. These findings correlate with a poor prognosis if left untreated. However, surgical decision-making must also incorporate patient-specific factors such as age, baseline function, comorbidities, and overall goals of care.

In contrast, conservative medical management —which includes blood pressure control, close neurological monitoring, and supportive care—is appropriate for smaller hemorrhages, deep lesions, or patients who are poor surgical candidates. Hyperosmolar therapy (e.g., mannitol or hypertonic saline) may be employed as a temporizing measure to reduce intracranial pressure, but it does not address the mass effect or source of bleeding. Similarly, intravenous antihypertensive therapy plays a crucial role in minimizing hematoma expansion but is not a definitive treatment for large ICHs causing mass effect.

Ultimately, the decision to operate should be individualized, balancing radiographic findings, clinical status, and patient-specific risks to optimize outcomes.

Key Characteristics of Intracerebral Hemorrhage:

- Volume: The volume of the hemorrhage is a critical factor in determining the need for surgery. Hematomas greater than 30 mL are generally considered for surgical intervention.
- Location: Lobar hemorrhages are more amenable to surgical evacuation compared to deep-seated hemorrhages.
- Neurological status: Deteriorating consciousness and evidence of increased intracranial pressure (e.g., midline shift) are indications for surgery.
- Midline shift: Significant midline shift (> 5 mm) is associated with poor outcomes and is an indication for surgical intervention.
- Patient factors: Age, comorbidities, and overall prognosis should be considered when deciding on surgical intervention.

(A) **Conservative medical management**, including blood pressure control and supportive care, is typically reserved for smaller hemorrhages or patients who are poor surgical candidates. **(B) Hyperosmolar therapy** (e.g., mannitol or hypertonic saline) may be used temporarily to reduce intracranial pressure but is not definitive treatment. **(D) Intravenous antihypertensive therapy** is important for managing blood pressure but does not address the mass effect of a large hemorrhage.[122,123]

▸▸ Question 56

A 65-year-old woman undergoes carotid endarterectomy for a symptomatic 70% stenosis of the left internal carotid artery. Postoperatively, she develops a hoarse voice and difficulty swallowing. Which cranial nerve is most likely affected?

- A. Hypoglossal nerve (CN XII)
- B. Vagus nerve (CN X)
- C. Glossopharyngeal nerve (CN IX)
- D. Accessory nerve (CN XI)
- E. Facial nerve (CN VII)

Correct answer is B

Postoperative hoarseness and difficulty swallowing following carotid endarterectomy are most commonly due to injury to the vagus nerve (CN X), which can result in vocal cord paralysis and dysphagia. The vagus nerve is located between the common carotid artery and internal jugular vein and should be identified and protected during surgery to avoid injury. Other potential complications include cranial nerve injuries, hematoma, and stroke (▸ Fig. 1.24).[124,125]

▸▸ Question 57

A 60-year-old woman with symptomatic carotid artery stenosis is considered for carotid stenting (▸ Fig. 1.25). Which of the following conditions is considered a contraindication for carotid artery stenting?

- A. Severe aortic stenosis
- B. Chronic kidney disease
- C. Severe calcification of the carotid artery
- D. Mild intracranial atherosclerosis
- E. Recent myocardial infarction

Correct answer is C

Severe calcification of the carotid artery, particularly concentric calcification, is a contraindication for carotid stenting due to the increased risk of embolization and technical difficulties during the procedure. Carotid endarterectomy is typically preferred in such cases. Other considerations for stenting include patient's vascular anatomy (including aortic arch and carotid bifurcation), comorbid conditions, and surgical risks.[126,127]

▸▸ Question 58

Which of the following best describes the mechanism by which middle meningeal artery embolization treats chronic subdural hematomas?

- A. Direct evacuation of hematoma contents
- B. Reduction of neovascularization and inflammatory response
- C. Promotion of reabsorption of the hematoma through osmotic effects
- D. Mechanical compression of the hematoma cavity
- E. Enhancement of cerebral venous drainage

Correct answer is B

Middle meningeal artery embolization treats chronic subdural hematomas primarily by reducing neovascularization and the associated inflammatory response. This mechanism helps prevent the reformation of the hematoma and stabilizes the existing hematoma, ultimately facilitating its reabsorption. Multiple embolic agents have been described in this technique, including Onyx, N-butyl cyanoacrylate glue, particles, and coils.[128]

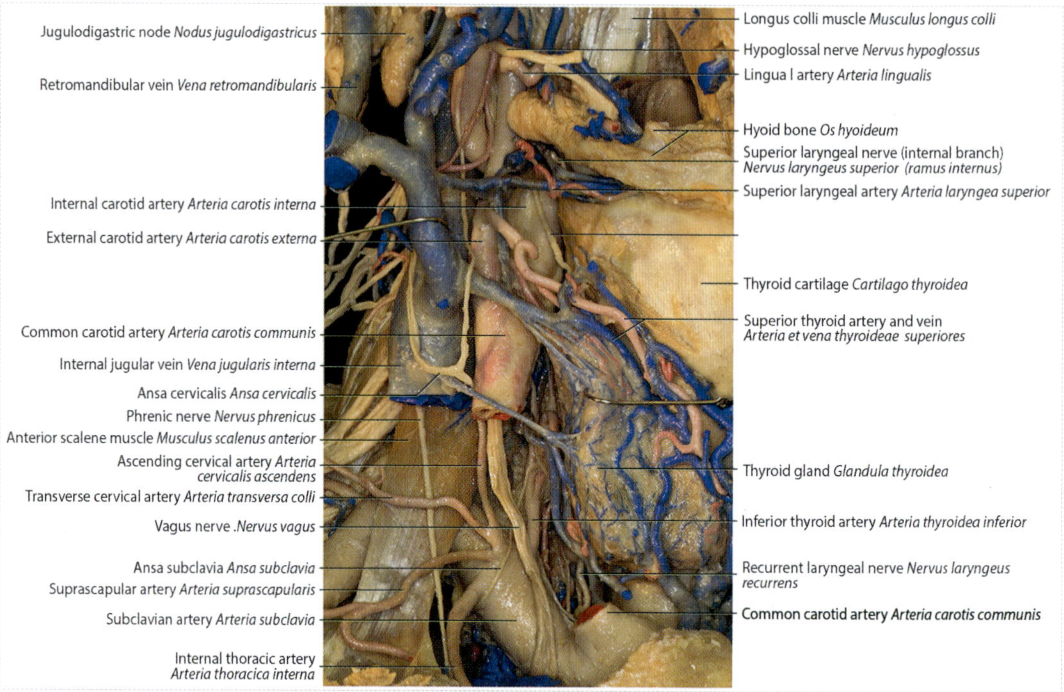

Fig. 1.24 (Source: Reproduced from 7 Anterior Aspect of the Neck: Deep Dissection. In: Peris-Celda M, Martinez-Soriano F, Rhoton A, ed. Rhoton's Atlas of Head, Neck, and Brain: 2D and 3D Images. 1st ed. New York: Thieme; 2017.)

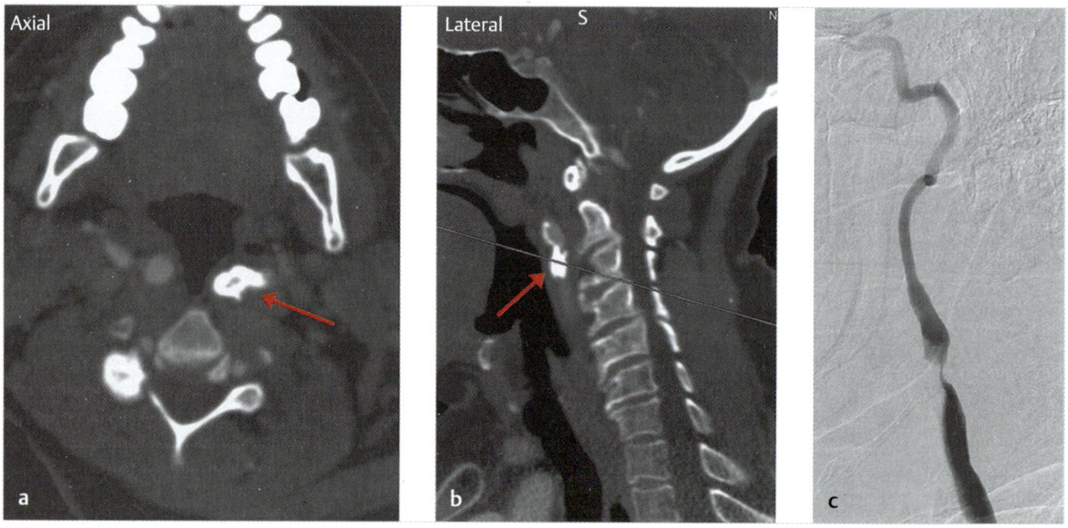

Fig. 1.25 (Source: Reproduced from Anatomical and Imaging Aspects. In: Mokin M, Levy E, Siddiqui A, eds. Video Atlas of Acute Ischemic Stroke Intervention. 1st ed. New York: Thieme; 2022.)

References

[1] Molyneux A, Kerr R, Stratton I, et al; International Subarachnoid Aneurysm Trial (ISAT) Collaborative Group. International Subarachnoid Aneurysm Trial (ISAT) of neurosurgical clipping versus endovascular coiling in 2143 patients with ruptured intracranial aneurysms: a randomized trial. Lancet 2002;360(9342):1267–1274

[2] Alkhaibary A, Alharbi A, Alnefaie N, et al. Spinal dural arteriovenous fistula: a comprehensive review of the history, classification systems, management, and prognosis. Chin Neurosurg J 2024;10(1):2

[3] Barnett HJM, Taylor DW, Eliasziw M, et al; North American Symptomatic Carotid Endarterectomy Trial Collaborators. Benefit of carotid endarterectomy in patients with symptomatic moderate or severe stenosis. N Engl J Med. 1998;339(20):1415–1425

[4] Brott TG, Hobson RW II, Howard G, et al. Stenting versus endarterectomy for treatment of carotid-artery stenosis. N Engl J Med 2010;363(1):11–23

[5] MRC Asymptomatic Carotid Surgery Trial (ACST) Collaborative Group. Prevention of disabling and fatal strokes by successful carotid endarterectomy in patients without recent neurological symptoms: randomised controlled trial. Lancet 2004;363(9420):1491–1502

[6] Yadav JS, Wholey MH, Kuntz RE, et al. Protected carotid-artery stenting versus endarterectomy in high-risk patients. N Engl J Med 2004;351(15):1493–1501

[7] Mantese VA, Timaran CH, Chiu D, Begg RJ, Brott TG; CREST Investigators. The Carotid Revascularization Endarterectomy versus Stenting Trial (CREST): stenting versus carotid endarterectomy for carotid disease. Stroke 2010;41(10 Suppl):S31–S34

[8] Einhäupl K, Stam J, Bousser MG, et al; European Federation of Neurological Societies. EFNS guideline on treating cerebral venous and sinus thrombosis in adult patients. Eur J Neurol 2010;17(10):1229–1235

[9] Ferro JM, Canhão P, Stam J, Bousser MG, Barinagarrementeria F; ISCVT Investigators. Prognosis of cerebral vein and dural sinus thrombosis: International Study on Cerebral Vein and Dural Sinus Thrombosis (ISCVT) results. Stroke 2004;35(3):664–670

[10] Connolly ES Jr, Rabinstein AA, Carhuapoma JR, et al. Guidelines for the management of aneurysmal subarachnoid hemorrhage: a guideline for healthcare professionals from the American Heart Association/American Stroke Association. Stroke 2012;43(6):1711–1737

[11] Pickard JD, Murray GD, Illingworth R, et al. Effect of oral nimodipine on cerebral infarction and outcome after subarachnoid haemorrhage: British aneurysm nimodipine trial. BMJ 1989;298(6674):636–642

[12] Dorhout Mees SM, Rinkel GJ, Feigin VL, et al. Calcium antagonists for aneurysmal subarachnoid haemorrhage. Cochrane Database Syst Rev 2007;(3):CD000277

[13] Wong GK, Poon WS, Chan MTV, et al. Intravenous magnesium sulphate for aneurysmal subarachnoid hemorrhage (IMASH): a randomized, double-blinded, placebo-controlled, multicenter phase III trial. Stroke 2010;41(5):921–926

[14] Helbok R, Schiefecker AJ, Delazer M, et al. Cerebral vasospasm and early brain injury after aneurysmal subarachnoid hemorrhage: new preventive strategies and early treatment options. J Neurol 2015;357(1–2):147–153

[15] Bennett MH, Trytko B, Jonker B. Hyperbaric oxygen therapy for the adjunctive treatment of traumatic brain injury. Cochrane Database of Systematic Reviews 2012, Issue 12. Art. No.: CD004609. DOI: 10.1002/14651858.CD004609.pub3. Accessed 06 December 2025

[16] Anderson CS, Heeley E, Huang Y, et al. Rapid blood-pressure lowering in patients with acute intracerebral hemorrhage. N Engl J Med 2013;368(25):2355–65

[17] Morgenstern LB, Hemphill JC III, Anderson C, et al. Guidelines for the management of spontaneous intracerebral hemorrhage: a guideline for healthcare professionals from the American Heart Association/American Stroke Association. Stroke 2010;41(9):2108–2129

[18] Scott RM, Smith ER. Moyamoya disease and moyamoya syndrome. N Engl J Med 2009;360(12):1226–1237

[19] Miyamoto S, Yoshimoto T, Hashimoto N, et al. Effects of extracranial-intracranial bypass for patients with hemorrhagic moyamoya disease: results of the Japan Adult Moyamoya Trial. Stroke 2014;45(5):1415–1421

[20] Stupp R, Mason WP, van den Bent MJ, et al. Radiotherapy plus concomitant and adjuvant temozolomide for glioblastoma. N Engl J Med 2005;352(10):987–996

[21] Brandes AA, Tosoni A, Spagnolli F, et al. Disease progression or pseudoprogression after concomitant radiochemotherapy treatment: pitfalls in neurooncology. Neuro Oncol 2008;10(3):361–367

[22] Etz CD, Plestis KA, Kari FA, et al. Thoracoabdominal aortic aneurysm repair in the elephant trunk era: the impact of spinal cord protection strategies on perioperative outcomes. J Thorac Cardiovasc Surg 2014;148(6):2911–2918

[23] Safi HJ, Miller CC, Huynh TT, et al. Distal aortic perfusion and cerebrospinal fluid drainage for thoracoabdominal and descending thoracic aortic repair: ten years of organ protection. Ann Surg 2003;238(3):372–380

[24] Meyer-Heim AD, Boltshauser E. Spontaneous intracranial haemorrhage in children: aetiology, presentation and outcome. Brain Dev 2003;25(6):416–421

[25] Robertson F, Kallmes D, Cloft HJ. Neurovascular manifestations of connective-tissue diseases: a review. Interv Neuroradiol 2011;17(3):271–278

[26] Pierot L, Cognard C, Anxionnat R, Ricolfi F. Endovascular treatment of ruptured intracranial aneurysms: factors affecting midterm quality anatomic results: analysis in a prospective, multicenter series of patients (CLARITY). AJNR 2012; 33(8):1475–1480

[27] Mocco J, Snyder KV, Albuquerque FC, Bendok BR, Boulos AS, Carpenter JS, Fiorella DJ, Hoh BL, Howington JU, Jankowitz BT, Liebma NKM, Rai AT, Rodriguez-Mercado R, Siddiqui AH, Veznedaroglu E, Hopkins LN, Levy EI. Treatment of intracranial aneurysms with the enterprise stent: a multicenter registry: Clinical article. JNS 2009; 110(1):35-39

[28] Kim JS. Pure lateral medullary infarction: clinical-radiological correlation of 130 acute, consecutive patients. Brain 2003;126(Pt 8):1864–1872

[29] Norrving B, Magnusson M, Holtås S. Isolated acute vertigo in the elderly; vestibular or vascular disease? Acta Neurol Scand 1995;91(1):43–48

[30] Salvarani C, Brown RD Jr., Calamia KT, et al. Primary central nervous system vasculitis: analysis of 101 patients. Ann Neurol 2007;62(5):442–451

[31] De Boysson H, Zuber M, Naggara O, et al. Primary angiitis of the central nervous system: description of the first fifty-two adults enrolled in the French cohort of patients

with primary vasculitis of the central nervous system. Arthritis Rheumatol 2014;66(5):1315–1326
[32] Krings T, Geibprasert S, terBrugge KG. Spinal dural arteriovenous fistulas. AJNR Am J Neuroradiol 2009;30(4):639–648
[33] Jellema K, Canta LR, Tijssen CC, et al. Spinal dural arteriovenous fistulas: a congestive myelopathy that initially mimics a peripheral nerve disorder. Brain 2006;129(Pt 12):3150–3164
[34] Macdonald RL, Higashida RT, Keller E, et al. Randomized trial of clazosentan in patients with aneurysmal subarachnoid hemorrhage undergoing endovascular coiling. Stroke 2012;43(6):1463–1469
[35] Dorsch NWC. Therapeutic approaches to vasospasm in subarachnoid hemorrhage. Curr Opin Crit Care 2002;8 (2):128–133
[36] Becske T, Kallmes DF, Saatci I, et al. Pipeline for uncoilable or failed aneurysms: results from a multicenter clinical trial. Radiology 2013;267(3):858–868
[37] Siddiqui AH, Abla AA, Kan P, et al. Panacea or problem: flow diverters in the treatment of symptomatic large or giant fusiform, dissecting, and thrombosed intracranial aneurysms. Neurosurgery 2012;70(6):1348–1359; discussion 1359
[38] Spetzler RF, Martin NA. A proposed grading system for arteriovenous malformations. J Neurosurg 1986;65(4):476–483
[39] Lawton MT, Kim H, McCulloch CE, Mikhak B, Young WL. A supplementary grading scale for selecting patients with brain arteriovenous malformations for surgery. Neurosurgery 2010;66(4):702–713; discussion 713
[40] Starke RM, Komotar RJ, Otten ML, Hahn DK, Fischer I, Palmese CA, Connolly ES Jr. Endovascular and microsurgical treatment of cerebral arteriovenous malformations: current recommendations. Surg Neurol Intern 2011;2:1
[41] Mohr JP, Parides MK, Stapf C, et al. Medical management with or without interventional therapy for unruptured brain arteriovenous malformations (ARUBA): a multicentre, non-blinded, randomised trial. Lancet 2014;383 (9917):614–621
[42] Connolly ES Jr, Rabinstein AA, Carhuapoma JR, et al. Guidelines for the management of aneurysmal subarachnoid hemorrhage: a guideline for healthcare professionals from the American Heart Association/American Stroke Association. Stroke 2012;43(6):1711–1737
[43] Rinkel GJE, Djibuti M, Algra A, van Gijn J. Prevalence and risk of rupture of intracranial aneurysms: a systematic review. Stroke 1998;29(1):251–256
[44] Frontera JA, Lewin JJ III, Rabinstein AA, et al. Guideline for reversal of antithrombotics in intracranial hemorrhage: a statement for healthcare professionals from the Neurocritical Care Society and Society of Critical Care Medicine. Neurocrit Care 2016;24(1):6–46
[45] Steiner T, Poli S, Griebe M, et al. Fresh frozen plasma versus prothrombin complex concentrate in patients with intracranial haemorrhage related to vitamin K antagonists (INCH): a randomised trial. Lancet Neurol 2016;15 (6):566–573
[46] Powers WJ, Rabinstein AA, Ackerson T, et al. 2018 Guidelines for the early management of patients with acute ischemic stroke: a guideline for healthcare professionals from the American Heart Association/American Stroke Association. Stroke 2018;49(3):e46–e110
[47] Bushnell C, McCullough LD, Awad IA, et al. Guidelines for the prevention of stroke in women: a statement for healthcare professionals from the American Heart Association/American Stroke Association. Stroke 2014;45 (5):1545–1588
[48] Sloan MA, Haley EC Jr, Kassell NF, et al. Sensitivity and specificity of transcranial Doppler ultrasonography in the diagnosing of vasospasm following subarachnoid hemorrhage. Neurology 1989;39(11):1514–1518
[49] Aaslid R, Markwalder TM, Nornes H. Noninvasive transcranial Doppler ultrasound recording of flow velocity in basal cerebral arteries. J Neurosurg 1982;57(6):769–774
[50] Raymond J, Guilbert F, Weill A, et al. Long-term angiographic recurrences after selective endovascular treatment of aneurysms with detachable coils. Stroke 2003;34 (6):1398–1403
[51] Fernandez Zubillaga A, Guglielmi G, Viñuela F, Duckwiler GR. Endovascular occlusion of intracranial aneurysms with electrically detachable coils: correlation of aneurysm neck size and treatment results. AJNR Am J Neuroradiol 1994;15(5):815–820
[52] Kawanabe Y, Sadato A, Taki W, Hashimoto N. Endovascular occlusion of intracranial aneurysms with Guglielmi detachable coils: correlation between coil packing density and coil compaction. Acta Neurochir (Wien) 2001;143 (5):451–455
[53] Tamatani S, Ito Y, Abe H, Koike T, Takeuchi S, Tanaka R. Evaluation of the stability of aneurysms after embolization using detachable coils: correlation between stability of aneurysms and embolized volume of aneurysms. AJNR Am J Neuroradiol 2002;23(5):762–767
[54] Stapf C, Mohr JP, Choi JH, Hartmann A, Mast H. Arteriovenous malformations of the brain. N Engl J Med 2003;348 (25):2543–2546
[55] Al-Shahi Salman R, White PM, Counsell CE, et al. Outcome after conservative management or intervention for unruptured brain arteriovenous malformations. JAMA 2014;311 (16):1661–1669
[56] Stapf C, Mast H, Sciacca RR, et al. Predictors of hemorrhage in patients with untreated brain arteriovenous malformation. Neurology 2006;66(9):1350–1355
[57] Borden JA, Wu JK, Shucart WA. A proposed classification for spinal and cranial dural arteriovenous fistulous malformations and implications for treatment. J Neurosurg 1995;82(2):166–179
[58] Cognard C, Gobin YP, Pierot L, et al. Cerebral dural arteriovenous fistulas: clinical and angiographic correlation with a revised classification of venous drainage. Radiology 1995;194(3):671–680
[59] Hye RJ, Cikrit DF, Gewertz BL. Carotid endarterectomy: strategies for managing intraoperative complications. J Vasc Surg 1994;19(6):993–999
[60] Fearn SJ, Parry AD, Picton AJ, Mortimer AJ, McCollum CN. The use of phenylephrine to maintain blood pressure during carotid endarterectomy under regional anaesthesia. Eur J Vasc Endovasc Surg 1996;12(4):424–429
[61] Bogniotti LAC, Teivelis MP, Cardozo FAM, et al. Hemodynamic depression after carotid surgery: incidence, risk factors and outcomes. Clinics (Sao Paulo) 2022;77:100090
[62] Ekberg O, Bergqvist D, Takolander R, Uddman R, Kitzing P. Pharyngeal function after carotid endarterectomy. Dysphagia 1989;4(3):151–154
[63] Müller MD, Lyrer P, Brown MM, Bonati LH. Carotid artery stenting versus endarterectomy for treatment of carotid artery stenosis. Cochrane Database Syst Rev 2020;2(2): CD000515

[64] Howard G, Roubin GS, Jansen O, et al.; Carotid Stenting Trialists' Collaboration. Association between age and risk of stroke or death from carotid endarterectomy and carotid stenting: a meta-analysis of pooled patient data from four randomised trials. Lancet 2016;387(10025):1305–1311[Erratum in: Lancet. 2016;387(10025):1276. doi: 10.1016/S0140-6736(16)00623-1. PMID: 26880122]

[65] House JW, Brackmann DE. Facial nerve grading system. Otolaryngol Head Neck Surg 1985;93(2):146–147

[66] Tien RD, Felsberg GJ, Chhem RK. MR imaging of facial nerve enhancement in Bell's palsy and in other facial nerve disorders. AJR Am J Roentgenol 1990;155(2):573–579

[67] Chimowitz MI, Lynn MJ, Derdeyn CP, et al. Stenting versus aggressive medical therapy for intracranial arterial stenosis. N Engl J Med 2011;365(11):993–1003

[68] Gorelick PB, Wong KS, Bae HJ, Pandey DK. Large artery intracranial occlusive disease: a large worldwide burden but a relatively neglected frontier. Stroke 2008;39(8):2396–2399

[69] Powers WJ, Clarke WR, Grubb RL Jr, Videen TO, Adams HP Jr, Derdeyn CP; COSS Investigators. Extracranial-intracranial bypass surgery for stroke prevention in hemodynamic cerebral ischemia: the Carotid Occlusion Surgery Study randomized trial. JAMA 2011;306(18):1983–1992 (Erratum in: JAMA. 2011;306(24):2672. Obviagele, Bruce [corrected to Ovbiagele, Bruce]. PMID: 22068990; PMCID: PMC3601825)

[70] Barrow DL, Spector RH, Braun IF, et al. Classification and treatment of spontaneous carotid-cavernous sinus fistulas. J Neurosurg 1985;62(2):248–256

[71] Ellis JA, Goldstein H, Connolly ES Jr, Meyers PM. Carotid-cavernous fistulas. Neurosurg Focus 2012;32(5):E9

[72] Shen CC, Tsuei YS, Yang MY, et al. Gamma Knife radiosurgery for indirect dural carotid-cavernous fistula: long-term ophthalmological outcome. Life (Basel) 2022;12 (8):1175

[73] Park SH, Park KS, Kang DH, Hwang JH, Hwang SK. Stereotactic radiosurgery for dural carotid cavernous sinus fistulas. World Neurosurg 2017;106:836–843

[74] Schievink WI. Spontaneous dissection of the carotid and vertebral arteries. N Engl J Med 2001;344(12):898–906

[75] Biousse V, D'Anglejan-Chatillon J, Massiou H, et al. Head pain in non-traumatic carotid artery dissections: a series of 65 patients. Cephalalgia 1994;14(1):33–36

[76] van Gijn J, Kerr RS, Rinkel GJ. Subarachnoid haemorrhage. Lancet 2007;369(9558):306–318

[77] Juvela S, Porras M, Poussa K. Natural history of unruptured intracranial aneurysms: probability of and risk factors for aneurysm rupture. J Neurosurg 2000;93(3):379–387

[78] Wermer MJ, van der Schaaf IC, Algra A, Rinkel GJ. Risk of rupture of unruptured intracranial aneurysms in relation to patient and aneurysm characteristics: an updated meta-analysis. Stroke 2007;38(4):1404–1410

[79] Wiebers DO, Whisnant JP, Huston J III, et al; International Study of Unruptured Intracranial Aneurysms Investigators. Unruptured intracranial aneurysms: natural history, clinical outcome, and risks of surgical and endovascular treatment. Lancet 2003;362(9378):103–110

[80] Brott TG, Hobson RW II, Howard G, et al. Stenting versus endarterectomy for treatment of carotid-artery stenosis. N Engl J Med 2010;363(1):11–23

[81] Barnett HJM, Taylor DW, Eliasziw M, et al; North American Symptomatic Carotid Endarterectomy Trial Collaborators. Benefit of carotid endarterectomy in patients with symptomatic moderate or severe stenosis. N Engl J Med 1998;339(20):1415–1425

[82] MRC Asymptomatic Carotid Surgery Trial (ACST) Collaborative Group. Prevention of disabling and fatal strokes by successful carotid endarterectomy in patients without recent neurological symptoms: randomised controlled trial. Lancet 2004;363(9420):1491–1502

[83] Yadav JS, Wholey MH, Kuntz RE, et al. Protected carotid-artery stenting versus endarterectomy in high-risk patients. N Engl J Med 2004;351(15):1493–1501

[84] Mantese VA, Timaran CH, Chiu D, Begg RJ, Brott TG; CREST Investigators. The Carotid Revascularization Endarterectomy versus Stenting Trial (CREST): stenting versus carotid endarterectomy for carotid disease. Stroke 2010;41(10, Suppl):S31–S34

[85] Brott TG, Halperin JL, Abbara S, et al. 2011 ASA/ACCF/AHA/AANN/AANS/ACR/ASNR/CNS/SAIP/SCAI/SIR/SNIS/SVM/SVS guideline on the management of patients with extracranial carotid and vertebral artery disease. Stroke 2011;42(8): e464–e540

[86] Barnett HJM, Taylor DW, Eliasziw M, et al. Benefit of carotid endarterectomy in patients with symptomatic moderate or severe stenosis. N Engl J Med 1998;339(20):1415–1425

[87] Wang J, Bai X, Wang T, Dmytriw AA, Patel AB, Jiao L. Carotid stenting versus endarterectomy for asymptomatic carotid artery stenosis: a systematic review and meta-analysis. Stroke 2022;53(10):3047–3054 [Erratum in: Stroke. 2023 Mar;54(3):e122. doi: 10.1161/STR.0000000000000 426. PMID: 35730457]

[88] Ringleb PA, Allenberg J, Bruckmann H, et al. 30 day results from the SPACE trial of stent-protected angioplasty versus carotid endarterectomy in symptomatic patients: a randomised non-inferiority trial. Lancet 2006;368(9543):1239–1247

[89] Bonati LH, Dobson J, Featherstone RL, et al. Long-term outcomes after stenting versus endarterectomy for treatment of symptomatic carotid stenosis: the International Carotid Stenting Study (ICSS) randomised trial. Lancet 2015;385 (9967):529–538

[90] van Dijk JM, terBrugge KG, Willinsky RA, et al. Clinical course of cranial dural arteriovenous fistulas with cortical venous reflux. Stroke 2002;33(5):1233–1236

[91] Awad IA, Little JR, Akarawi WP, et al. Intracranial dural arteriovenous malformations: factors predisposing to an aggressive neurological course. J Neurosurg 1990;72 (6):839–850

[92] Wiebers DO, Whisnant JP, Huston J, et al. Unruptured intracranial aneurysms: natural history, clinical outcome, and risks of surgical and endovascular therapy. Lancet 2003;362(9378):103–110

[93] Connolly ES Jr, Rabinstein AA, Carhuapoma JR, et al. Guidelines for the management of aneurysmal subarachnoid hemorrhage. Stroke 2012;43(6):1711–1737

[94] Molyneux AJ, Kerr RS, Yu LM, et al. International subarachnoid aneurysm trial (ISAT) of neurosurgical clipping versus endovascular coiling in 2143 patients with ruptured intracranial aneurysms: a randomised comparison of effects on survival, dependency, seizures, rebleeding, subgroups, and aneurysm occlusion. Lancet 2005;366 (9488):809–817

[95] van Rooij WJ, Sluzewski M, Beute GN. Procedural morbidity and mortality of elective coiling of unruptured intracranial aneurysms. AJNR Am J Neuroradiol 2006;27 (8):1678–1680

[96] Bond KM, Brinjikji W, Murad MH, Kallmes DF, Cloft HJ, Lanzino G. Diffusion-weighted imaging-detected ischemic lesions following endovascular treatment of cerebral aneurysms: a systematic review and meta-analysis. AJNR Am J Neuroradiol 2017;38(2):304–309
[97] Habtezghi AB, Ghozy S, Bilgin C, Kobeissi H, Kadirvel R, Kallmes DF. DWI-detected ischemic lesions after endovascular treatment for cerebral aneurysms: an updated systematic review and meta-analysis. AJNR Am J Neuroradiol 2023;44(11):1256–1261
[98] Bederson JB, Connolly ES Jr, Batjer HH, et al. Guidelines for the management of aneurysmal subarachnoid hemorrhage. Stroke 2009;40(3):994–1025
[99] Connolly ES Jr, Rabinstein AA, Carhuapoma JR, et al. Guidelines for the management of aneurysmal subarachnoid hemorrhage: a guideline for healthcare professionals from the American Heart Association/American Stroke Association. Stroke 2012;43(6):1711–1737.
[100] Allen GS, Ahn HS, Preziosi TJ, et al. Cerebral arterial spasm – a controlled trial of nimodipine in patients with subarachnoid hemorrhage. N Engl J Med 1983;308(11):619–624
[101] Connolly ES Jr, Rabinstein AA, Carhuapoma JR, et al. Guidelines for the management of aneurysmal subarachnoid hemorrhage. Stroke 2012;43(6):1711–1737
[102] Fisher CM, Kistler JP, Davis JM. Relation of cerebral vasospasm to subarachnoid hemorrhage visualized by computerized tomographic scanning. Neurosurgery 1980;6(1):1–9
[103] Connolly ES Jr, Rabinstein AA, Carhuapoma JR, et al. Guidelines for the management of aneurysmal subarachnoid hemorrhage. Stroke 2012;43(6):1711–1737
[104] Spetzler RF, Martin NA. A proposed grading system for arteriovenous malformations. J Neurosurg 1986;65 (4):476–483
[105] Lawton MT, Rutledge WC, Kim H, et al. Brain arteriovenous malformations. Nat Rev Dis Primers 2015;1:15008
[106] Mohr JP, Parides MK, Stapf C, et al. Medical management with or without interventional therapy for unruptured brain arteriovenous malformations (ARUBA): a multicentre, non-blinded, randomised trial. Lancet 2014;383 (9917):614–621
[107] Brown RD Jr, Flemming KD, Meyer FB, et al. Natural history, evaluation, and management of intracranial vascular malformations. Mayo Clin Proc 2005;80(2):269–281
[108] Kondziolka D, McLaughlin MR, Kestle JR. Simple risk predictions for arteriovenous malformation hemorrhage. Neurosurgery 1995;37(5):851–855
[109] Mohr JP, Kejda-Scharler J, Pile-Spellman J. Diagnosis and treatment of arteriovenous malformations. Curr Neurol Neurosci Rep 2013;13(2):324
[110] Lawton MT, Rutledge WC, Kim H, et al. Brain arteriovenous malformations. Nat Rev Dis Primers 2015;1:15008
[111] DeLuca J, Diamond BJ. Aneurysm of the anterior communicating artery: a review of neuroanatomical and neuropsychological sequelae. J Clin Exp Neuropsychol 1995;17 (1):100–121
[112] Connolly ES Jr, Rabinstein AA, Carhuapoma JR, et al. Guidelines for the management of aneurysmal subarachnoid hemorrhage: a guideline for healthcare professionals from the American Heart Association/American Stroke Association. Stroke 2012;43(6):1711–1737
[113] Al-Shahi R, Bhattacharya JJ, Currie DG, et al. Prospective, population-based detection of intracranial vascular malformations in adults: the Scottish Intracranial Vascular Malformation Study (SIVMS). Stroke 2003;34(5):1163–1169
[114] Friedlander RM. Clinical practice. Arteriovenous malformations of the brain. N Engl J Med 2007;356(26):2704–2712
[115] Pollock BE, Flickinger JC, Lunsford LD, et al. Factors associated with successful arteriovenous malformation radiosurgery. Neurosurgery 1998;42(6):1239–1247
[116] Stapf C, Mast H, Sciacca RR, et al. Predictors of hemorrhage in patients with untreated brain arteriovenous malformation. Neurology 2006;66(9):1350–1355
[117] Broderick JP, Brott TG, Duldner JE, et al. Volume of intracerebral hemorrhage. A powerful and easy-to-use predictor of 30-day mortality. Stroke 1993;24(7):987–993
[118] Qureshi AI, Mendelow AD, Hanley DF. Intracerebral haemorrhage. Lancet 2009;373(9675):1632–1644
[119] Hemphill JC III, Greenberg SM, Anderson CS, et al. Guidelines for the management of spontaneous intracerebral hemorrhage: a guideline for healthcare professionals from the American Heart Association/American Stroke Association. Stroke 2015;46(7):2032–2060
[120] Steiner T, Al-Shahi Salman R, Beer R, et al. European Stroke Organisation (ESO) guidelines for the management of spontaneous intracerebral hemorrhage. Int J Stroke 2014;9(7):840–855
[121] Connolly SJ, Milling TJ Jr, Eikelboom JW, et al. Andexanet alfa for acute major bleeding associated with factor Xa inhibitors. N Engl J Med 2016;375(12):1131–1141
[122] Mendelow AD, Gregson BA, Fernandes HM, et al. Early surgery versus initial conservative treatment in patients with spontaneous supratentorial intracerebral hematomas in the International Surgical Trial in Intracerebral Haemorrhage (STICH): a randomised trial. Lancet 2005;365 (9457):387–397
[123] Morgenstern LB, Hemphill JC III, Anderson C, et al. Guidelines for the management of spontaneous intracerebral hemorrhage: a guideline for healthcare professionals from the American Heart Association/American Stroke Association. Stroke 2010;41(9):2108–2129
[124] Sundt TM Jr, Sandok BA, Whisnant JP. Carotid endarterectomy. Complications and preoperative assessment of risk. Mayo Clin Proc 1975;50(5):301–306
[125] Ballotta E, Da Giau G, Baracchini C, et al. Cranial and cervical nerve injuries after carotid endarterectomy: a prospective study. Surgery 1999;125(1):85–91
[126] Brott TG, Hobson RW II, Howard G, et al. Stenting versus endarterectomy for treatment of carotid-artery stenosis. N Engl J Med 2010;363(1):11–23.
[127] Gurm HS, Yadav JS, Fayad P, et al. Long-term results of carotid stenting versus endarterectomy in high-risk patients. N Engl J Med 2008;358(15):1572–1579
[128] Link TW, Rapoport BI, Paine SM, et al. Middle meningeal artery embolization for chronic subdural hematoma: a series of 60 cases. Neurosurgery 2019;85(6):801–807

2 Neuro-Oncology

Syed I. Khalid, Lei Liu, Maciej S. Lesniak

▸▸ Question 1

A 45-year-old man presents with a history of progressive headaches and seizures. MRI reveals an infiltrative mass in the frontal lobe exhibiting ring enhancement with central necrosis. Histopathology shows pleomorphic astrocytic cells, microvascular proliferation, and areas of necrosis with pseudopalisading tumor cells. Molecular studies reveal a wild-type *IDH1* gene. Which of the following genetic alterations is most likely associated with this tumor?

- A. 1p/19q co-deletion
- B. EGFR amplification
- C. BRAF V600E mutation
- D. *NF2* gene mutation
- E. Histone H3 K27 M mutation

Correct answer is B

The patient has a glioblastoma, which is the most aggressive astrocytic tumor (WHO Grade IV). Histological features include necrosis with pseudopalisading cells and microvascular proliferation. Primary (de novo) glioblastomas typically occur in older adults and often have **EGFR amplification** and **PTEN mutations** with a wild-type *IDH1* gene. Secondary glioblastomas arise from lower-grade astrocytomas, usually in younger patients, and often have IDH1 mutations. A 1p/19q co-deletion is characteristic of oligodendrogliomas. BRAF V600E mutations are associated with pilocytic astrocytomas and certain pediatric gliomas. NF2 mutations are linked to schwannomas and meningiomas. Histone H3 K27 M mutations are characteristic of diffuse midline gliomas, such as diffuse intrinsic pontine gliomas.[1,2]

▸▸ Question 2

A 50-year-old woman undergoes resection of a parasagittal brain tumor. Histopathology reveals meningothelial cells arranged in whorls with numerous psammoma bodies. Immunohistochemistry is positive for epithelial membrane antigen (EMA) and progesterone receptors. Which chromosome abnormality is most commonly associated with this tumor?

- A. Deletion of chromosome 1p
- B. Monosomy of chromosome 22
- C. Trisomy of chromosome 21
- D. Deletion of chromosome 17p
- E. Translocation t(11;22)

Correct answer is B

Meningiomas are common intracranial tumors derived from arachnoid cap cells. Histological features include whorls and psammoma bodies. Immunohistochemistry often shows positivity for EMA and progesterone receptors. The most frequent cytogenetic abnormality is **monosomy of chromosome 22**, which leads to the loss of the *NF2* gene located on 22q12. Deletion of chromosome 1p is associated with oligodendrogliomas. Trisomy 21 is linked to Down syndrome. Deletion of 17p involves the p53 gene, often mutated in astrocytic tumors. Translocation t(11;22) is characteristic of Ewing sarcoma.[3,4,5]

▸▸ Question 3

A 30-year-old woman presents with a slowly enlarging, painless mass at the cerebellopontine angle, causing hearing loss and tinnitus. The resected tumor shows Antoni A and Antoni B patterns with Verocay bodies on histology. Which immunohistochemical marker is most likely positive in this tumor (▸ Fig. 2.1)?

- A. Glial fibrillary acidic protein (GFAP)
- B. S-100 protein
- C. Synaptophysin
- D. Cytokeratin
- E. Epithelial membrane antigen (EMA)

Correct answer is B

Vestibular schwannomas (acoustic neuromas) are benign nerve sheath tumors arising from Schwann cells of the vestibulocochlear nerve (CN VIII). Histologically, they display Antoni A regions (dense cellular areas) and Antoni B regions (loosely cellular areas), with Verocay bodies (aligned nuclei). **S-100 protein** is a marker for neural crest-derived cells, including Schwann cells, and is typically positive. GFAP is positive in glial tumors. Synaptophysin is a marker for neuronal and neuroendocrine cells. Cytokeratin is found in epithelial cells. EMA is positive in meningiomas.[6]

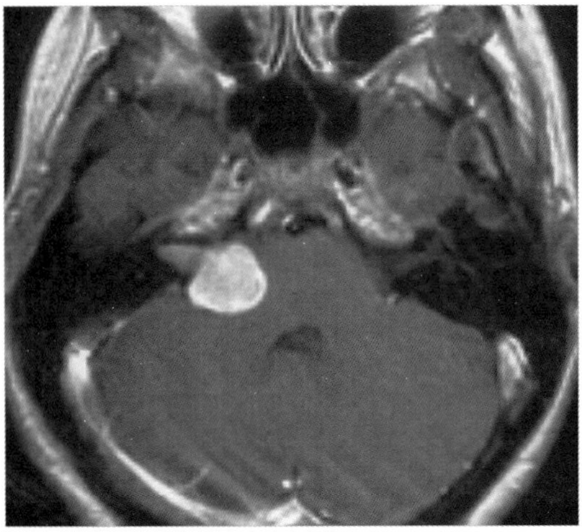

Fig. 2.1 (Source: Reproduced from Valvassori G. Vestibular schwannomas. In: Mafee M, Valvassori G, Becker M, eds. Valvassori's Imaging of the Head and Neck. 2nd ed. Stuttgart: Thieme; 2004.)

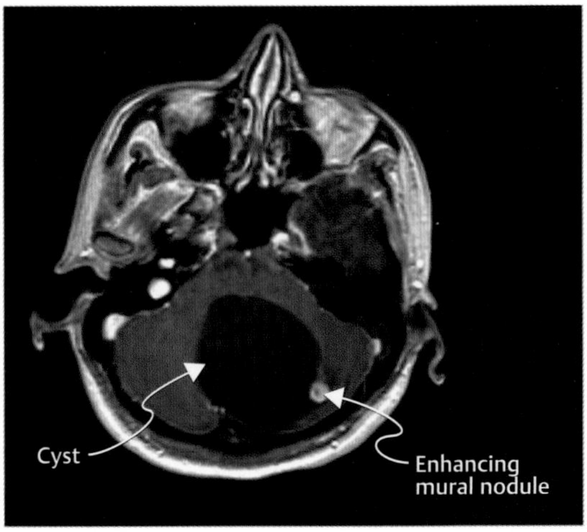

Fig. 2.2 (Source: Reproduced from Imaging. In: Greenberg M, ed. Greenberg's Handbook of Neurosurgery. 10th ed. New York: Thieme; 2023.)

▸▸ Question 4

A 6-year-old boy presents with headache, vomiting, and gait instability. MRI reveals a cystic cerebellar mass with an enhancing mural nodule. Histology shows bipolar cells with elongated hair-like processes and Rosenthal fibers. Which genetic disorder is most commonly associated with this type of tumor?

- A. Neurofibromatosis type 1
- B. Tuberous sclerosis complex
- C. Von Hippel–Lindau (VHL) disease
- D. Li–Fraumeni syndrome
- E. Sturge–Weber syndrome

Correct answer is C

The tumor described is a **pilocytic astrocytoma**, the most common benign brain tumor in children, typically located in the cerebellum. Histology shows Rosenthal fibers and hair-like (pilocytic) astrocytes. **VHL disease** is associated with hemangioblastomas, but patients with VHL can also develop pilocytic astrocytomas. Neurofibromatosis type 1 is associated with optic pathway gliomas. Tuberous sclerosis complex is linked to subependymal giant cell astrocytomas. Li–Fraumeni syndrome involves p53 mutations and various tumors. Sturge–Weber syndrome is characterized by leptomeningeal angiomas. ▸ Fig. 2.2 shows a pilocytic astrocytoma of the posterior fossa.[7]

Note the characteristic nonenhancing cyst wall with an enhancing mural nodule.

Image: axial T1 MRI with contrast.

▸▸ Question 5

A 4-year-old girl presents with obstructive hydrocephalus. MRI reveals a heterogeneous mass in the fourth ventricle extending into the foramina of Luschka and Magendie. Surgical resection is performed. Histopathology shows perivascular pseudorosettes and ependymal canals. Which of the following is the most likely diagnosis (▸ Fig. 2.3)?

- A. Medulloblastoma
- B. Ependymoma
- C. Choroid plexus papilloma
- D. Pilocytic astrocytoma
- E. Diffuse intrinsic pontine glioma

Correct answer is B

Ependymomas are tumors arising from ependymal cells lining the ventricles and central canal of the spinal cord. In children, they commonly occur in the fourth ventricle, causing hydrocephalus. Histologically, they exhibit perivascular pseudorosettes (tumor cells arranged around blood vessels)

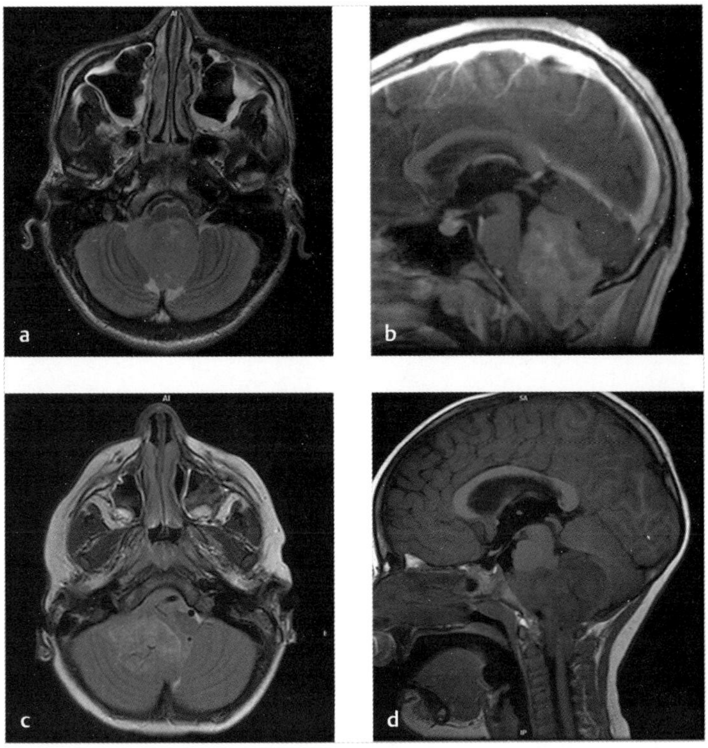

Fig. 2.3 (Source: Reproduced from Diagnosis and assessment. In: Jean W, ed. Skull Base Surgery: Strategies. 1st ed. New York: Thieme; 2019.)

and true ependymal rosettes. Medulloblastomas also occur in the posterior fossa but consist of small round blue cells and Homer Wright rosettes. Choroid plexus papillomas arise from choroid plexus epithelium. Pilocytic astrocytomas are cystic cerebellar tumors with Rosenthal fibers. Diffuse intrinsic pontine gliomas are brainstem tumors with a poor prognosis.[8,9]

▸▸ Question 6

A 35-year-old man presents with seizures and a slowly growing frontal lobe mass. MRI shows a calcified cortical tumor with heterogeneous enhancement. Histopathology reveals uniform cells with round nuclei surrounded by a clear halo (perinuclear clearing) and a delicate branching capillary network ("chicken-wire" vasculature). Which chromosomal alteration is most characteristic of this tumor?

- A. Deletion of chromosomes 1p and 19q
- B. Amplification of *EGFR* gene
- C. BRAF V600E mutation
- D. Monosomy of chromosome 22
- E. Mutation of the *TSC1* gene

Correct answer is A

The tumor described is an **oligodendroglioma**, which often presents in middle-aged adults with seizures. Histological features include cells with a "fried-egg" appearance due to perinuclear clearing and a "chicken-wire" capillary pattern. The most characteristic genetic alteration is the **co-deletion of chromosomes 1p and 19q**, associated with a better prognosis and responsiveness to chemotherapy. EGFR amplification is common in primary glioblastomas. BRAF mutations are seen in pilocytic astrocytomas and pleomorphic xanthoastrocytomas. Monosomy 22 is associated with meningiomas. Mutations in *TSC1* or *TSC2* genes are linked to tuberous sclerosis complex. ▸ Fig. 2.4 shows (**a**) Oligodendroglioma: highly cellular tumor composed of cells with round to oval nuclei and prominent perinuclear halos. (**b**) Diffuse astrocytoma: moderately cellular tumor composed of astrocytic cells with pleomorphic hyperchromatic nuclei, pink cytoplasm, and fibrillary processes.[10]

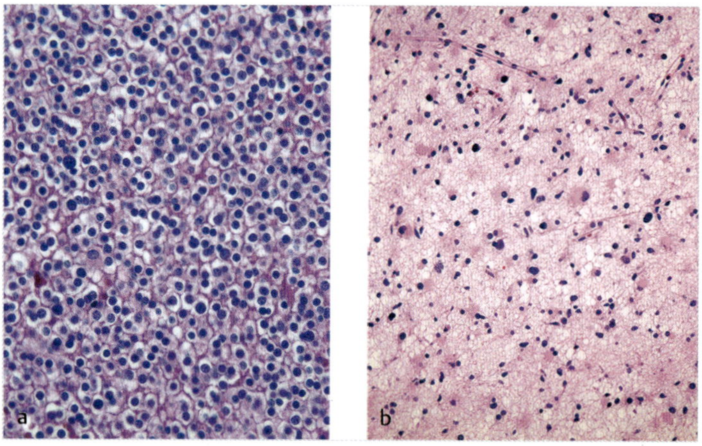

Fig. 2.4 (Source: Reproduced from Oligodendroglioma (WHO Grade II or III). In: Cataltepe O, Jallo G, eds. Pediatric Epilepsy Surgery: Preoperative Assessment and Surgical Treatment. 2nd ed. New York: Thieme; 2019.)

▸▸ Question 7

A 28-year-old woman with neurofibromatosis type 2 (NF2) presents with bilateral hearing loss and tinnitus. Imaging reveals bilateral cerebellopontine angle tumors. The *NF2* gene product, merlin (schwannomin), is involved in which cellular process?

- A. Regulation of the cell cycle
- B. Signal transduction at the neuromuscular junction
- C. Maintenance of cytoskeletal integrity
- D. DNA repair mechanisms
- E. Apoptosis regulation

Correct answer is C

The ***NF2* gene** encodes **merlin (also known as schwannomin)**, a tumor suppressor protein involved in the maintenance of cytoskeletal integrity and cell-to-cell adhesion. Loss of Merlin function leads to uncontrolled cell proliferation, particularly in Schwann cells, resulting in schwannomas. NF2 is characterized by bilateral vestibular schwannomas and other intracranial and spinal tumors. Regulation of the cell cycle is more associated with p53. Signal transduction at the neuromuscular junction involves proteins such as acetylcholine receptors. DNA repair mechanisms involve genes such as BRCA1/2. Apoptosis regulation is associated with Bcl-2 family proteins (▸ Fig. 2.5).[6]

▸▸ Question 8

A 5-year-old boy presents with precocious puberty and Parinaud syndrome (upward gaze palsy). MRI reveals a mass in the pineal region. Serum markers show elevated beta-human chorionic gonadotropin (β-hCG). Which of the following is the most likely diagnosis?

- A. Pineocytoma
- B. Pineoblastoma
- C. Germinoma
- D. Teratoma
- E. Astrocytoma

Correct answer is C

Germinomas are the most common pineal region tumors in children and can secrete **β-hCG**, leading to precocious puberty in boys. Parinaud syndrome results from compression of the dorsal midbrain. Germinomas are sensitive to radiation therapy. Pineocytomas and pineoblastomas are pineal parenchymal tumors but are less likely to produce β-hCG. Teratomas may also occur in this region but have different clinical and radiological features. Astrocytomas in the pineal region are rare (▸ Fig. 2.6).[11,12,13]

▸▸ Question 9

A 40-year-old man with a history of AIDS presents with progressive confusion and focal neurological deficits. MRI reveals multiple,

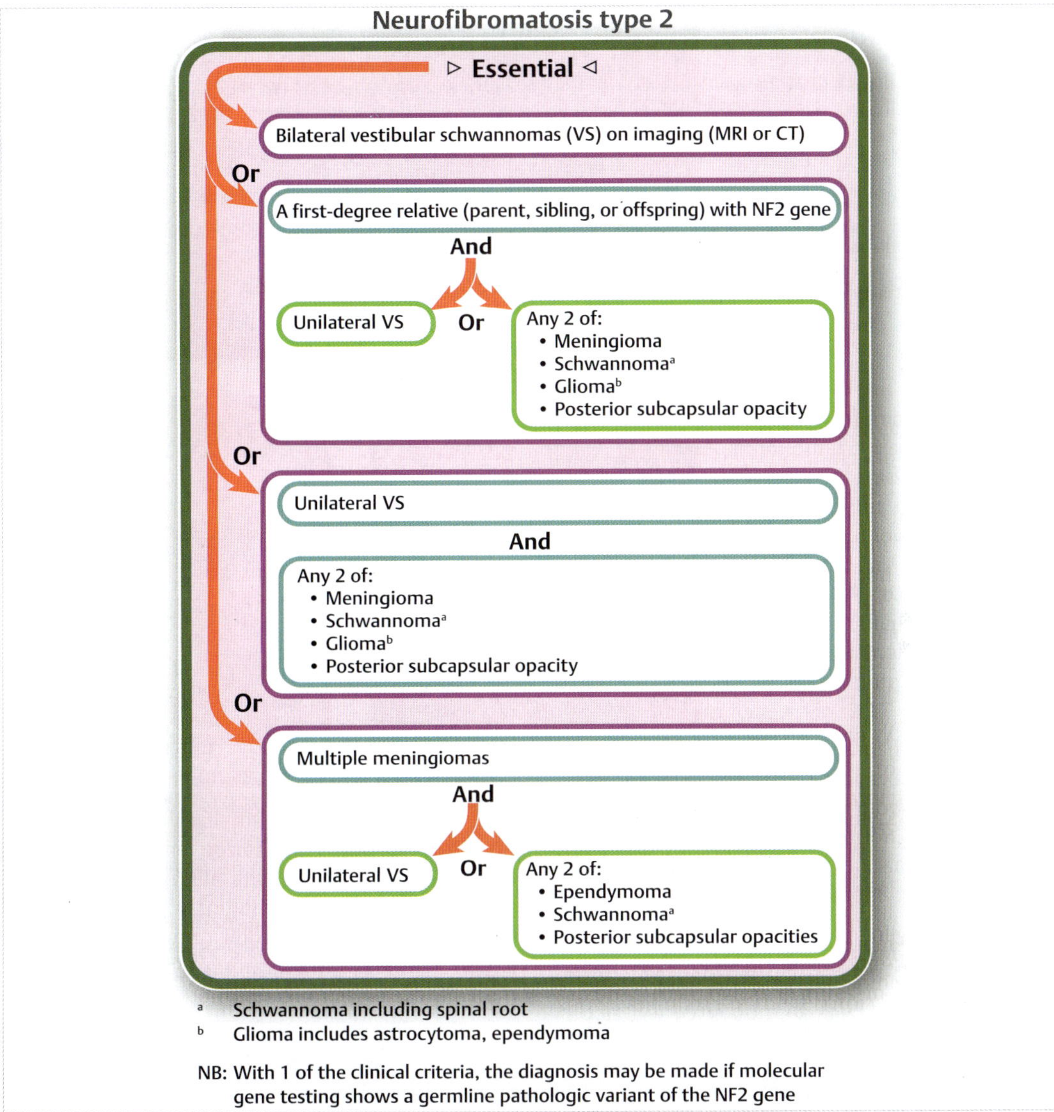

Fig. 2.5 (Source: Reproduced from Diagnostic criteria for neurofibromatosis type 2 (NF2). In: Greenberg M, ed. Greenberg's Handbook of Neurosurgery. 10th ed. New York: Thieme; 2023.)

bilateral, asymmetric white matter lesions without significant mass effect or contrast enhancement. Stereotactic biopsy demonstrates demyelination with oligodendrocyte loss and enlarged nuclei containing viral inclusions. Which virus is most likely responsible for these findings?

- A. Epstein–Barr virus (EBV)
- B. John Cunningham (JC) virus
- C. Cytomegalovirus (CMV)
- D. Herpes simplex virus type 1 (HSV-1)
- E. Human herpesvirus 6 (HHV-6)

Correct answer is B

The patient has **progressive multifocal leukoencephalopathy (PML)**, a demyelinating disease caused by the **JC virus**, a polyomavirus that infects oligodendrocytes. It occurs in immunosuppressed individuals, such as those with AIDS. MRI shows

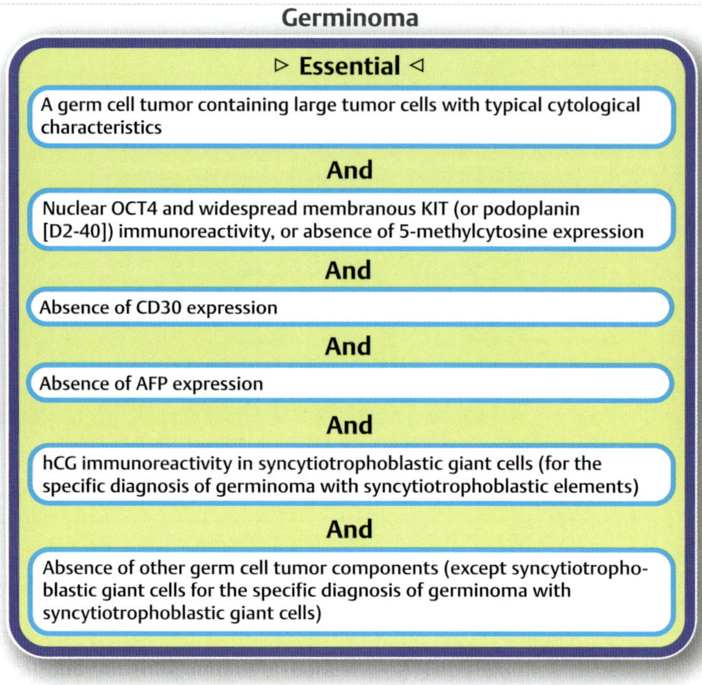

Fig. 2.6 (Source: Reproduced from Diagnostic criteria for germinoma. In: Greenberg M, ed. Greenberg's Handbook of Neurosurgery. 10th ed. New York: Thieme; 2023.)

multifocal white matter lesions without mass effect. EBV is associated with primary CNS lymphoma. CMV can cause encephalitis in immunocompromised patients but has different histological features. HSV-1 causes temporal lobe encephalitis. HHV-6 is linked to roseola infantum and may reactivate in immunosuppressed patients but is less commonly associated with PML-like symptoms. ▶ Fig. 2.7 shows a patient with acquired immunodeficiency syndrome with PML. PML lesions involve the subcortical white matter bilaterally and asymmetrically. There are hyperintensity lesions on (**a**) T2, (**b**) fluid-attenuated inversion recovery, (**c**) diffusion-weighted imaging (DWI), and (**d**) apparent diffusion coefficient map images. On DWI, the periphery of the lesions is hyperintense when compared to their central portions (*arrows*). (**e**) No contrast enhancement is seen on T1-weighted images postgadolinium.[14]

▸▸ Question 10

A 7-year-old girl presents with seizures. MRI reveals cortical thickening and a dysplastic lesion in the temporal lobe. Histopathology shows disorganized cortical architecture with large dysmorphic neurons and balloon cells. Which of the following is the most likely diagnosis?

- A. Focal cortical dysplasia (FCD) Type IIb
- B. Tuberous sclerosis complex
- C. Ganglioglioma
- D. Dysembryoplastic neuroepithelial tumor (DNET)
- E. Rasmussen encephalitis

Correct answer is A

FCD Type IIb is characterized by cortical dyslamination, dysmorphic neurons, and balloon cells. It

Table 2.1 ILAE classification of FCD

FCD type 1 (isolated)	FCD with abnormal radial cortical lamination (type Ia)	FCD with abnormal tangential cortical lamination (type Ib)	FCD with abnormal radial and tangential cortical lamination (type Ic)	
FCD type 2	FCD with dysmorphic neurons (type IIa)		FCD with dysmorphic neurons and balloon cells (type IIb)	
FCD type 3 (associated with principal lesion)	Cortical lamination abnormalities in the temporal lobe associated with hippocampal sclerosis (type IIIa)	Cortical lamination abnormalities adjacent to a glia or glioneuronal tumor (type IIIb)	Cortical lamination abnormalities adjacent to vascular malformation (type IIIc)	Cortical lamination abnormalities adjacent to any other lesion acquired during early life, e.g., trauma, ischemic injury, encephalitis (type IIId)

Abbreviation: FCD, focal cortical dysplasia.
Source: Reproduced from Cataltepe O, Jallo G, eds. Pediatric Epilepsy Surgery: Preoperative Assessment and Surgical Treatment. 2nd ed. New York: Thieme Medical Publishers, Inc.; 2019.

is a common cause of intractable epilepsy in children. The presence of balloon cells distinguishes Type IIb from other types. Tuberous sclerosis also shows cortical tubers with similar cells but is associated with other systemic findings. Gangliogliomas are tumors containing both neuronal and glial components. DNETs are benign tumors causing epilepsy but have different histology. Rasmussen encephalitis is a chronic inflammatory disease leading to progressive neurological deficits (▶ Table 2.1).[15,16]

▸▸ Question 11

A 60-year-old man presents with rapidly progressive dementia and myoclonus. MRI shows hyperintensities in the basal ganglia on diffusion-weighted imaging. EEG demonstrates periodic sharp wave complexes. Which histopathological finding is most likely in this patient?

- A. Neurofibrillary tangles composed of tau protein
- B. Cytoplasmic Lewy bodies containing alpha-synuclein
- C. Spongiform changes in the gray matter
- D. Demyelination with preservation of axons
- E. Lymphocytic infiltration with perivascular cuffing

Correct answer is C

The patient likely has **Creutzfeldt–Jakob disease**, a prion disease characterized by rapidly progressive dementia, myoclonus, and EEG changes. Histopathology shows **spongiform changes** due to vacuolation of neurons and neuropil in the gray matter. Neurofibrillary tangles are seen in Alzheimer disease. Lewy bodies are found in Parkinson disease and Lewy body dementia. Demyelination with preserved axons is characteristic of multiple sclerosis. Lymphocytic infiltration with perivascular cuffing is seen in viral encephalitis (▶ Fig. 2.8).[17]

▸▸ Question 12

A 3-year-old boy presents with macrocephaly and developmental delay. MRI reveals multiple cortical and subcortical tubers, subependymal nodules along the lateral ventricles, and a mass obstructing the foramen of Monro. Which genetic mutations are most commonly associated with this condition?

- A. Mutations in *NF1* gene
- B. Mutations in *NF2* gene
- C. Mutations in *TSC1* or *TSC2* genes
- D. Deletion of chromosome 22q11
- E. Expansion of CGG repeats in *FMR1* gene

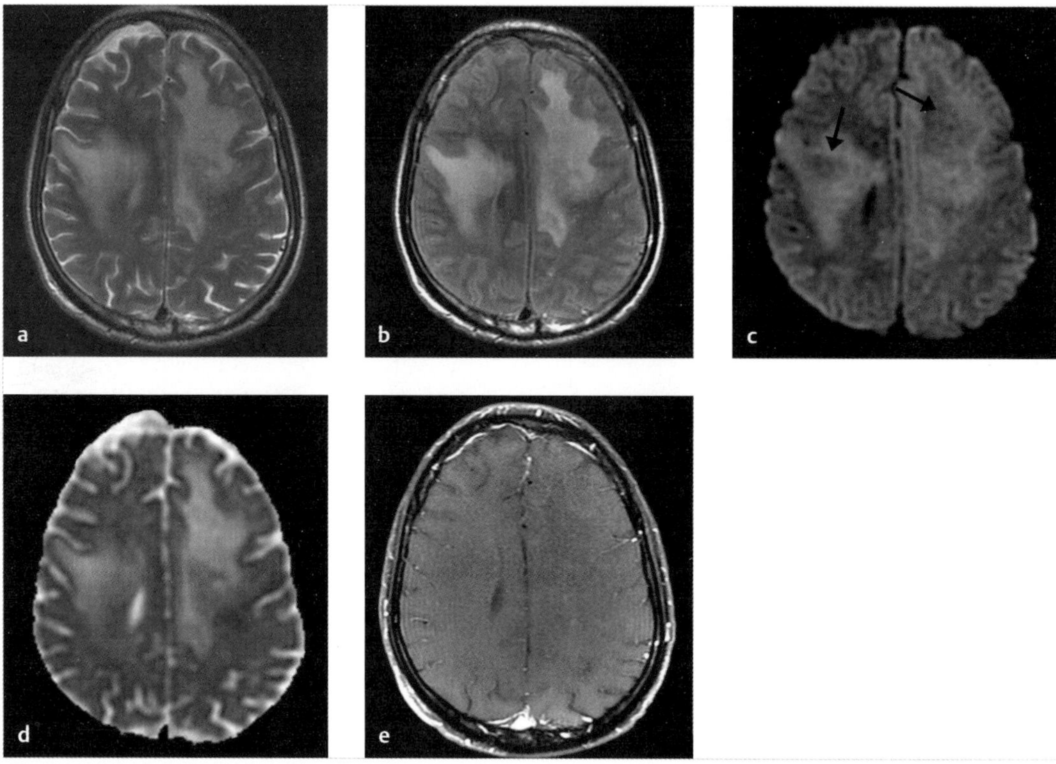

Fig. 2.7 (Source: Reproduced from Viral infections. In: Leite C, Castillo M, eds. Diffusion Weighted and Diffusion Tensor Imaging: A Clinical Guide. 1st ed. New York: Thieme; 2016.)

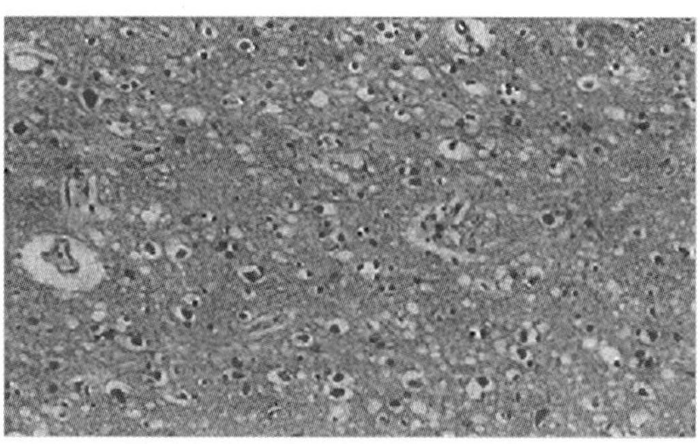

Fig. 2.8 (Source: Reproduced from Citow J, Macdonald R, Puffer R, et al., eds. Comprehensive Neurosurgery Board Review. 3rd ed. New York: Thieme; 2019.)

Correct answer is C

The patient has **tuberous sclerosis complex (TSC)**, a neurocutaneous disorder caused by mutations in the ***TSC1*** (hamartin) or ***TSC2*** (tuberin) genes. Features include cortical tubers, subependymal nodules, and subependymal giant cell astrocytomas (SEGAs) near the foramen of Monro, leading to hydrocephalus. NF1 mutations cause neurofibromatosis type 1. NF2 mutations lead to neurofibromatosis type 2. Deletion of 22q11 is seen in DiGeorge syndrome. CGG repeat expansion in FMR1 causes fragile X syndrome (▶ Table 2.2).[18]

▸▸ Question 13

A 50-year-old woman presents with painful ophthalmoplegia and proptosis of the right eye. MRI shows an enhancing mass in the right cavernous sinus extending into the orbital apex. Biopsy reveals spindle-shaped cells with whorled patterns and psammoma bodies. Which artery is most likely encased by this tumor?

- A. Anterior cerebral artery
- B. Middle cerebral artery

Table 2.2 Clinical diagnostic criteria of tuberous sclerosis complex

Definitive diagnosis: 2 major criteria, or 1 major *and* ≥ 2 minor
Possible diagnosis: 1 major or ≥ 2 minor
Major criteria
≥ 3 hypomelanotic macules ≥ 5 mm diameter
≥ 3 angiofibromas or fibrous cephalic plaque
≥ 2 ungual fibroma
Shagreen patch
Multiple retinal hamartomas
Cortical dysplasias (including tubers and cerebral white matter radial migration lines)
Subependymal nodules
Subependymal giant cell astrocytoma (SEGA)
Cardiac rhabdomyoma
Lymphangioleiomyomatosis
≥ 2 angiomyolipomas
Minor criteria
"Confetti" skin lesions
≥ 4 pits in dental enamel
≥ 2 intraoral fibromas
Achromic retinal patch
Multiple renal cysts
Nonrenal hamartomas

Source: Reproduced from Greenberg's Handbook of Neurosurgery. Greenberg M, ed. 10th ed. New York: Thieme; 2023.

- C. Internal carotid artery (ICA)
- D. Posterior communicating artery
- E. Ophthalmic artery

Correct answer is C

The tumor is a **meningioma** located in the cavernous sinus. The **ICA** passes through the cavernous sinus and can be encased by tumors in this location. Meningiomas often show spindle cells, whorls, and psammoma bodies on histology. The anterior and middle cerebral arteries are intracranial and not within the cavernous sinus. The posterior communicating artery branches from the ICA but comes off after the cavernous sinus. The ophthalmic artery arises from the ICA after it exits the cavernous sinus.[3,4,5]

▸▸ Question 14

A 65-year-old man presents with back pain and lower extremity weakness. MRI of the spine shows a destructive lesion in the vertebral body with an associated soft tissue mass compressing the spinal cord. Biopsy reveals malignant glands forming irregular structures with mucin production. Immunohistochemistry is positive for carcinoembryonic antigen (CEA). Which primary cancer is most likely?

- A. Prostate adenocarcinoma
- B. Lung adenocarcinoma
- C. Renal cell carcinoma
- D. Multiple myeloma
- E. Non-Hodgkin lymphoma

Correct answer is B

Metastatic **lung adenocarcinoma** commonly involves the spine and can produce gland-forming malignant cells with mucin production. **CEA positivity** supports the diagnosis. Prostate cancer typically produces small glands without mucin and is PSA positive. Renal cell carcinoma often shows clear cells and is associated with hemorrhagic lesions. Multiple myeloma is a plasma cell neoplasm that produces lytic bone lesions but has different histology. Non-Hodgkin lymphoma involves lymphoid cells.[19,20]

▸▸ Question 15

A 2-year-old boy presents with increasing head circumference and hydrocephalus. MRI shows a large, enhancing mass within the lateral ventricle. Histology reveals papillary structures lined by cuboidal epithelial cells with a fibrovascular core. Which of the following is the most likely diagnosis (▸ Fig. 2.9)?

- A. Central neurocytoma
- B. Choroid plexus papilloma

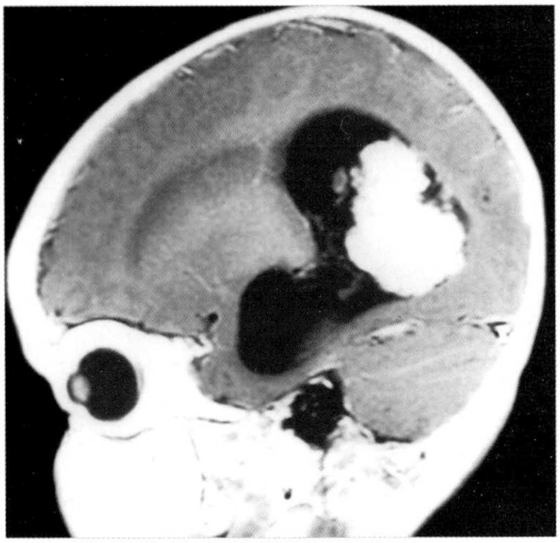

Fig. 2.9 (Source: Reproduced from Pathology and differential diagnosis. In: Keating R, Goodrich J, Packer R, eds. Tumors of the Pediatric Central Nervous System. 2nd ed. New York: Thieme; 2013.)

- C. Ependymoma
- D. Subependymal giant cell astrocytoma
- E. Medulloblastoma

Correct answer is B

Choroid plexus papillomas are intraventricular tumors that can overproduce cerebrospinal fluid, leading to hydrocephalus, especially in children. They are characterized histologically by papillary fronds lined with a single layer of epithelial cells over a fibrovascular core. Central neurocytomas occur in young adults and have neurocytic features. Ependymomas can occur in ventricles but have perivascular pseudorosettes. Subependymal giant cell astrocytomas are associated with tuberous sclerosis and occur near the foramen of Monro. Medulloblastomas are posterior fossa tumors.[21]

▸▸ Question 16

A 55-year-old woman presents with back pain and lower limb weakness. MRI shows an intradural extramedullary mass at the thoracic level. Surgical resection is performed. Histology reveals clusters of uniform spindle cells with elongated nuclei, dense eosinophilic cytoplasm, and occasional nuclear palisading. Which tumor marker is most likely positive?

- A. Cytokeratin
- B. EMA
- C. S-100 protein
- D. GFAP
- E. CD20

Correct answer is C

The patient has a **spinal schwannoma**, an intradural extramedullary tumor arising from Schwann cells. Histology shows spindle cells and nuclear palisading (Antoni A pattern). **S-100 protein** is positive in Schwann cells. Cytokeratin is found in epithelial cells. EMA is positive in meningiomas. GFAP is expressed in glial tumors. CD20 is a B-cell marker.[6]

▸▸ Question 17

A 45-year-old woman presents with headaches and visual disturbances. MRI reveals a homogenously enhancing mass arising from the sella turcica. Endocrine studies show elevated prolactin levels. Histology shows monotonous sheets of cells with uniform round nuclei and a “salt and pepper” chromatin pattern. Which of the following treatments is most appropriate?

- A. Surgical resection via transsphenoidal approach
- B. Radiation therapy
- C. Chemotherapy with temozolomide
- D. Dopamine agonist therapy
- E. Somatostatin analogs

Correct answer is D

The patient has a **prolactin-secreting pituitary adenoma** (prolactinoma). Elevated prolactin levels cause headaches and visual disturbances due to mass effect. First-line treatment is medical management with **dopamine agonists** (e.g., bromocriptine or cabergoline), which inhibit prolactin secretion and can reduce tumor size. Surgical resection is reserved for refractory cases. Radiation therapy and chemotherapy are not first-line treatments. Somatostatin analogs are used for growth hormone-secreting adenomas.[22,23]

▸▸ **Question 18**

A 30-year-old man presents with bitemporal hemianopsia. MRI shows a suprasellar mass with cystic and solid components, calcifications, and enhancement. Histology reveals stratified squamous epithelium with peripheral palisading and "wet" keratin. Which embryological structure is the origin of this tumor?

- A. Rathke pouch
- B. Neural tube
- C. Neural crest
- D. Remnants of the notochord
- E. Diencephalon

Correct answer is A

Craniopharyngiomas arise from epithelial remnants of **Rathke pouch**, an embryonic precursor to the anterior pituitary gland. They are commonly located in the suprasellar region, can cause visual field defects, and often contain calcifications and cystic components. Histology shows features resembling adamantinomatous epithelium with "wet" keratin. The neural tube gives rise to the CNS structures. The neural crest forms peripheral nerves and other structures. Remnants of the notochord can give rise to chordomas. The diencephalon develops into structures including the thalamus and hypothalamus.[24]

▸▸ **Question 19**

A 25-year-old woman presents with headaches and seizures. MRI reveals a well-circumscribed cortical mass in the temporal lobe with cystic and solid components. Histology shows both neoplastic neurons and glial cells, with occasional calcifications. Which of the following is the most likely diagnosis?

- A. Dysembryoplastic neuroepithelial tumor (DNET)
- B. Ganglioglioma
- C. Pleomorphic xanthoastrocytoma
- D. Oligodendroglioma
- E. Pilocytic astrocytoma

Correct answer is B

Gangliogliomas are rare, typically low-grade tumors composed of mixed neuronal and glial elements, often presenting with seizures in young adults. They are well-circumscribed and may have cystic components. Histology shows mature ganglion cells (neurons) and neoplastic glial cells. DNETs also cause seizures but have a different histological pattern with mucin-rich pools and floating neurons. Pleomorphic xanthoastrocytomas have lipidized astrocytes and are often superficial. Oligodendrogliomas have "fried-egg" cells and a chicken-wire vasculature. Pilocytic astrocytomas are more common in children.[25,26]

▸▸ **Question 20**

A 38-year-old man presents with a history of polycythemia and cerebellar symptoms. MRI reveals a cystic cerebellar mass with an enhancing mural nodule. Genetic testing confirms a mutation in the *VHL* gene. Which of the following additional findings is most likely in this patient?

- A. Renal cell carcinoma
- B. Optic nerve glioma
- C. Acoustic neuroma
- D. Café-au-lait spots
- E. Lisch nodules on the iris

Correct answer is A

Von Hippel–Lindau (VHL) disease is an autosomal dominant disorder caused by mutations in the *VHL* gene. It is characterized by **hemangioblastomas** in the CNS, especially the cerebellum and retina, and an increased risk of **clear cell renal cell carcinoma**. Polycythemia can occur due to erythropoietin production by hemangioblastomas. Optic nerve gliomas and café-au-lait spots are associated with neurofibromatosis type 1. Acoustic neuromas (vestibular schwannomas) are linked to neurofibromatosis type 2. Lisch nodules are pigmented iris hamartomas seen in NF1.[27]

▸▸ **Question 21**

A 62-year-old woman with a history of breast cancer presents with a sudden onset of headache and altered mental status. CT scan shows a lobar intracerebral hemorrhage in the parietal lobe. There is no history of hypertension. Which of the following is the most likely underlying cause?

- A. Hypertensive arteriolar sclerosis
- B. Cerebral amyloid angiopathy (CAA)
- C. Ruptured arteriovenous malformation
- D. Hemorrhagic transformation of an ischemic stroke
- E. Coagulopathy due to chemotherapy

Correct answer is B

CAA involves deposition of β-amyloid protein in the walls of cerebral blood vessels, leading to vessel fragility and hemorrhage, typically in the elderly and often in lobar regions. It is associated with Alzheimer disease but can occur independently. Hypertension causes deep brain hemorrhages (e.g., basal ganglia, thalamus, pons, cerebellum). Arteriovenous malformations are more common in younger patients. Hemorrhagic transformation occurs in ischemic strokes but is less likely without prior ischemia. Coagulopathy could cause bleeding but is less specific and would affect multiple sites.[28,29]

▸▸ Question 22

A 48-year-old man presents with lower back pain and radiculopathy. MRI shows a well-demarcated intradural extramedullary lesion at the level of L2. Histology reveals clusters of epithelioid cells with foamy cytoplasm and numerous blood vessels. Immunohistochemistry is positive for inhibin A. Which genetic condition is associated with this type of tumor?

- A. Neurofibromatosis type 1
- B. Tuberous sclerosis complex
- C. Von Hippel–Lindau (VHL) disease
- D. Cowden syndrome
- E. Li–Fraumeni syndrome

Correct answer is C

The tumor is a **hemangioblastoma**, which can occur in the spinal cord and is associated with **VHL disease**. Histology shows vascular tumors with stromal cells (inhibin A positive). Hemangioblastomas are a hallmark of VHL disease, along with retinal angiomas and the risk of renal cell carcinoma. Neurofibromatosis type 1 involves neurofibromas and optic gliomas. Tuberous sclerosis features cortical tubers and subependymal giant cell astrocytomas. Cowden syndrome involves PTEN mutations and hamartomas. Li–Fraumeni syndrome is associated with p53 mutations.[27]

▸▸ Question 23

A 6-year-old boy presents with ataxia and signs of increased intracranial pressure. MRI reveals a midline cerebellar mass. Histology shows small blue cells with hyperchromatic round nuclei and scant cytoplasm forming Homer Wright rosettes. Which molecular marker is associated with a better prognosis in this tumor?

- A. MYC amplification
- B. WNT pathway activation
- C. p53 mutation
- D. Isochromosome 17q
- E. SHH pathway activation

Correct answer is B

The tumor is a **medulloblastoma**, a malignant cerebellar tumor common in children. Histology shows small round blue cells and Homer Wright rosettes. Molecular subgrouping is important for prognosis. **WNT pathway activation** (e.g., β-catenin mutations) is associated with the best prognosis among medulloblastoma subtypes. MYC amplification and isochromosome 17q are associated with a poorer prognosis. SHH pathway activation has an intermediate prognosis. p53 mutations also indicate a worse outcome. ▸ Fig. 2.10 shows medulloblastoma histology: (**a**) Hematoxylin and eosin (H&E) stain of classic medulloblastoma, which is a highly cellular, small, round-cell tumor; (**b**) Immunohistochemistry for neurofilament protein (structural elements of neuronal axons and dendrites) demonstrates tumor cells infiltrating normal brain tissue; (**c**) Desmoplastic medulloblastoma as seen by reticulin staining (*left, blue*) and by H&E staining (*right, pink*). The reticulin-rich areas, which can be seen, result in the firm consistency of the tumor. The pale regions are reticulin free. H&E staining demonstrates a nodular architecture; (**d**) H&E stain of a large-cell or anaplastic medulloblastoma. Nuclear pleomorphism and a high rate of mitotic activity can be seen (▸ Table 2.3).[30,31,32]

▸▸ Question 24

A 70-year-old man presents with rapidly progressive weakness and sensory loss in the lower extremities. MRI of the spine shows a longitudinally extensive lesion involving the thoracic spinal cord with contrast enhancement. Cerebrospinal fluid (CSF) analysis reveals elevated protein and the presence of malignant lymphoid cells. What is the most likely diagnosis?

- A. Multiple sclerosis
- B. Transverse myelitis
- C. Primary central nervous system (CNS) lymphoma
- D. Metastatic carcinoma
- E. Sarcoidosis

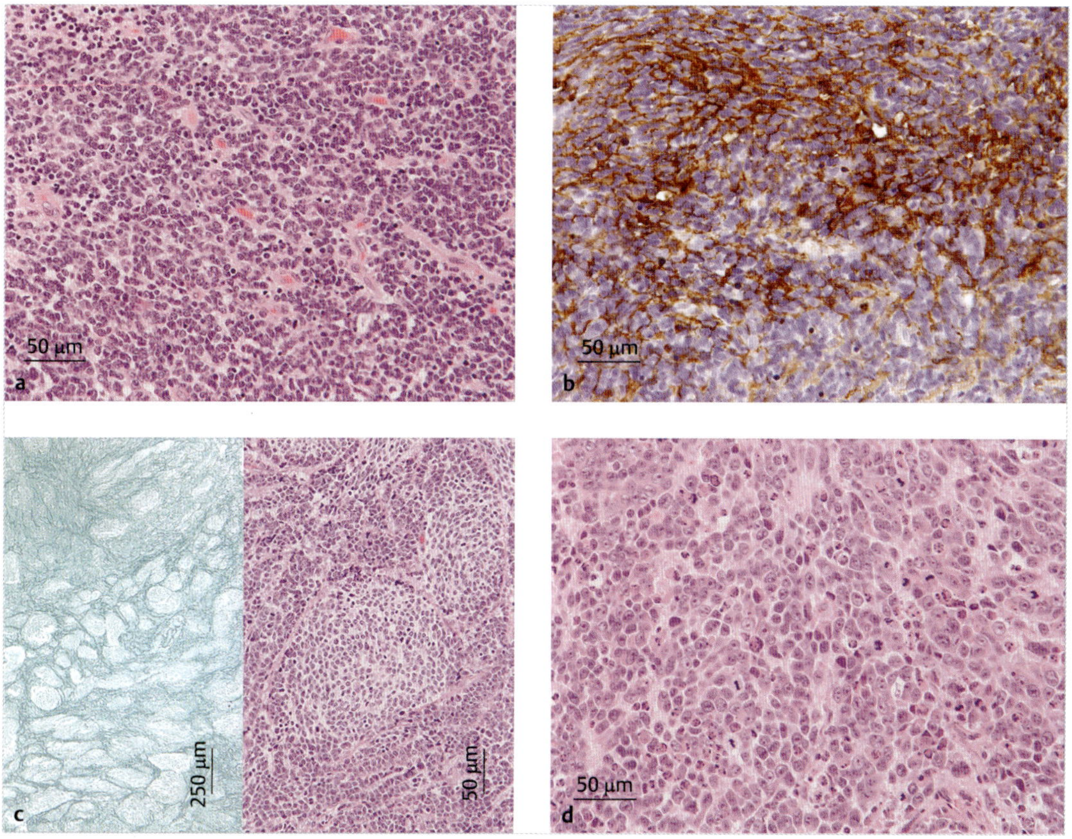

Fig. 2.10 (Source: Reproduced from Pathophysiology. In: Spetzler R, Kalani M, Lawton M, eds. Surgery of the Brainstem. 1st ed. New York: Thieme; 2019.)

Correct answer is C

Primary CNS lymphoma can involve the spinal cord and present with rapidly progressive neurological deficits. It is a diffuse large B-cell lymphoma confined to the CNS. CSF findings include malignant lymphoid cells. Multiple sclerosis typically presents with relapsing-remitting lesions. Transverse myelitis is inflammatory but not neoplastic. Metastatic carcinoma is less likely to produce CSF lymphoid cells. Sarcoidosis can involve the CNS but would show noncaseating granulomas.[33]

▸▸ Question 25

A 55-year-old man presents with lower back pain and signs of spinal cord compression. Imaging reveals a destructive lesion of the sacrum extending into adjacent soft tissues. Biopsy shows physaliphorous cells with bubbly cytoplasm embedded in a myxoid matrix. Which immunohistochemical marker is most likely positive?

- A. S-100 protein
- B. Epithelial membrane antigen (EMA)
- C. Cytokeratin
- D. GFAP
- E. CD68

Correct answer is C

The tumor is a **chordoma**, a malignant tumor arising from notochordal remnants, commonly in the sacrum or clivus. Histology shows physaliphorous cells (cells with vacuolated cytoplasm). **Chordomas are positive for cytokeratin** and EMA, reflecting their epithelial characteristics. S-100 may be variably positive. GFAP is expressed in glial cells. CD68 is a marker for

Table 2.3 Characteristics of genetically defined medulloblastoma variants[a]

Feature	*WNT*-activated	*SHH*-activated	Group 3	Group 4
TP53 status	–	*TP53* mutant *TP53* WT	–	–
Incidence	10%	30%	25%	35%
Age	Older children and adolescents (median age, 10 y)	Bimodal Infants (< 3 y) Adolescents or young adults (> 16 y)	Infants and children	Peak age: 10 y 50% of MBs in children 25% of MBs in adults
Sex ratio	M:F = 1:1	M:F = 1:1	M:F = 2:1	M:F = 3:1
Location	Midline of the fourth ventricle, may infiltrate the dorsal brainstem	Pediatric: midline or vermis Adults: cerebellar hemispheres	Midline of the fourth ventricle	Midline of the fourth ventricle
Histology	Classic Large-cell or anaplastic (rare)	Classic Large-cell or anaplastic Desmoplastic or nodular (rare in TP53 mutant) Extensive nodularity (only in *TP53* WT)	Classic Large-cell or anaplastic	Classic Large-cell or anaplastic (rare)
Metastasis	5–10%	15–20%	40–50%	30–40%
Recurrence	Rare	Local	Leptomeningeal	Leptomeningeal
Prognosis	Classic histology: low risk Large-cell or anaplastic: uncertain significance	*TP53* mutant: high risk *TP53* WT: standard or low risk	Classic histology: standard risk Large-cell or anaplastic: high risk	Classic histology: standard risk Large-cell or anaplastic: uncertain significance
5-y survival	> 90%	75%	45–55%	75%

Abbreviations: F, female; M, male; MB, medulloblastoma; *SHH*, sonic hedgehog; *TP53*, tumor protein 53; *WNT*, wingless activated; WT, wild type.
Source: Data from Louis et al (2016) and Coluccia et al (2016).[3,4]
[a]Molecular subgroups of medulloblastoma have been shown to correspond to different patient demographics and clinical features. Histology and molecular genetics in combination are now used to inform prognosis.

macrophages. ► Fig. 2.11 shows magnetic resonance imaging scan in short tau inversion recovery (STIR) sequence showing a regular hypodense mass ventral to the sacrum (sacral chordoma), in (**A**) sagittal and (**B**) axial views; ► Fig. 2.12 shows hematoxylin and eosin stained sections showing a tumoral proliferation composed of cells with (**A**) vacuolated cytoplasm and (**B**) areas resembling cartilage. (**C**) Cytokeratin immunohistochemistry was strongly positive. (**D**) There was nuclear positivity for brachyury. Final pathology was consistent with chordoma.[19,20]

►► Question 26

A 12-year-old boy presents with headaches, nausea, and papilledema. MRI reveals a well-circumscribed mass in the fourth ventricle, causing hydrocephalus. Histopathology shows sheets of small blue cells with hyperchromatic nuclei and scant cytoplasm. Immunohistochemistry is positive for synaptophysin and neuron-specific enolase (NSE). Which of the following is the most likely diagnosis?

- A. Ependymoma
- B. Medulloblastoma

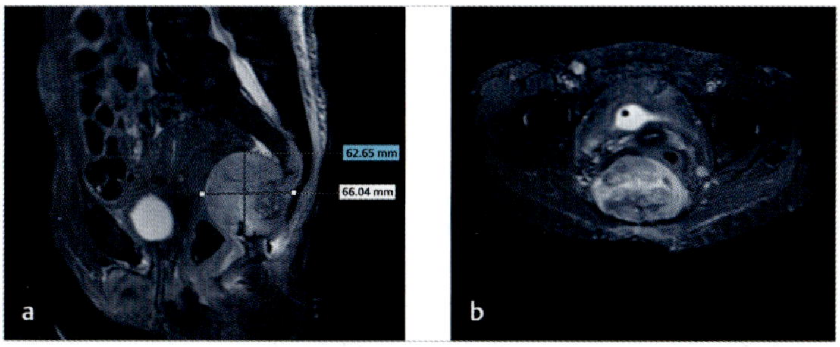

Fig. 2.11 (Source: Reproduced from Santos NA, Maximiano ML, Cortez PR. Partial sacrectomy in the management of sacral chordoma: case report and literature review. Arquivos Brasileiros de Neurocirurgia: Brazilian Neurosurgery 2024;43(04):343–346)

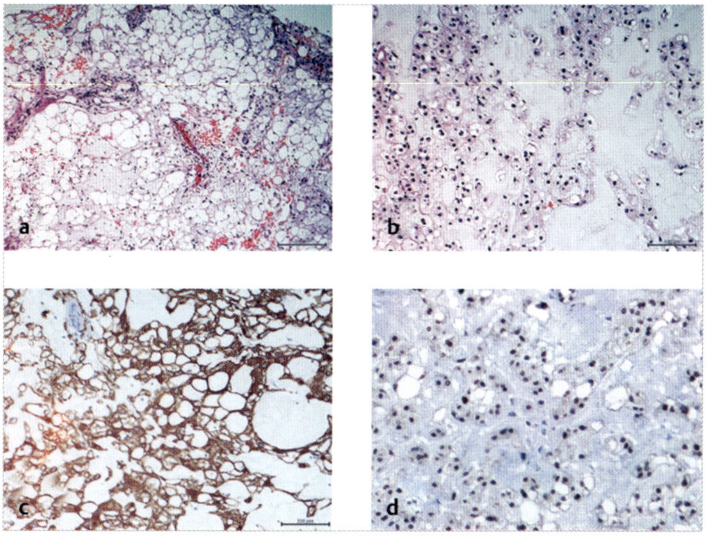

Fig. 2.12 (Source: Reproduced from AlOtaibi F, Guiot M, Muanza T, et al. Giant petroclival primary intradural chordoma: case report and systematic review of the literature. J Neurol Surg Rep 2014;75(01):160–169)

- C. Pilocytic astrocytoma
- D. Choroid plexus papilloma
- E. Brainstem glioma

Correct answer is B

Medulloblastomas are highly malignant cerebellar tumors common in children, often arising in the midline and can fill the fourth ventricle, leading to hydrocephalus. Histologically, they are composed of densely packed small round blue cells with high nuclear-to-cytoplasmic ratios. Immunohistochemistry is positive for neuronal markers like synaptophysin and NSE. Ependymomas also occur in the fourth ventricle but have perivascular pseudorosettes. Pilocytic astrocytomas are characterized by Rosenthal fibers. Choroid plexus papillomas arise from the choroid plexus epithelium. Brainstem gliomas are typically diffuse intrinsic pontine gliomas.[30,32]

▸▸ Question 27

A 35-year-old woman presents with seizures. MRI shows a temporal lobe mass with cystic and solid components that enhance with contrast. Histology reveals a tumor composed of astrocytic cells with abundant reticulin deposition and pleomorphic, lipid-laden cells. Which molecular alteration is commonly associated with this tumor?

- A. BRAF V600E mutation
- B. IDH1 mutation
- C. 1p/19q co-deletion
- D. EGFR amplification
- E. *NF2* gene deletion

Correct answer is A

The tumor described is a **pleomorphic xanthoastrocytoma (PXA)**, a rare astrocytic tumor that occurs in young adults, often presenting with seizures. Histology shows pleomorphic astrocytes with lipidized (xanthomatous) cytoplasm and reticulin deposition. **BRAF V600E mutations** are commonly found in PXAs. IDH1 mutations are typical of lower-grade astrocytomas and oligodendrogliomas. 1p/19q co-deletion is characteristic of oligodendrogliomas. EGFR amplification is common in primary glioblastomas. *NF2* gene deletion is associated with meningiomas and schwannomas.[7,19,20]

►► Question 28

A 29-year-old woman with a history of systemic lupus erythematosus presents with new-onset seizures. MRI shows a ring-enhancing lesion in the parietal lobe with surrounding edema. Stereotactic biopsy reveals septate hyphae branching at acute angles. Which of the following organisms is most likely responsible?

- A. *Candida albicans*
- B. *Aspergillus fumigatus*
- C. *Mucor* species
- D. *Cryptococcus neoformans*
- E. *Staphylococcus aureus*

Correct answer is B

Aspergillus fumigatus is a mold that forms septate hyphae branching at 45-degree angles (acute angles). It can cause brain abscesses, especially in immunocompromised patients such as those with lupus on immunosuppressive therapy. Candida forms yeast and pseudohyphae. *Mucor* species have broad, nonseptate hyphae with right-angle branching. *Cryptococcus neoformans* is a yeast with a thick capsule. *Staphylococcus aureus* is a common bacterial cause of brain abscesses but does not produce hyphae.[34,35]

►► Question 29

A 42-year-old man presents with chronic headaches and visual disturbances. MRI reveals an extra-axial mass along the convexity of the brain with a dural tail sign. Surgical resection is performed. Histology shows meningothelial cells with high cellularity, mitotic figures, and small foci of necrosis. The Ki-67 labeling index is elevated. What is the WHO grade of this tumor?

- A. Grade I (benign)
- B. Grade II (atypical)
- C. Grade III (anaplastic)
- D. Grade IV (malignant)
- E. Not applicable

Correct answer is B

An **atypical meningioma (WHO Grade II)** is characterized by increased cellularity, higher mitotic activity (4–19 mitoses per 10 high-power fields), and may have small foci of necrosis. An elevated Ki-67 index indicates increased proliferation. Grade I meningiomas are benign with low mitotic activity. Grade III (anaplastic) meningiomas have overtly malignant features, including > 20 mitoses per 10 high-power fields, and are considered malignant (WHO Grade III). There is no WHO Grade IV for meningiomas.[3,4,5]

►► Question 30

An 18-year-old male presents with progressive lower limb weakness and urinary retention. MRI of the spine shows an intramedullary tumor in the conus medullaris region. Histology reveals elongated bipolar cells with processes forming perivascular pseudorosettes. Which tumor marker is most likely positive?

- A. Glial fibrillary acidic protein (GFAP)
- B. S-100 protein
- C. Synaptophysin
- D. Epithelial membrane antigen (EMA)
- E. CD68

Correct answer is A

The tumor is likely an **ependymoma**, the most common intramedullary spinal cord tumor in adults and young adults. Histology shows cells forming perivascular pseudorosettes and true ependymal rosettes. **GFAP positivity** indicates glial origin. S-100 protein is positive in Schwann cells and melanocytic tumors. Synaptophysin is a neuronal marker. EMA may be positive in meningiomas. CD68 is a marker for macrophages.[8,9]

►► Question 31

A 55-year-old woman presents with a history of seizures. MRI shows a heterogeneously enhancing mass in the parietal lobe with areas of calcification. Histology reveals malignant cells with high

mitotic activity and endothelial proliferation. Fluorescence in situ hybridization (FISH) shows amplification of the *PDGFRA* gene. Which type of glioblastoma does this most likely represent?
- A. Classical subtype
- B. Mesenchymal subtype
- C. Proneural subtype
- D. Neural subtype
- E. Giant cell glioblastoma

Correct answer is C

The **proneural subtype** of glioblastoma is characterized by amplification or mutation of the ***PDGFRA*** gene and is more common in younger patients. It often arises from lower-grade gliomas and may have a slightly better prognosis than other subtypes. The classical subtype is associated with EGFR amplification. The mesenchymal subtype often shows NF1 mutations. The neural subtype expresses neuronal markers. Giant cell glioblastoma is a histological variant with multinucleated giant cells.[1,2]

▸▸ Question 32

A 65-year-old man presents with progressive cognitive decline and gait disturbances. MRI shows enlarged ventricles with normal sulci. Cerebrospinal fluid (CSF) opening pressure is normal. Which of the following is the most likely underlying pathophysiology?
- A. Obstructive hydrocephalus due to aqueductal stenosis
- B. Overproduction of CSF by a choroid plexus papilloma
- C. Impaired CSF absorption at the arachnoid granulations
- D. Increased CSF viscosity due to meningitis
- E. Atrophy of the brain parenchyma

Correct answer is C

The patient has normal-pressure hydrocephalus (NPH), characterized by the triad of gait disturbance, dementia, and urinary incontinence. Ventricles are enlarged despite normal or intermittently elevated CSF pressure on lumbar puncture. The underlying mechanism is impaired CSF absorption at the arachnoid granulations. Obstructive hydrocephalus would result in persistently increased CSF pressure. Choroid plexus papilloma overproduces CSF but is rare in adults. Increased CSF viscosity is seen in meningitis. Brain atrophy leads to ex-vacuo ventriculomegaly, which also shows enlarged sulci, unlike NPH.[36]

▸▸ Question 33

A 50-year-old woman presents with symptoms of increased intracranial pressure. MRI shows a cystic lesion in the pineal region with peripheral enhancement. Surgical resection reveals an epithelial-lined cyst with keratin debris. Which of the following is the most likely diagnosis?
- A. Pineocytoma
- B. Germinoma
- C. Epidermoid cyst
- D. Dermoid cyst
- E. Arachnoid cyst

Correct answer is C

An **epidermoid cyst** is a benign lesion lined by stratified squamous epithelium and contains keratin debris. It can occur in the pineal region and appear cystic on imaging. Epidermoid cysts can cause symptoms due to mass effect. Dermoid cysts also contain skin appendages like hair and sebaceous glands. Pineocytomas are pineal parenchymal tumors. Germinomas are germ cell tumors. Arachnoid cysts are cerebrospinal fluid–filled sacs within the arachnoid membrane.[11,12,13]

▸▸ Question 34

A 40-year-old man presents with trigeminal neuralgia. MRI reveals an extra-axial mass at the cerebellopontine angle compressing the trigeminal nerve. Histology shows elongated cells with wavy nuclei embedded in a collagenous stroma. Which of the following is the most likely diagnosis?
- A. Schwannoma
- B. Neurofibroma
- C. Meningioma
- D. Epidermoid tumor
- E. Hemangioblastoma

Correct answer is B

A **neurofibroma** is a benign nerve sheath tumor composed of Schwann cells, fibroblasts, and perineurial cells. Histology shows a mix of cells with wavy nuclei in a collagenous matrix. While schwannomas are also nerve sheath tumors, they are typically encapsulated and composed solely of Schwann cells. Neurofibromas are associated with neurofibromatosis type 1. Meningiomas arise from meningothelial cells. Epidermoid tumors contain keratin debris. Hemangioblastomas are vascular tumors.

▸▸ Question 35

A 28-year-old woman presents with visual disturbances and is found to have an optic nerve glioma. She also has multiple café-au-lait spots and axillary freckling. Which of the following additional findings is most likely present?

- A. Bilateral vestibular schwannomas
- B. Lisch nodules on the iris
- C. Ash-leaf spots
- D. Retinal angiomas
- E. Cutaneous hemangiomas

Correct answer is B

The patient has **neurofibromatosis type 1 (NF1)**, characterized by optic nerve gliomas, café-au-lait spots, axillary freckling, and **Lisch nodules** (pigmented iris hamartomas). Bilateral vestibular schwannomas are seen in NF2. Ash-leaf spots are hypopigmented macules seen in tuberous sclerosis complex. Retinal angiomas are associated with Von Hippel–Lindau disease. Cutaneous hemangiomas are common but not specific (▸ Fig. 2.13).[37]

▸▸ Question 36

A 6-year-old boy presents with refractory epilepsy. MRI shows a nonenhancing cortical lesion in the temporal lobe. Histology reveals columns of dysplastic neurons in a mucin-rich matrix with floating neurons. Which of the following is the most likely diagnosis?

- A. Ganglioglioma
- B. Dysembryoplastic neuroepithelial tumor (DNET)
- C. Cortical dysplasia
- D. Oligodendroglioma
- E. Pilocytic astrocytoma

Correct answer is B

DNETs are benign cortical tumors presenting with epilepsy in children and young adults. Histology shows dysplastic neurons ("floating neurons") in a mucin-rich background and columns of glial cells. Gangliogliomas have both neuronal and glial components but lack the mucinous matrix. Cortical dysplasia is a developmental anomaly. Oligodendrogliomas have "fried-egg" cells and a chicken-wire vasculature. Pilocytic astrocytomas are more common in the cerebellum.[25,26]

▸▸ Question 37

A 45-year-old man presents with back pain and weakness in the lower limbs. Imaging shows an expansile lesion in the thoracic vertebral body with a "soap-bubble" appearance on X-ray. Biopsy reveals multinucleated giant cells and mononuclear stromal cells. Which of the following is the most likely diagnosis?

- A. Osteoblastoma
- B. Giant cell tumor of bone
- C. Chordoma
- D. Eosinophilic granuloma
- E. Hemangioma

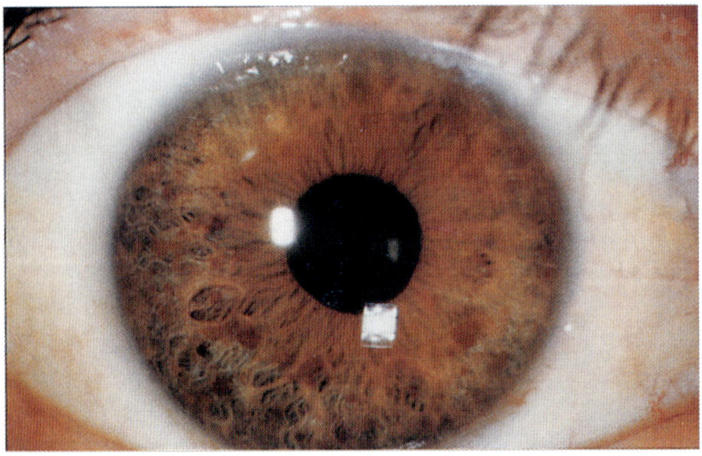

Fig. 2.13 (Source: Reproduced from Borsody M, ed. Comprehensive Board Review in Neurology. 2nd ed. New York: Thieme; 2012.)

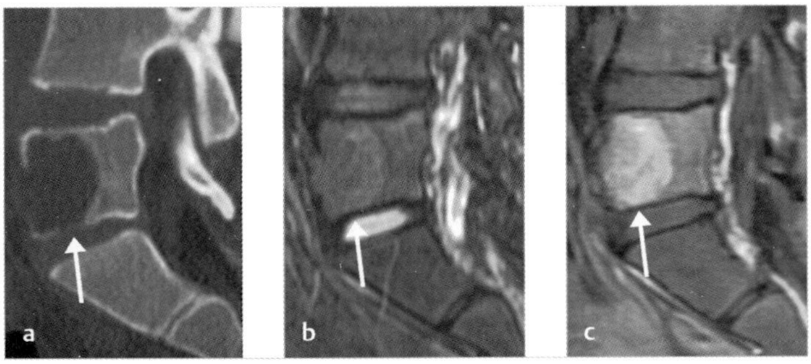

Fig. 2.14 (Source: Reproduced from Solitary osseous lesions involving the spine. In: Meyers S, ed. Differential Diagnosis in Neuroimaging: Spine. 1st ed. New York: Thieme; 2016.)

Correct answer is B

Giant cell tumor of bone is a benign but locally aggressive tumor, often affecting the epiphysis of long bones and vertebral bodies. Radiographically, it has a lytic "soap-bubble" appearance. Histology shows numerous multinucleated giant cells (osteoclast-like) and mononuclear stromal cells. Osteoblastomas are similar but typically smaller and affect the posterior elements of the spine. Chordomas arise from notochordal remnants. Eosinophilic granulomas are Langerhans cell histiocytosis lesions. Hemangiomas are vascular lesions. ▶ Fig. 2.14 is a (**a**) sagittal CT of a 13-year-old female that shows a radiolucent giant cell tumor (*arrow*) involving the anterior portion of the L5 vertebral body that has (**b**) intermediate signal on sagittal T2-weighted imaging (*arrow*) and (**c**) gadolinium contrast enhancement on sagittal fat-suppressed T1-weighted imaging (*arrow*). The tumor erodes the anterior cortical margin of the vertebral body.[38,39,40]

▸▸ Question 38

A 60-year-old woman presents with facial pain and muscle weakness. Electrophysiological studies show a decremental muscle response with repetitive nerve stimulation. Imaging reveals a mass in the anterior mediastinum. Which of the following antibodies is most likely present?

- A. Antiacetylcholine receptor antibodies
- B. Anti-voltage-gated calcium channel antibodies
- C. Anti-MuSK antibodies
- D. Anti-NMDA receptor antibodies
- E. Anti-GAD antibodies

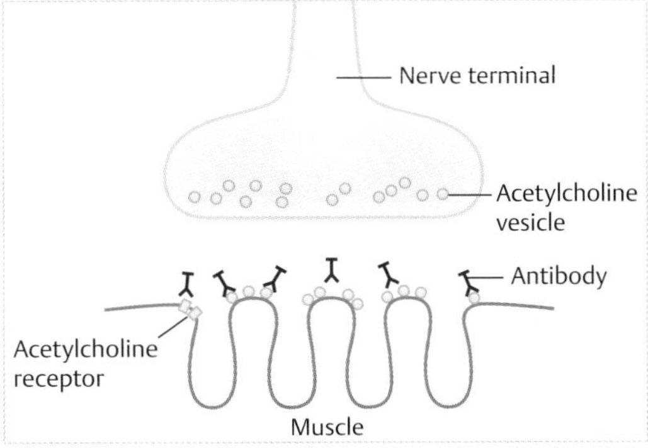

Fig. 2.15 (Source: Reproduced from Receptors. In: Dhikav V, Anand K, eds. Principles and Practice of Neuropsychopharmacology. 1st ed. Noida: Thieme; 2021.)

Correct answer is A

The patient has **myasthenia gravis**, characterized by autoantibodies against **acetylcholine receptors** at the neuromuscular junction, leading to muscle weakness that worsens with activity. The association with a **thymoma** (anterior mediastinal mass) is common. Anti-voltage-gated calcium channel antibodies are seen in Lambert-Eaton myasthenic syndrome. Anti-MuSK antibodies are another cause of myasthenia gravis but are less common and often in patients without thymoma. Anti-NMDA receptor antibodies are associated with encephalitis. Anti-GAD antibodies are seen in stiff-person syndrome (▶ Fig. 2.15).[41]

▸▸ Question 39

A 70-year-old man with a history of atrial fibrillation presents with a sudden onset of left-sided weakness. MRI shows an area of restricted diffusion in the right internal capsule. What is the most likely pathological finding in the affected area after 12 hours?

- A. Neutrophil infiltration
- B. Liquefactive necrosis
- C. Eosinophilic neurons (red neurons)
- D. Microglial proliferation
- E. Reactive astrocytosis

Correct answer is C

In the first 12 to 24 hours after an ischemic stroke, histopathology shows **eosinophilic (red) neurons** due to irreversible neuronal injury. Neutrophil infiltration occurs at 24 to 48 hours. Liquefactive necrosis develops over days. Microglial proliferation and phagocytosis occur at 3 to 5 days. Reactive astrocytosis and glial scar formation happen weeks later.[28,29]

▸▸ Question 40

A 65-year-old woman presents with progressive memory loss and difficulty performing daily tasks. MRI shows cortical atrophy, particularly in the temporal and parietal lobes. Histology of a brain biopsy shows neurofibrillary tangles composed of hyperphosphorylated tau protein and extracellular amyloid plaques. Which enzyme is responsible for the abnormal cleavage of amyloid precursor protein, leading to amyloid-beta accumulation?

- A. Alpha-secretase
- B. Beta-secretase
- C. Gamma-secretase
- D. Acetylcholinesterase
- E. Monoamine oxidase

Correct answer is B

In **Alzheimer disease**, abnormal cleavage of amyloid precursor protein (APP) by **beta-secretase** and gamma-secretase leads to the formation of amyloid-beta peptides, which accumulate as extracellular plaques. Alpha-secretase cleavage is part of the nonamyloidogenic pathway. Acetylcholinesterase breaks down acetylcholine. Monoamine oxidase metabolizes monoamines like serotonin and dopamine.[42]

▸▸ Question 41

A 50-year-old man presents with headaches and anosmia. MRI reveals a mass in the olfactory groove region with hyperostosis of the underlying bone. Histology shows spindle cells in whorled patterns with psammoma bodies. Which surgical approach is most appropriate for complete resection?

- A. Transsphenoidal approach
- B. Pterional (frontotemporal) craniotomy
- C. Bifrontal craniotomy
- D. Suboccipital craniotomy
- E. Retrosigmoid approach

Correct answer is C

An **olfactory groove meningioma** is best approached via a **bifrontal craniotomy**, which provides direct access to the anterior cranial fossa and allows for en bloc resection of the tumor and involved bone. The transsphenoidal approach is for sellar lesions. The pterional approach is for lesions in the anterior and middle cranial fossae but not optimal for midline anterior skull base tumors. Suboccipital and retrosigmoid approaches are for posterior fossa lesions.[3,4,5]

▸▸ Question 42

A 45-year-old man with AIDS presents with seizures and cognitive decline. MRI shows multiple nonenhancing lesions in the white matter. Brain biopsy reveals abnormal oligodendrocytes with enlarged nuclei and ground-glass chromatin. Which of the following is the most appropriate antiviral therapy?

- A. Acyclovir
- B. Ganciclovir
- C. Cidofovir
- D. Highly active antiretroviral therapy (HAART)
- E. Foscarnet

Correct answer is D

The patient has **progressive multifocal leukoencephalopathy** (PML) caused by reactivation of the **John Cunningham (JC) virus** in immunocompromised individuals. There is no effective antiviral therapy against the JC virus; **HAART** improves immune function and is the best approach to halt disease progression. Acyclovir is for herpesviruses. Ganciclovir and foscarnet are for cytomegalovirus. Cidofovir has activity against some DNA viruses but not effective for PML.[14]

▸▸ **Question 43**

A 7-year-old girl presents with early-onset puberty and gelastic (laughing) seizures. MRI reveals a hypothalamic mass. Which of the following is the most likely diagnosis?

- A. Hypothalamic hamartoma
- B. Craniopharyngioma
- C. Pilocytic astrocytoma
- D. Germinoma
- E. Optic pathway glioma

Correct answer is A

Hypothalamic hamartomas are benign malformations causing precocious puberty due to gonadotropin-releasing hormone secretion and gelastic seizures (involuntary laughing). MRI shows a nonenhancing mass in the hypothalamus. Craniopharyngiomas can cause endocrine disturbances but are cystic and calcified. Pilocytic astrocytomas are more common in the cerebellum. Germinomas may occur in the hypothalamic region but typically in older children. Optic pathway gliomas affect the optic nerves and chiasm.[15,16]

▸▸ **Question 44**

A 30-year-old man presents with headaches and visual field defects. MRI reveals an enhancing mass in the third ventricle, causing hydrocephalus. Histology shows monotonous small cells with round nuclei and scant cytoplasm, and immunohistochemistry is positive for synaptophysin and negative for GFAP. Which of the following is the most likely diagnosis?

- A. Central neurocytoma
- B. Subependymoma
- C. Ependymoma
- D. Choroid plexus papilloma
- E. Colloid cyst

Correct answer is A

Central neurocytomas are rare intraventricular tumors in young adults, often located in the lateral or third ventricles. Histology shows neuronal differentiation (synaptophysin positive) without glial markers (GFAP negative). Subependymomas are slow-growing tumors in the ventricles but have different histology. Ependymomas express GFAP. Choroid plexus papillomas arise from choroid plexus epithelium. Colloid cysts are gelatinous cysts in the third ventricle but lack solid tumor cells (▸ Table 2.4). ▸ Fig. 2.16 shows a central neurocytoma. Axial T2-weighted (**a**) and corresponding postcontrast T1-weighted (**b**) images show a heterogeneous, partially enhancing, lobular right lateral ventricular mass, which abuts the septum pellucidum. There is a predominant T2 isointensity with cystic foci. ▸ Fig. 2.17 shows a central neurocytoma viewed at 200 × (**a**) and 400 × (**b**) magnification, with small- to medium-sized, round, bland tumor cells with lightly eosinophilic cytoplasm growing in patternless sheets.[21]

Table 2.4 Central neurocytoma: pathological features

Composed of small, uniform cells of glial-neural origin with a "fried-egg" appearance
Alternating cellular and fibrillary background
Immunohistochemical staining:
GFAP, NSE, and synaptophysin positive
Abbreviations: GFAP, glial fibrillary acidic protein; NSE, neuron-specific enolase.

▸▸ **Question 45**

A 65-year-old woman presents with a sudden onset of vertigo, nausea, and left-sided ataxia. MRI shows an infarct in the territory of the left posterior inferior cerebellar artery (PICA). Which of the following symptoms is also expected?

- A. Right-sided hemiparesis
- B. Left-sided loss of pain and temperature sensation in the face
- C. Loss of vibration and proprioception on the left side
- D. Bilateral visual field defects
- E. Aphasia

Correct answer is B

An infarct in the **PICA** territory causes **lateral medullary (Wallenberg) syndrome**, which includes ipsilateral loss of pain and temperature sensation in the face (due to trigeminal nucleus involvement), contralateral loss in the body, ipsilateral Horner syndrome, ataxia, vertigo, and

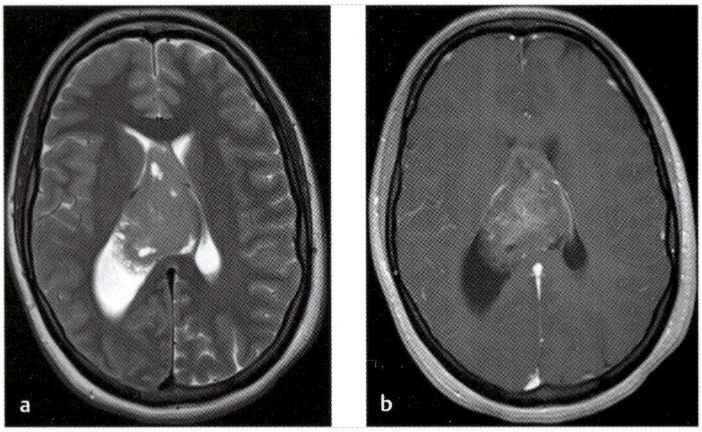

Fig. 2.16 (Source: Reproduced from Central Neurocytoma. In: Jain R, Essig M, eds. Brain Tumor Imaging. 1st ed. New York: Thieme; 2015.)

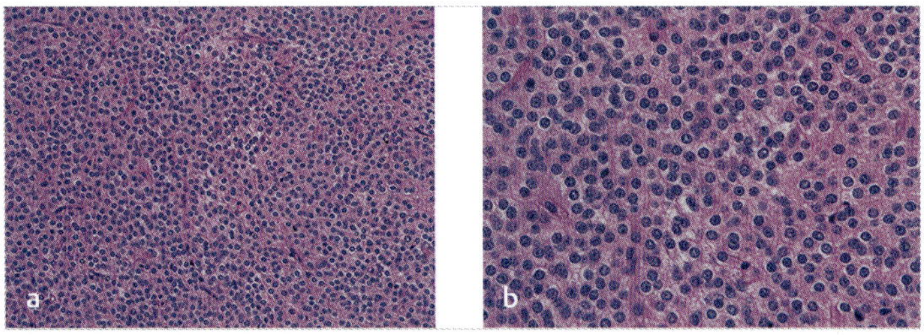

Fig. 2.17 (Source: Reproduced from Central Neurocytoma. In: Jain R, Essig M, eds. Brain Tumor Imaging. 1st ed.. New York: Thieme; 2015.)

dysphagia. Motor pathways are typically spared, so hemiparesis is uncommon. Loss of vibration and proprioception indicates medial lemniscus involvement, not typical in PICA strokes. Visual field defects and aphasia are associated with cortical strokes (▶ Fig. 2.18).[43]

▸▸ Question 46

A 4-year-old boy presents with a large head and developmental delays. MRI shows dilation of the lateral ventricles due to aqueductal stenosis. Which of the following is the most appropriate surgical treatment?

- A. Ventriculoperitoneal shunt placement
- B. Third ventriculostomy
- C. Endoscopic fenestration of the aqueduct
- D. Placement of a subdural drain
- E. Temporal lobectomy

Correct answer is A

Aqueductal stenosis is a common cause of noncommunicating (obstructive) hydrocephalus, particularly in children. It leads to dilation of the lateral and third ventricles, with a normal or small fourth ventricle.

Endoscopic third ventriculostomy is often the preferred surgical option, especially in older children, as it creates a bypass for cerebrospinal fluid from the third ventricle to the subarachnoid space, avoiding the need for permanent shunt hardware.[36]

▸▸ Question 47

A 70-year-old man presents with dementia, urinary incontinence, and ataxic gait. MRI shows enlarged ventricles without significant cortical atrophy. Which of the following cerebrospinal fluid (CSF) findings is expected?

- A. Elevated opening pressure
- B. Decreased glucose concentration
- C. Elevated protein levels
- D. Normal opening pressure
- E. Presence of oligoclonal bands

Correct answer is D

In **normal-pressure hydrocephalus** (NPH), the CSF opening pressure is **normal** despite ventricular enlargement. CSF glucose and protein levels are typically normal. Oligoclonal bands are seen in multiple sclerosis.[36]

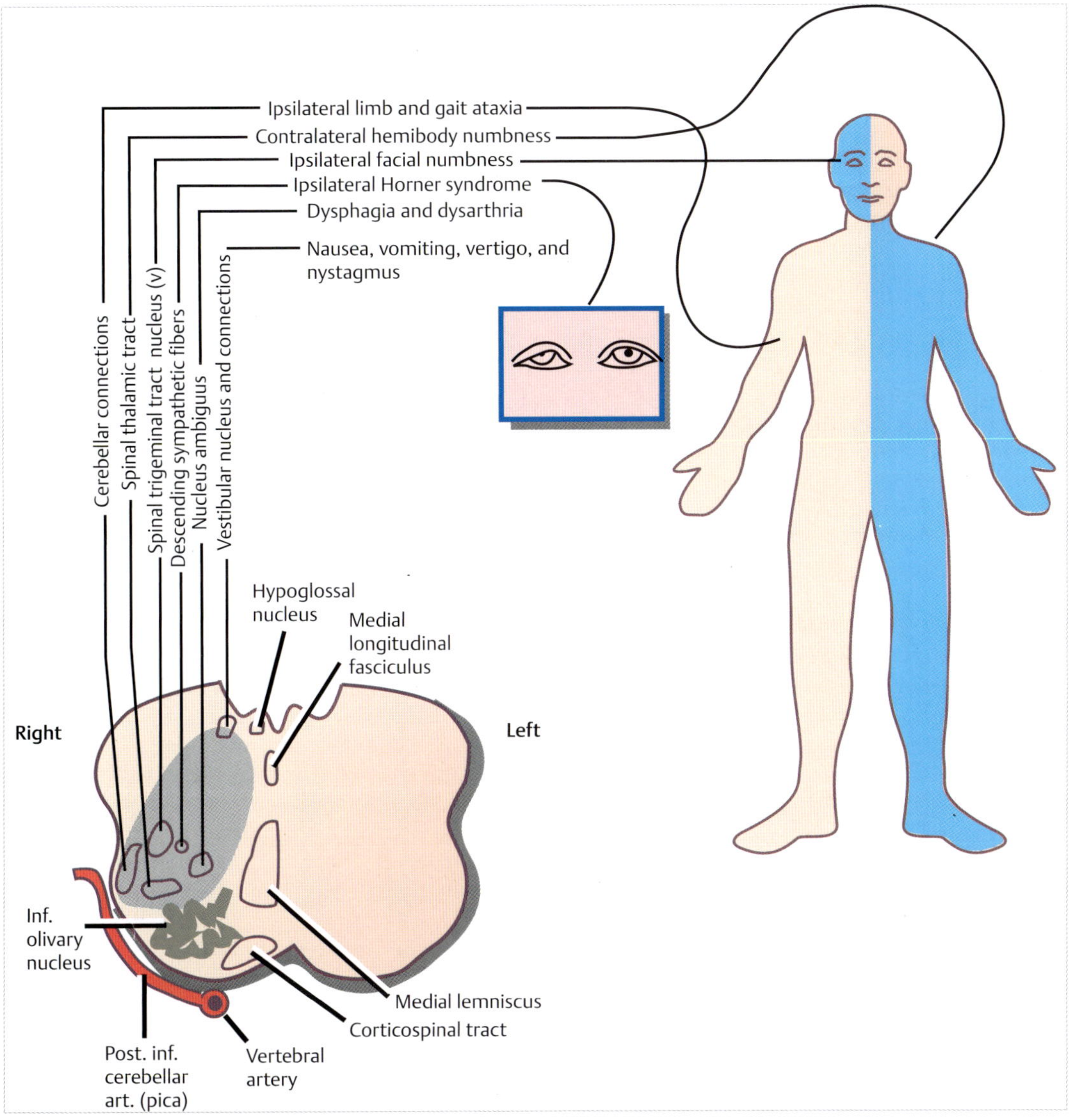

Fig. 2.18 (Source: Reproduced from Alberstone C, Benzel E, Jones S, Wang Z, Steinmetz M, eds. Anatomic Basis of Neurologic Diagnosis. 2nd ed. New York: Thieme Medical Publishers, Inc.; 2023.)

▸▸ Question 48

A 25-year-old woman presents with weakness and paresthesia in her right arm and leg. MRI shows multiple demyelinating lesions in the brain and spinal cord. CSF analysis reveals oligoclonal bands. Which of the following findings is most specific for multiple sclerosis (MS)?

- A. Bilateral optic neuritis
- B. Internuclear ophthalmoplegia (INO)
- C. Positive Babinski sign
- D. Spasticity
- E. Fatigue

Correct answer is B

INO is a disorder of horizontal gaze caused by a lesion in the medial longitudinal fasciculus and is highly specific for **MS** in young adults. Bilateral optic neuritis can occur in MS but is not specific. Positive Babinski sign, spasticity, and fatigue are common neurological symptoms but not specific to MS.[44,45]

▸▸ Question 49

A 3-year-old boy presents with macrocephaly and seizures. He has port-wine stains on the left side of his face. MRI shows leptomeningeal angiomas over the left cerebral hemisphere. Which of the following is the most likely diagnosis?

- A. Tuberous sclerosis complex
- B. Sturge–Weber syndrome
- C. Neurofibromatosis type 1
- D. Von Hippel–Lindau disease
- E. Ataxia-telangiectasia

Correct answer is B

Sturge–Weber syndrome is a neurocutaneous disorder characterized by facial port-wine stains (nevus flammeus), leptomeningeal angiomas, seizures, and intellectual disability. Tuberous sclerosis involves cortical tubers and ash-leaf spots. Neurofibromatosis type 1 has café-au-lait spots and neurofibromas. Von Hippel–Lindau disease features hemangioblastomas and renal cell carcinoma. Ataxia-telangiectasia involves cerebellar ataxia and telangiectasias.[46]

▸▸ Question 50

A 45-year-old woman presents with progressive weakness and muscle wasting in her hands and arms. She has fasciculations and increased deep tendon reflexes. Which of the following pathological findings is most likely present?

- A. Loss of upper motor neurons in the motor cortex and lower motor neurons in the anterior horns
- B. Demyelination of peripheral nerves with onion bulb formation
- C. Degeneration of the dorsal columns and corticospinal tracts
- D. Loss of GABAergic neurons in the caudate nucleus
- E. Wallerian degeneration of the spinothalamic tract

Correct answer is A

The patient has **amyotrophic lateral sclerosis**, characterized by degeneration of both upper motor neurons (UMNs) in the motor cortex and lower motor neurons (LMNs) in the anterior horns of the spinal cord. This leads to mixed UMN and LMN signs (e.g., weakness, atrophy, fasciculations, hyperreflexia). Demyelination with onion bulb formation is seen in Charcot–Marie–Tooth disease. Degeneration of the dorsal columns and corticospinal tracts occurs in vitamin B12 deficiency. Loss of GABAergic neurons in the caudate nucleus is seen in Huntington disease. Wallerian degeneration of the spinothalamic tract is not typical of any common disease.[47]

▸▸ Question 51

A 34-year-old woman presents with hearing loss and tinnitus on the right side. MRI reveals an enhancing mass in the internal auditory canal extending into the cerebellopontine angle. She is diagnosed with a vestibular schwannoma. Which genetic syndrome is most likely if she also has similar tumors on the left side?

- A. Neurofibromatosis type 1
- B. Neurofibromatosis type 2 (NF2)
- C. Tuberous sclerosis complex
- D. Von Hippel–Lindau disease
- E. Li–Fraumeni syndrome

Correct answer is B

NF2 is characterized by **bilateral vestibular schwannomas** leading to hearing loss, tinnitus, and balance issues. NF2 results from mutations in the *NF2* gene encoding merlin. Neurofibromatosis type 1 features neurofibromas, café-au-lait spots, and Lisch nodules but not bilateral vestibular schwannomas. Tuberous sclerosis involves cortical tubers and skin findings. Von Hippel–Lindau disease includes hemangioblastomas and renal cell carcinoma. Li–Fraumeni syndrome involves various cancers due to p53 mutations.[6]

▸▸ Question 52

A 25-year-old man presents with severe back pain and is found to have an osteoblastic lesion in the vertebral body of L1. Biopsy reveals small round blue cells that are CD99 positive and t(11;22)(q24;q12) translocation is detected. What is the most likely diagnosis?

- A. Osteosarcoma
- B. Ewing sarcoma
- C. Lymphoma
- D. Multiple myeloma
- E. Chordoma

Correct answer is B

Ewing sarcoma is a malignant bone tumor affecting young individuals. It is characterized by small round blue cells on histology, positivity for CD99 (MIC2), and a specific translocation t(11;22)(q24;q12) leading to the EWS–FLI1 fusion gene. Osteosarcoma produces osteoid matrix and occurs in metaphyses of long bones. Lymphoma involves lymphoid cells. Multiple myeloma shows plasma cell proliferation. Chordomas arise from notochordal remnants and typically occur in the sacrum or clivus.[38,39,40]

▸▸ Question 53

A 6-year-old boy presents with developmental delay and seizures. Physical examination reveals ash-leaf hypopigmented macules on the skin and periungual fibromas. MRI shows cortical tubers and subependymal nodules. Which of the following cardiac abnormalities is commonly associated with this condition?

- A. Ventricular septal defect
- B. Cardiac rhabdomyoma
- C. Atrial myxoma
- D. Patent ductus arteriosus
- E. Coarctation of the aorta

Correct answer is B

Tuberous sclerosis complex is associated with cortical tubers, subependymal giant cell astrocytomas, skin findings (ash-leaf spots, periungual fibromas), and **cardiac rhabdomyomas**. These benign cardiac tumors are often asymptomatic and may regress over time. Ventricular septal defects and patent ductus arteriosus are common congenital heart defects but not specifically associated with tuberous sclerosis. Atrial myxomas are seen in adults. Coarctation of the aorta is associated with Turner syndrome.[18]

▸▸ Question 54

A 7-year-old girl presents with headaches and is found to have a mass in the posterior fossa compressing the fourth ventricle. Histology shows biphasic patterns with areas of dense cellularity and loose myxoid regions. Which tumor is most consistent with these findings?

- A. Medulloblastoma
- B. Pilocytic astrocytoma
- C. Ependymoma
- D. Schwannoma
- E. Hemangioblastoma

Correct answer is D

While **schwannomas** are rare in the posterior fossa of children, the histological description of **Antoni A and Antoni B areas** is characteristic of schwannomas. In the cerebellopontine angle, they typically arise from cranial nerve VIII. Medulloblastomas are malignant small blue cell tumors. Pilocytic astrocytomas have Rosenthal fibers. Ependymomas have perivascular pseudorosettes. Hemangioblastomas are vascular tumors associated with Von Hippel–Lindau disease. ▸ Fig. 2.19 shows a **schwannoma**. (**a**) Encapsulated tumor with attached nerve ("N"). Cut surface is light tan, glistening, with interspersed yellow areas and prominent cystic areas. (**b**) Antoni A area: compact spindle cells with nuclear palisades forming Verocay bodies (H&E × 100). (**c**) Antoni B area: loosely arranged cobweb-like network of tumor cells (H&E × 40). (**d**) Diffuse strong S100 immunopositivity (S100 IHC, × 40). (**e**, **f**) *Cellular schwannoma*. (**e**) Cellular, compact cells, with no Verocay bodies or Antoni B areas (H&E × 40). (**f**) Increased mitoses (*encircled*), which may prompt consideration of a malignant peripheral nerve sheath tumor (H&E × 200), which can be distinguished by diffuse S100 positivity in cellular schwannoma (*inset*: S100 IHC × 40) as opposed to patchy in malignant peripheral nerve sheath tumor.

▸▸ Question 55

A 28-year-old man from Central America presents with seizures and headaches. MRI shows multiple cystic lesions with surrounding edema and some calcifications. The most likely causative agent is (▸ Fig. 2.20):

- A. *Taenia solium*
- B. *Toxoplasma gondii*
- C. *Echinococcus granulosus*
- D. *Schistosoma mansoni*
- E. *Naegleria fowleri*

Correct answer is A

The patient has **neurocysticercosis**, caused by the larval form of ***Taenia solium***, the pork tapeworm. Ingestion of eggs leads to cyst formation in the central nervous system. Imaging shows cystic lesions that may calcify. *Toxoplasma gondii* causes ring-enhancing lesions in immunocompromised patients. *Echinococcus* causes hydatid cysts, typically in the liver and lungs. *Schistosoma* affects the spinal cord. *Naegleria fowleri* causes primary amebic meningoencephalitis.[48]

▸▸ Question 56

A 60-year-old man with a history of seizures undergoes surgical resection of a low-grade astrocytoma. Histology shows cytological atypia without mitotic figures, necrosis, or vascular

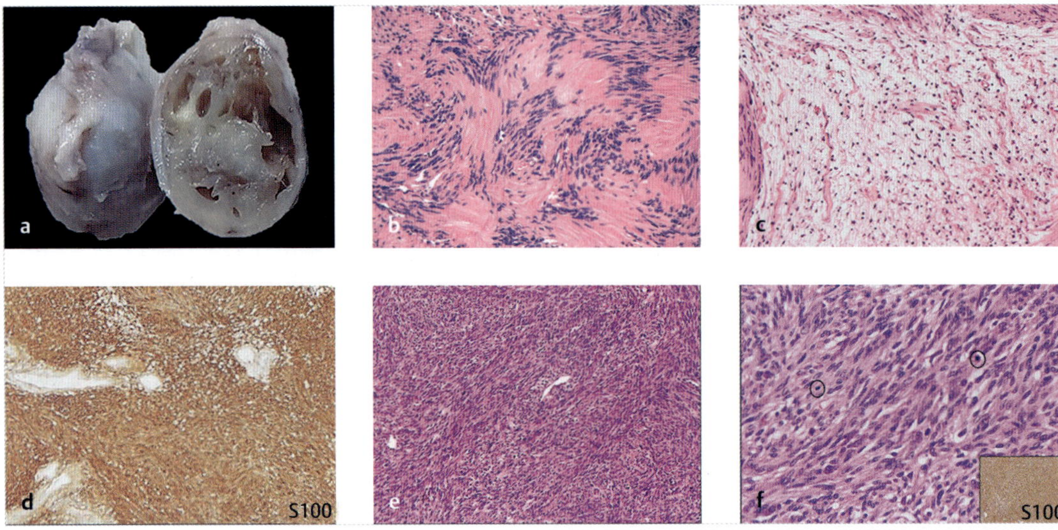

Fig. 2.19 (Source: Reproduced from Essential and desirable diagnostic criteria. In: Sarkar C, Santosh V, Chacko G, eds. Essentials of Diagnostic Surgical Neuropathology. 2nd ed. Noida: Thieme; 2022.)

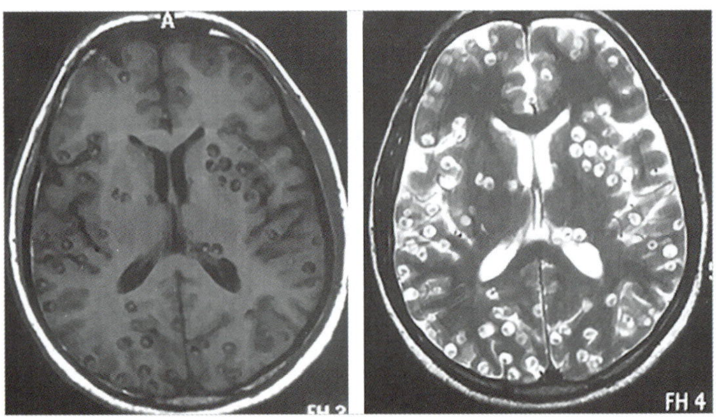

Fig. 2.20 (Source: Reproduced from Prajapati HP. Diffuse parenchymal neurocysticercosis: a case report and review of literature. Ind J Neurotrauma 2020;17(02):149–152)

proliferation. According to the WHO classification, what is the grade of this tumor?

- A. Grade I
- B. Grade II
- C. Grade III
- D. Grade IV
- E. Grade 0

Correct answer is B

A **WHO Grade II astrocytoma** shows cytological atypia but lacks mitotic activity, endothelial proliferation, or necrosis. Grade I tumors are typically pilocytic astrocytomas and are more circumscribed. Grade III (anaplastic astrocytoma) shows increased mitotic activity. Grade IV (glioblastoma) includes necrosis and/or microvascular proliferation. There is no Grade 0.

▸▸ Question 57

A 55-year-old man presents with back pain and bowel dysfunction. MRI shows a destructive sacral mass. Biopsy reveals cells with bubbly, vacuolated cytoplasm (physaliphorous cells) and immunohistochemistry positive for cytokeratin. From which embryonic structure does this tumor originate?

- A. Neural crest cells
- B. Notochord remnants
- C. Primitive neuroectoderm
- D. Mesenchymal stem cells
- E. Surface ectoderm

Correct answer is B

The tumor is a **chordoma**, which arises from **notochord remnants**. Chordomas commonly occur in the sacrum and clivus. Histology shows physaliphorous cells with vacuolated cytoplasm. They express cytokeratin and brachyury. Neural crest cells give rise to peripheral nervous system structures. Primitive neuroectoderm forms central nervous system neurons. Mesenchymal stem cells give rise to sarcomas. Surface ectoderm forms skin and related structures.[19,20]

▸▸ Question 58

A 45-year-old woman with poorly controlled diabetes mellitus presents with facial pain, orbital swelling, and black eschar on the nasal turbinates. MRI reveals sinusitis with extension into the orbit and brain. Biopsy shows broad, nonseptate hyphae branching at right angles. What is the most likely causative organism?
- A. *Aspergillus fumigatus*
- B. *Mucor* species
- C. *Candida albicans*
- D. *Cryptococcus neoformans*
- E. *Histoplasma capsulatum*

Correct answer is B
The patient has **rhinocerebral mucormycosis**, a serious fungal infection caused by ***Mucor* species**, which are opportunistic fungi affecting immunocompromised individuals, especially diabetics with ketoacidosis. Histology shows broad, nonseptate hyphae with right-angle branching. *Aspergillus* has septate hyphae with acute-angle branching. *Candida* is a yeast-forming pseudohyphae. *Cryptococcus* is a yeast with a thick capsule. Histoplasma is a dimorphic fungus that causes pulmonary infections.[34,35]

▸▸ Question 59

A 45-year-old woman presents with neck pain and difficulty swallowing. Imaging reveals a foramen magnum meningioma compressing the medulla. During a far lateral approach to resect the lesion, which intradural structure can be safely divided to widen the surgical corridor?
- A. Anterior spinal artery
- B. Posterior inferior cerebellar artery
- C. Dentate ligament
- D. Accessory nerve
- E. Hypoglossal nerve

Correct answer is C
In a **far lateral approach** to the foramen magnum, division of the **dentate ligament** allows mobilization of the spinal cord and provides better access to anterior and lateral lesions. The dentate ligament is a pial extension anchoring the spinal cord laterally. Dividing it does not cause neurological deficits. The anterior spinal artery and posterior inferior cerebellar artery are vital structures and should be preserved. The accessory and hypoglossal nerves should also be preserved to maintain function.[3,4,5]

▸▸ Question 60

A 55-year-old man with a nonfunctioning pituitary macroadenoma undergoes stereotactic radiosurgery. Six months later, he develops fatigue, weight gain, and cold intolerance. Laboratory tests reveal low cortisol and thyroid hormone levels. What is the most common complication after pituitary adenoma radiosurgery?
- A. Visual field defects
- B. Cranial nerve palsies
- C. Anterior pituitary insufficiency
- D. Radiation-induced neoplasm
- E. Cerebral edema

Correct answer is C
The most common complication after **pituitary adenoma radiosurgery** is **anterior pituitary insufficiency**, resulting from radiation damage to normal pituitary tissue. Hormone deficiencies can include cortisol, thyroid hormone, and gonadotropins. Visual complications are less common if radiation doses to the optic apparatus are kept below safe thresholds. Cranial nerve palsies and radiation-induced neoplasms are rare. Cerebral edema can occur but is less common.[22,23]

▸▸ Question 61

A 6-year-old boy with neurofibromatosis type 1 (NF1) presents with decreased visual acuity and proptosis of the right eye. MRI reveals an optic pathway glioma involving the optic nerve and chiasm. Which tumor is most commonly associated with NF1 in children?
- A. Meningioma
- B. Optic pathway glioma
- C. Acoustic neuroma
- D. Pilocytic astrocytoma
- E. Ependymoma

Correct answer is B
In children with **NF1**, the most common tumor is an **optic pathway glioma**, which is typically a

low-grade pilocytic astrocytoma. These tumors can affect the optic nerves, chiasm, and tracts, leading to visual deficits. Meningiomas and acoustic neuromas are more associated with NF2. Pilocytic astrocytomas can occur sporadically but are not specifically associated with NF1 in this context. Ependymomas are less common in NF1.[37]

▸▸ **Question 62**

A 35-year-old man presents with low back pain and leg weakness. MRI reveals a well-circumscribed intradural extramedullary mass at the conus medullaris. Surgical resection confirms a myxopapillary ependymoma. What is the most appropriate management for this tumor?

- A. Observation with serial imaging
- B. Radiation therapy alone
- C. Laminectomy and tumor resection
- D. Chemotherapy
- E. Stereotactic radiosurgery

Correct answer is C

Myxopapillary ependymomas are WHO Grade I tumors commonly located in the conus medullaris and filum terminale. The treatment of choice is **surgical resection via laminectomy**. Gross total resection offers the best prognosis. Radiation therapy may be considered for residual or recurrent tumors but is not the first-line treatment. Chemotherapy and stereotactic radiosurgery have limited roles. Observation is not appropriate due to the potential for neurological deterioration.[38,39,40]

▸▸ **Question 63**

A 50-year-old man presents with a seizure and is found to have a calcified frontal lobe mass. Biopsy reveals cells with round nuclei, clear cytoplasm, and a delicate capillary network. Genetic analysis shows loss of heterozygosity of chromosomes 1p and 19q. What is the most likely diagnosis?

- A. Astrocytoma
- B. Oligodendroglioma
- C. Ependymoma
- D. Meningioma
- E. Metastatic carcinoma

Correct answer is B

The patient's tumor is an **oligodendroglioma**, characterized histologically by "fried-egg" appearing cells (round nuclei with clear cytoplasm) and a "chicken-wire" capillary pattern. The **loss of heterozygosity of 1p/19q** is a genetic hallmark of oligodendrogliomas and is associated with better prognosis and responsiveness to therapy. Astrocytomas lack these features. Ependymomas typically arise in ventricular locations. Meningiomas are extra-axial tumors. Metastatic carcinomas have different histologies.[10]

▸▸ **Question 64**

During intraoperative monitoring of brainstem auditory evoked responses (BAERs), which parameter is the most sensitive indicator of compromise to the auditory pathway?

- A. Decrease in amplitude of wave I
- B. Increase in latency of wave V
- C. Increase in interpeak latency of waves I–III
- D. Increase in interpeak latency of waves I–V
- E. Absence of wave II

Correct answer is D

The **interpeak latency of waves I–V** in BAER monitoring represents the conduction time from the auditory nerve through the brainstem auditory pathway to the midbrain. An **increase in the I–V interpeak latency** is the most sensitive parameter indicating compromise of the auditory pathway during surgery. Wave I reflects the distal auditory nerve, while wave V is generated near the inferior colliculus. Changes in the I–III interpeak latency are less sensitive. A decrease in amplitude is less specific.[49,50]

▸▸ **Question 65**

An MRI spectroscopy of a cerebral mass shows a reduced N-acetylaspartate (NAA) peak and an increased choline peak relative to creatine. Which type of tumor is most consistent with these findings?

- A. Meningioma
- B. Low-grade glioma
- C. High-grade glioma
- D. Metastatic carcinoma
- E. Abscess

Correct answer is C

In **MR spectroscopy**, a **reduced NAA peak**, indicates neuronal loss or dysfunction, while an **increased choline peak** reflects increased cellular membrane turnover and proliferation, as seen in high-grade tumors such as **glioblastomas**. The choline-to-creatine ratio is elevated. Low-grade gliomas may show less pronounced changes. Meningiomas and metastatic carcinomas have different spectroscopic profiles. An abscess may show elevated lactate and lipid peaks. ▶ Fig. 2.21 shows (**a**) axial brain magnetic resonance imaging, T1-weighted image with gadolinium showing a ring-enhancing lesion involving the right thalamus. (**b**) Magnetic resonance spectroscopy spectrum showing prominent Cho peak, decreased NAA peak, very high Cho:NAA ratio, and also high Cho: Cr ratio. All these findings favor a preoperative diagnosis of a high-grade glioma. (**c**) Axial contrast-enhanced stereotactic brain computed tomography scan showing the target site for stereotactic biopsy. Histopathologic examination of the tissues obtained via stereotactic biopsy confirmed the diagnosis of glioblastoma multiforme (World Health Organization Grade IV). Cho, choline; Cr, creatine; NAA, N-acetylaspartate.[51,52]

▸▸ Question 66

A neurosurgeon plans a transcondylar approach to resect a foramen magnum meningioma. How much of the occipital condyle can be safely resected without causing craniovertebral instability?

- A. Up to 25%
- B. Up to 33%
- C. Up to 50%
- D. Up to 75%
- E. Complete resection is safe

Correct answer is C

Resection of up to **50% of the occipital condyle** is generally considered safe and does not typically result in **craniovertebral instability**. Resection beyond 50% increases the risk of instability and may necessitate occipitocervical fusion. Careful preoperative planning and intraoperative assessment are essential to balance surgical exposure with structural preservation.[3,4,5]

▸▸ Question 67

A 40-year-old woman presents with signs of Cushing syndrome. Which diagnostic test is the most specific for confirming endogenous hypercortisolism?

- A. Random serum cortisol measurement
- B. Midnight salivary cortisol
- C. Low-dose dexamethasone suppression test
- D. 24-hour urinary free cortisol
- E. Adrenocorticotropic hormone (ACTH) stimulation test

Correct answer is D

The **24-hour urinary free cortisol** measurement is the most specific test for diagnosing **Cushing syndrome** as it reflects the integrated cortisol secretion over an entire day, eliminating the variability seen with diurnal rhythm and stress. Random serum cortisol levels and salivary cortisol can be affected by stress and time of day. The low-dose dexamethasone suppression test is a screening tool but can have false positives. The ACTH stimulation test assesses adrenal insufficiency.[53,54]

▸▸ Question 68

A 28-year-old woman presents with progressive diplopia. On examination, she has a right hypertropia that increases when tilting her head to the right, and she tilts her head to the left to compensate. Which cranial nerve palsy is most consistent with this presentation?

- A. Right oculomotor nerve (CN III) palsy
- B. Right trochlear nerve (CN IV) palsy
- C. Right abducens nerve (CN VI) palsy
- D. Left trochlear nerve (CN IV) palsy
- E. Left abducens nerve (CN VI) palsy

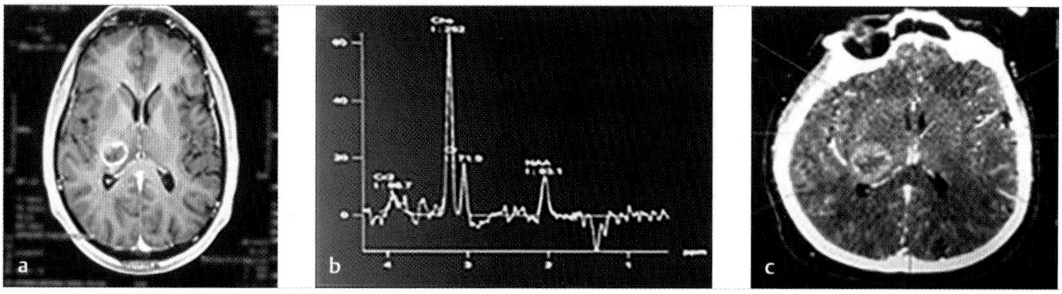

Fig. 2.21 (Source: Reproduced from Abdelaziz O, Eshra M, Belal A, et al. Diagnostic value of magnetic resonance spectroscopy compared with stereotactic biopsy of intra-axial brain lesions. J Neurol Surg A Cent Eur Neurosurg 2016;77(04):283–290.)

Correct answer is B

A **trochlear nerve (CN IV) palsy** causes vertical diplopia, with the affected eye deviating upward (hypertropia). The **Bielschowsky head tilt test** is positive when tilting the head toward the side of the lesion worsens the diplopia. Patients often tilt their head away from the lesion to minimize symptoms. In this case, the right CN IV is affected (▶ Fig. 2.22).[44,45]

▸▸ Question 69

A 45-year-old man presents with severe retro-orbital pain and ophthalmoplegia affecting cranial nerves III, IV, and VI on the right side. MRI reveals inflammation in the right cavernous sinus without evidence of infection or mass lesion. Which of the following is the most likely diagnosis?

- A. Tolosa–Hunt syndrome
- B. Cavernous sinus thrombosis
- C. Carotid-cavernous fistula
- D. Orbital apex syndrome
- E. Giant cell arteritis

Correct answer is A

Tolosa–Hunt syndrome is characterized by **painful ophthalmoplegia** due to idiopathic granulomatous inflammation of the cavernous sinus or superior orbital fissure. It presents with acute orbital pain and multiple cranial nerve palsies (III, IV, VI, and sometimes V1). Corticosteroid therapy typically results in rapid symptom improvement. Cavernous sinus thrombosis is usually septic and presents with signs of infection. Carotid-cavernous fistula presents with pulsatile exophthalmos and bruit (▶ Fig. 2.23).[55,56]

▸▸ Question 70

A 60-year-old man with chronic alcoholism presents with confusion, ataxia, and ophthalmoplegia. He is diagnosed with Wernicke encephalopathy. Which of the following is the most consistent pathologic finding in this condition?

- A. Hemorrhagic lesions in the mammillary bodies
- B. Demyelination of the posterior columns

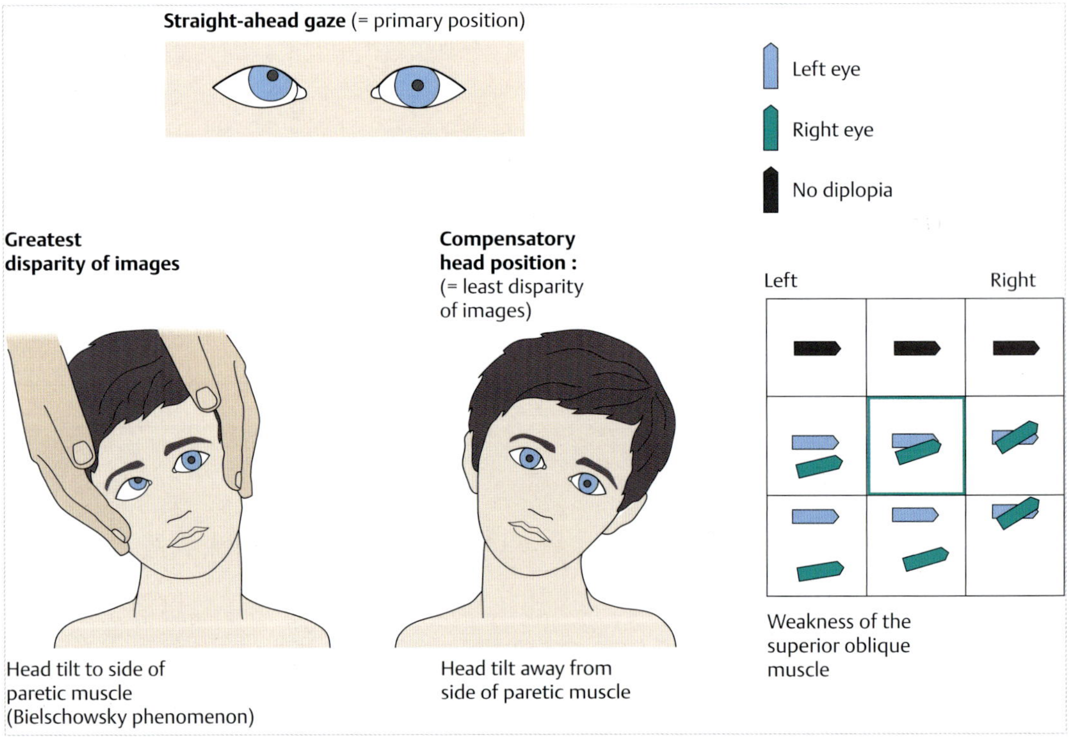

Fig. 2.22 (Source: Reproduced from Mattle H, Mumenthaler M, Taub E, eds. Fundamentals of Neurology: An Illustrated Guide. 2nd ed. Stuttgart: Georg Thieme Verlag KG; 2016)

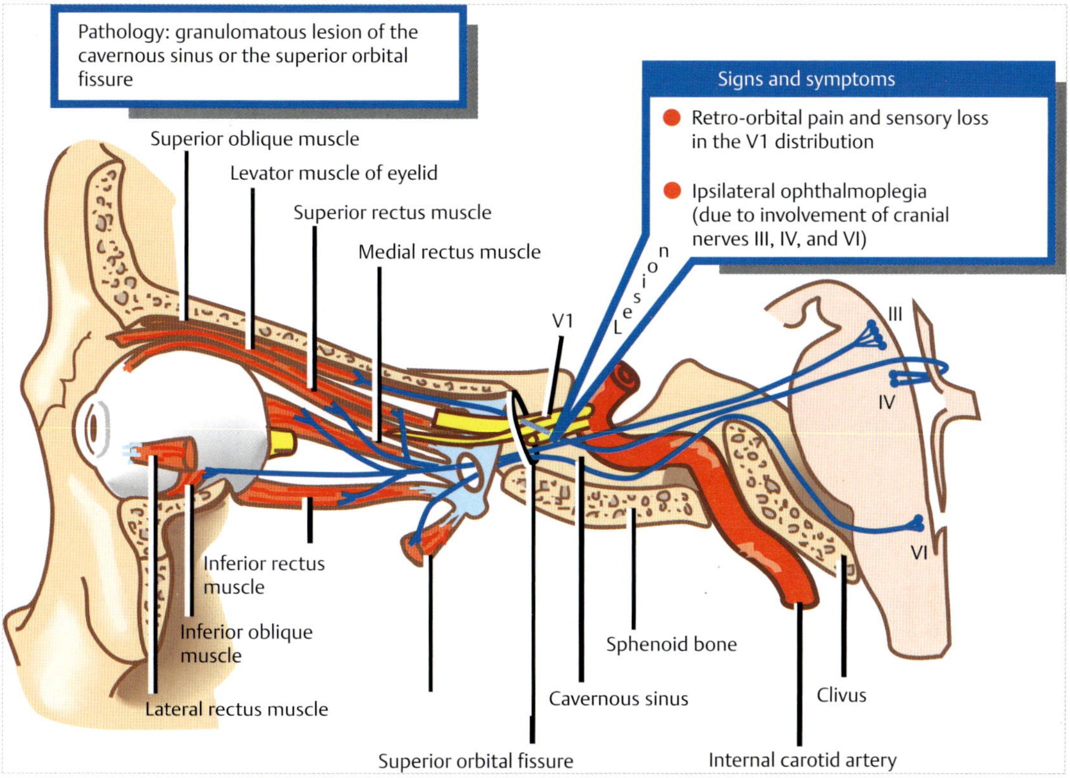

Fig. 2.23 (Source: Reproduced from Alberstone C, Benzel E, Jones S, Wang Z, Steinmetz M, eds. Anatomic Basis of Neurologic Diagnosis. 2nd ed. New York: Thieme Medical Publishers, Inc.; 2023.)

- C. Neuronal loss in the substantia nigra
- D. Cortical amyloid plaques
- E. Demyelination of the optic nerves

Correct answer is A

Wernicke encephalopathy is caused by **thiamine (vitamin B1) deficiency**, leading to damage in regions of the brain with high metabolic demand. Pathologically, it is characterized by **hemorrhagic lesions and neuronal loss in the mammillary bodies**, thalamus, periaqueductal gray matter, and cerebellar vermis. Demyelination of the posterior columns is seen in subacute combined degeneration due to B12 deficiency. Neuronal loss in the substantia nigra is seen in Parkinson disease. Cortical amyloid plaques are characteristic of Alzheimer disease.[57]

▸▸ Question 71

A 45-year-old woman is evaluated for progressive weight gain, central obesity, moon facies, and insulin-resistant type 2 diabetes mellitus. She is neurologically intact. An MR image of the brain is normal. Chest imaging reveals a small lung mass. Which of the following tests is most appropriate to distinguish between an adrenocorticotropic hormone (ACTH)-secreting pituitary adenoma and ectopic ACTH production?

- A. Low-dose dexamethasone suppression test
- B. High-dose dexamethasone suppression test
- C. Inferior petrosal sinus sampling
- D. Random ACTH measurement
- E. Corticotropin-releasing hormone (CRH) stimulation test

Correct answer is C

When imaging does not reveal a pituitary source in a patient with **ACTH-dependent Cushing syndrome**, **inferior petrosal sinus sampling** is the gold standard to differentiate between a pituitary adenoma (Cushing disease) and ectopic ACTH production. A central-to-peripheral ACTH gradient indicates a pituitary source, while a lack of gradient suggests ectopic production. High-dose dexamethasone suppression tests can be helpful but are less definitive. Random ACTH levels may not provide sufficient diagnostic information.[22,23,54,53]

▸▸ Question 72

A 65-year-old man with a known pituitary macroadenoma presents with worsening peripheral vision, fatigue, weight gain, and decreased libido. Laboratory studies reveal low cortisol and low free thyroxine levels. Which of the following hormone replacement strategies should be initiated prior to surgery?

- A. Start thyroid hormone replacement only
- B. Start cortisol replacement only
- C. Start cortisol replacement before thyroid hormone
- D. Start both cortisol and thyroid hormone simultaneously
- E. Defer hormone replacement until after surgery

Correct answer is C

In patients with **secondary adrenal insufficiency and hypothyroidism** due to pituitary insufficiency, it is critical to **replace cortisol before starting thyroid hormone**. Thyroid hormone replacement increases metabolic demand and can precipitate an **adrenal crisis** if cortisol levels are not sufficient. Therefore, cortisol replacement is initiated first, followed by thyroid hormone replacement once cortisol levels are adequate.[22,23]

▸▸ Question 73

A 38-year-old male patient with HIV presents with progressive neurological symptoms. Imaging reveals multiple ring-enhancing lesions. Before initiating corticosteroid therapy, the neurosurgeon plans a biopsy. Which of the following is a primary reason to perform the biopsy prior to steroid administration?

- A. Steroids may worsen the infection
- B. Steroids can reduce imaging contrast enhancement
- C. Steroids may interfere with histopathological diagnosis
- D. Steroids increase bleeding risk during biopsy
- E. Steroids have no effect on central nervous system (CNS) lymphomas

Correct answer is C

Corticosteroids can cause a rapid reduction in the size of CNS lymphomas, potentially leading to nondiagnostic biopsy results. Therefore, it is crucial to obtain a tissue diagnosis before administering steroids to ensure accurate identification and appropriate treatment planning.[33]

References

[1] Nakasu S, Deguchi S, Nakasu Y. IDH wild-type lower-grade gliomas with glioblastoma molecular features: a systematic review and meta-analysis. Brain Tumor Pathol 2023;40 (3):143–157

[2] Kanderi T, Munakomi S, Gupta V. Glioblastoma multiforme. In: StatPearls. Treasure Island, FL: StatPearls Publishing; 2025

[3] Lee S, Karas PJ, Hadley CC, et al. The role of Merlin/NF2 loss in meningioma biology. Cancers (Basel) 2019;11(11):1633

[4] Campero A, Baldoncini M, Villalonga JF, Paíz M, Lucifero AG, Luzzi S. Transcondylar fossa approach for resection of anterolateral foramen magnum meningioma. World Neurosurg 2021;154:91–92

[5] Narayan V, Jumah F, Nanda A. Resection of foramen magnum meningioma through modified far lateral approach. J Neurol Surg B Skull Base 2020;82(Suppl 1):S22–S24

[6] Halliday D, et al. An introduction to the internal auditory canal and the vestibular schwannoma. Otolaryngol Clin North Am 2023;56(3):431–442

[7] Collins VP, Jones TW, Giannini C. Pilocytic astrocytoma: pathology, molecular mechanisms and markers. Acta Neuropathol 2015;129(6):775–788

[8] Pajtler KW, Witt H, Sill M, et al. Molecular Classification of Ependymal Tumors across All CNS Compartments, Histopathological Grades, and Age Groups. Cancer Cell 2015;27 (5):728–743

[9] Wang C, Nguyen NA, Reier L, et al. Extensive thoracolumbosacral myxopapillary ependymoma presenting with syncope. Cureus 2025;17(3):e95457

[10] Louis DN, Perry A, Wesseling P, et al. The 2021 WHO Classification of Tumors of the Central Nervous System: a summary. Neuro Oncol 2021;23(8):1231–1251

[11] Wong KK, Tsai ML, Chang H, et al. CNS germ cell tumors: comprehensive review. Pediatric Brain and Spinal Cord Tumors 2023;2:421–455

[12] Alosaimi HS, Hafiz BE, Tawfiq IA, et al. Extensive CPA epidermoid presenting solely as unilateral hearing loss. Cureus 2025;17(5):e84721

[13] Ramesh R, Quintana D, Osorio R, et al. Long-term outcomes of intracranial epidermoid cysts. Neurosurgery 2024;97 (2):351–360

[14] Cortese I, Reich DS, Nath A. Progressive multifocal leukoencephalopathy and the spectrum of JC virus-related disease. Nat Rev Neurol 2021;17(1):37–51

[15] Blümcke I, Thom M, Aronica E, et al. The clinicopathologic spectrum of focal cortical dysplasias: a consensus classification. Epilepsia 2011;52(1):158–174

[16] Mitrica OM, Manole AM, Toma M, et al. Comprehensive review of hypothalamic hamartomas. Biomedicines 2025;13 (2):371

[17] Zerr I, Parchi P. Sporadic Creutzfeldt–Jakob disease. Handb Clin Neurol 2018;153:155–174
[18] Northrup H, Aronow Mary E, Bebin EM, et al. Tuberous sclerosis complex diagnostic criteria update. Pediatr Neurol 2021;123:50–66
[19] Shor D, Louie AV, Zeng KL, et al. Molecular markers predicting local control in lung cancer spine metastases treated with SBRT. J Neurooncol 2024;167(2):275–283
[20] Stacchiotti S, Sommer J. Building a global consensus approach to chordoma. Lancet Oncol 2015;16(2):e71–e83
[21] Safaee M, et al. Choroid plexus tumors: a review of the literature. World Neurosurg 2013;80(5):e203–e212
[22] Bourhila C, Cotrutz C, Conti A, et al. Cyberknife radiosurgery for secreting pituitary adenomas: meta-analysis. J Clin Neurosci 2025;133:111043
[23] Estephan K, Charbonneau L, Chennou F, et al. The surgical management of Cushing disease: a case series from a Canadian tertiary center. Neurol Res 2025:1–13
[24] Elshazly K, AbdelFatah MAR, Youssef ME, et al. Extended endoscopic transtuberculum approach for pediatric craniopharyngiomas. Neurosurg Rev 2025;48:923
[25] Cases-Cunillera S, Müller P, Waardenberg AJV, et al. Single-nucleus RNA sequencing of BRAF-negative gangliogliomas. Brain Commun 2025;7(5):fcaf372
[26] Ku Y, Esfahanizadeh A. Epilepsy management in pediatric brain tumors. Semin Pediatr Neurol 2025;53:101187
[27] Lonser RR, Glenn GM, Walther M, et al. von Hippel-Lindau disease. Lancet 2003;361(9374):2059–2067
[28] Yasar S, et al. In-vivo/ex-vivo MRI correlation of cerebral microbleeds and CAA. Alzheimers Dement 2025;21(S8): e109912
[29] Wang H, Yiqiang Z, Cai J, et al. Immune-mediated blood-brain barrier disruption after ischemic stroke. Front Immunol 2025;16:1716041
[30] Northcott PA, Robinson GW, Kratz CP, et al. Medulloblastoma. Nat Rev Dis Primers 2019;5(1):11
[31] Louis DN, Perry A, Reifenberger G, von Deimling A, Figarella-Branger D, Cavenee WK, Ohgaki H, Wiestler OD, Kleihues P, Ellison DW. The 2016 World Health Organization Classification of Tumors of the Central Nervous System: a summary. Acta Neuropathol 2016; 131(6):803–820
[32] Coluccia D, Figuereido C, Isik S, Smith C, Rutka JT. Medulloblastoma: tumor biology and relevance to treatment and prognosis paradigm. Curr Neurol Neurosci Rep 2016; 16 (5):43
[33] Grommes C, DeAngelis LM. Primary CNS Lymphoma. J Clin Oncol 2017;35(21):2410–2418
[34] Samantaray S, Kumar D, Meena DS, et al. Invasive cerebral aspergillosis: CSF galactomannan diagnostic utility. J Mycol Med 2023;33(3):101380
[35] Nurtdinova GM, Suleymanov AM, Bayazitov II, et al. COVID-19-associated mucormycosis with diabetic ketoacidosis. Ter Arkh 2022;94(11):1320–1325
[36] Relkin N, Marmarou A, Klinge P, et al. Diagnosing idiopathic normal-pressure hydrocephalus. Neurosurgery 2005; 57(3 Suppl):S4–16
[37] Gutmann DH, Ferner RE, Listernick RH, et al. Neurofibromatosis type 1. Nat Rev Dis Primers 2017;3:17004
[38] Yang Y, Liu JR, Han YS, et al. TAM density/spatial distribution predicting GCTB prognosis and denosumab response. MedComm 2025
[39] Birch W, et al. Denosumab inducing woven bone formation in spinal GCTB. JBMR Plus 2025
[40] Fan H, et al. Primary Ewing's sarcoma with EWSR1-FLI1 fusion. Gynecol Oncol Rep 2025;57:101949
[41] Gilhus NE, et al. Myasthenia gravis. Nat Rev Dis Primers 2019;5(1):30. DOI
[42] Scheltens P, et al. Alzheimer's disease. Lancet 2021;397 (10284):1577–1590
[43] Canut P, et al. Lateral medullary syndrome presenting with dizziness to dysphagia. Cureus 2024;16(11):e73118
[44] Jayakumar D, et al. Internuclear ophthalmoplegia in Artery of Percheron infarct. Cureus 2024;16(8):e67485
[45] Yamadera M, et al. Head tilt test differentiating sagging eye syndrome from trochlear palsy. Graefes Arch Clin Exp Ophthalmol 2023
[46] Shirley MD, et al. Sturge-Weber syndrome and port-wine stains caused by somatic mutation in GNAQ. N Engl J Med 2013;368(21):1971–1979
[47] Brown RH, Al-Chalabi A. Amyotrophic Lateral Sclerosis. N Engl J Med 2017;377(2):162–172
[48] Garcia HH, et al. Neurocysticercosis: updated concepts about an old disease. Lancet Neurol 2014;13(12):1202–1215
[49] Kato T, et al. Reassessing the role of subarcuate artery in hearing preservation during microvascular decompression. Neurol Med Chir (Tokyo) 2025;65(12):560–567
[50] Stark KG, et al. BAEPs to guide minimally invasive decompression in Chiari 1.5. Neurodiagn J 2025;65(3):242–250
[51] Moreno-Acosta P, et al. MRS/MRSI in post-treatment glioma follow-up. Cancer Diagn Progn 2025
[52] Kishimoto A, et al. Band-selective IR PRESS for lactate detection in brain tumors. bioRxiv 2024
[53] Liu Y, et al. Morning spot urinary cortisol-to-creatinine ratio: a novel screening tool. Front Endocrinol (Lausanne) 2025;16:1663619
[54] Páez-Granda D, et al. Ultrasound-guided jugular vein access for inferior petrosal sinus sampling. Cureus 2025;17(11): e96167
[55] Reznikova OI, et al. Tolosa-Hunt syndrome: comprehensive review. Vestn Oftalmol 2025;141(6):114
[56] Rathod P, et al. Tolosa-Hunt syndrome with complete resolution on glucocorticoids. J Assoc Physicians India 2025;73:1127
[57] Sechi G, Serra A. Wernicke's encephalopathy: new clinical settings and recent advances in diagnosis. Lancet Neurol 2007;6(5):442–455

3 Spine

Zachary A. Pennington, Syed I. Khalid, Aladine Elsamadicy, John H. Shin

▸▸ Question 1

A 24-year-old man presents following a high-velocity motorcycle collision as a helmeted driver. Disoriented on examination with 4/5 bilateral upper extremity weakness and severe proximal right leg weakness. He denies neck pain but endorses significant right hip pain. What is the first step in the management of this patient?

- A. Application of a cervical collar or in-line stabilization followed by high-resolution CT imaging
- B. High-resolution CT imaging
- C. Proceed immediately to the operating room for surgical decompression and fusion
- D. Application of a cervical collar and admission to the floor for observation
- E. Toxicology screening

Correct answer is A

This patient has sustained a high-energy injury with concerning neurological findings suggestive of spinal cord injury. Despite denying neck pain, the presence of a significant distracting injury (e.g., potential hip or femur fracture) and possible intoxication makes an accurate neurological assessment unreliable.

The correct first step is to stabilize the cervical spine with a collar or in-line stabilization before obtaining high-resolution CT imaging to assess for bony injury. Failure to immobilize the spine before imaging risks further neurological damage. Thoracolumbar precautions should also be maintained until imaging rules out injury at other spinal levels. Toxicology screening is part of the overall trauma evaluation but does not alter the immediate need for spinal stabilization and imaging.[1]

▸▸ Question 2

An intoxicated young male presents following a high-speed motor vehicle collision with mild proximal upper extremity weakness and a concurrent femur fracture limiting evaluation of his lower extremities. He denies neck pain. Which of the following options represents the best, evidence-based approach for evaluation of this patient?

- A. High-resolution CT of the cervical spine
- B. High-resolution CT of the entire mobile spine
- C. MR and high-resolution CT of the cervical spine
- D. Upright cervical spine radiographs with flexion/extension, anteroposterior, lateral, and odontoid views
- E. Clinical examination alone is sufficient

Correct answer is B

Based on the 2013 cervical spine trauma guidelines put together by the joint CNS/AANS working group, high-resolution CT is the imaging modality of choice for assessing spinal injuries in patients who have sustained recent trauma. In the present patient, who was involved in a motorcycle accident at 100 mph, the high-energy nature of the injury mechanism raises the possibility that he has sustained injuries to other levels of the spine. Consequently, complete evaluation of the patient should include CT of the thoracolumbar spine as well. MR is not indicated at present in this patient, as it significantly prolongs the preoperative evaluation in the event that a bony injury is discovered. Should pan-neuraxis CT fail to demonstrate an injury capable of explaining the neuro deficits seen on the patient's examination, then MR should be pursued. The CNS/AANS joint thoracolumbar trauma guidelines additionally suggest that for thoracolumbar spine trauma, MR may be indicated as it may influence management in up to 25% of cases. Nevertheless, CT to evaluate for bony injury is the best first step. This patient has a significant distracting injury (femur fracture) and is intoxicated; so, clinical examination alone is insufficient to evaluate for potential cervical spine injuries.[2]

▸▸ Question 3

Following a high-speed motorcycle accident, a patient undergoes high-resolution CT, which shows the following injury (▸ Fig. 3.1). Which of the following options is the best approach to the management of the patient's injury?

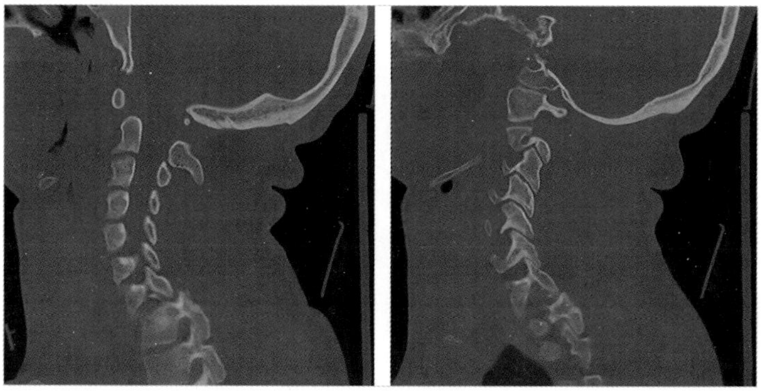

Fig. 3.1

- A. Cervical collar immobilization with an interval observation period and reimaging at 2 weeks
- B. Awake traction-reduction followed by external cervical immobilization if the facets reduce on imaging
- C. Posterior C5–T3 decompression and fusion
- D. Awake traction-reduction followed by C7/T1 anterior cervical diskectomy and fusion
- E. C7/T1 disk arthroplasty

Correct answer is D

The imaging above shows bilateral C7/T1 jumped facets. This results from a flexion-distraction injury, which leads to tearing of the capsular ligaments and translation of the cephalad vertebrae over the caudad vertebrae. Because the spine is misaligned and there is likely compression of the cervical nerve roots and potentially also spinal cord injury (MR was ultimately obtained by the treating physician and showed imaging findings consistent with central cord syndrome), spinal realignment is required. Initial management with closed reduction is reasonable and is practiced at many centers. The patient is positioned supine with Gardner-Wells tongs and shoulder pads to allow tension to be placed on the spinal column. Patients are imaged before the application of weight and then after every interval addition (generally a starting weight of 10–15 pounds is used with a maximum weight of 5–10 pounds per level). The patient's neurological examination is performed after every addition of weight and endpoints of traction are (1) the patient can no longer tolerate the examination due to pain, (2) the patient demonstrates a new neurological deficit, (3) the subluxation is successfully reduced, or (4) the maximum weight is reached without reduction of the subluxation. Prior to performing closed reduction, it is important to rule out occipitocervical injury, as the application of traction in such patients can lead to catastrophic injury or death due to occipitocervical dislocation (the so-called internal decapitation). Calvarial convexity fractures are also a contraindication to traction, as application of pressure from the Gardner-Wells tongs could worsen the fracture or cause concomitant intracranial injury. A final relative contraindication is the patient's inability to comply with repeat neurological examinations (e.g., due to intoxication), as neurological changes are an endpoint for closed reduction.

After performing reduction, surgical stabilization is merited as the present injury is due to injury of the capsular ligaments. Such capsular injury will not heal, and the patient will be left with a biomechanically unstable spine. In cases where successful reduction of the facet dislocation is achieved, an anterior or posterior approach can be pursued; the anterior approach is often considered acceptable as only a single motion segment requires fusion, and so the overall reduction in neck range of motion is less with an anterior approach. The anterior approach also has faster postoperative recovery, lower postoperative pain, and can remove any potentially retropulsed disk. In the case that traction fails to reduce the subluxation, an anterior approach can still be considered. In this approach, the Caspar pins are placed with a 10- to 20-degree convergent angle and brought together prior to distraction, creating a focal kyphosis that allows the inferior facet of the cephalad level to slip over the superior facet of the caudal level, reducing the fracture. An interbody spreader may also be placed in the disk space to

Table 3.1 Subaxial injury classification and severity scale

Characteristics	Points
Injury morphology	
No abnormality	0
Compression	1
Burst	2
Distraction	3
Translation	4
Integrity of the discoligamentous complex	
Intact	0
Indeterminate	1
Disrupted	2
Neurological status	
Intact	0
Nerve root injury	1
Complete	2
Incomplete	3
Persistent cord compression	+ 1
Total points	**Management**
1–3	Nonsurgical
4	Surgical or nonsurgical
5–10	Surgical

help maintain the distraction during reduction of the subluxation. A posterior approach can also be considered; however, in this case, the superior facet of the caudal level must often be drilled to reduce the subluxation, though the use of a curette to wedge the superior jumped facet over its caudal partner has also been described.

Finally, a helpful algorithm employed in cervical trauma for determining the need for surgical intervention is the subaxial injury classification and severity scale (SLICS), developed by Vaccaro and colleagues, which considers injury morphology, discoligamentous complex integrity, and neurological status to determine operative candidacy. In the present case, the patient had a translation injury (4), with a disrupted discoligamentous complex (2), and at minimum a bilateral nerve root injury (1), giving him a SLICS score of 7, which suggests operative intervention is merited (▶ **Table 3.1**).[3,4,5,6]

▸▸ Question 4

A 19-year-old male with past medical history significant for cigarette use presents with 18 months of progressive lower-back pain and intermittent bilateral leg pain worsened with upright posture and the lifting of heavy objects. Patient is intact on sensorimotor examination. Which of the following is the best next step in evaluating this patient?

- A. Plain radiographs of the lumbar spine
- B. Lumbar spine MRI
- C. Continued observation with conservative management (e.g., physical therapy)
- D. Interlaminar epidural steroid injection
- E. Lumbar spine CT

Correct answer is A

The patient presents with an 18-month history of progressive, primarily mechanical lower-back pain with only intermittent leg pain. While most cases of lower-back pain, especially in younger adults, are myofascial pain syndrome and are unlikely to demonstrate significant radiographic findings, this patient has been dealing with his symptoms for 18 months and so at minimal plain, radiograph is reasonable to evaluate for an underlying biomechanical explanation for his pain. As his main complaint is mechanical back pain, radiographs are more appropriate than MRI, which is better when evaluating for evidence of thecal sac or nerve root compression, which would present with radicular pain. Interlaminar epidural steroid injection can have some diagnostic utility in select patients, but its main role is as a nonoperative treatment for neurogenic claudication or lumbar radiculopathy by addressing nerve root inflammation. It is not an effective treatment for low-back pain. CT may be merited for evaluation of the bony spine in a patient undergoing surgical management but should not be performed before plain radiographs.

▸▸ Question 5

A young male with progressive mechanical back pain presents with the upright lumbar spine X-rays that show the following. Which of the following best describes the abnormality seen on the radiographs (▸ Fig. 3.2)?

- A. Congenital spondylolisthesis at L4/L5
- B. Degenerative spondylolisthesis at L5/S1
- C. Isthmic spondylolisthesis at L5/S1
- D. Acquired spondylolisthesis at L5/S1
- E. Pathologic spondylolisthesis at L4/L5

Correct answer is C

The imaging demonstrates an L5/S1 isthmic spondylolisthesis with a high sacral slope. Examination of the radiographs shows bilateral fractures between the superior and inferior articulating processes of the L5 vertebrae (the pars interarticularis), creating the pars defect that characterizes isthmic spondylolisthesis.

Spondylolisthesis can, in general, be characterized along two axes. The Wiltse classification system divides spondylolisthesis into five categories. Type 1 (dysplastic) results from congenital sacral dysplasia with rounding of the anterior-superior border of the S1 endplate, allowing the L5 vertebra to translate anteriorly. Type 2 (isthmic) results from fractures of the pars interarticularis of the cephalad vertebrae. Most common at L5/S1; type A results from a pars stress fracture (presumed etiology of present case) and type B results from repetitive fracture and healing with resultant elongation of the pars. Type 3 (degenerative) results from arthritic changes to the facet joints with weakening of the ligamentum flavum and resultant anterior translation. This is the **most common type**. Type 4 encompasses traumatic spondylolisthesis and type 5 is pathologic, often due to erosion by lytic bone tumors. A sixth type—iatrogenic spondylolisthesis—can also be described and may result from laminectomy with resultant destabilization of the motion segment.

The second means of classifying spondylolisthesis is the Meyerding system, which categorizes spondylolisthesis by the degree of slippage: grade 1 ≤ 25% anterior translation of the cephalad vertebra over the caudal vertebra, grade 2 = 25 to 50% slippage, grade 3 = 50 to 75% slippage, grade 4 = 76 to 100% slippage, and grade V (spondyloptosis) is > 100% translation.[7,8]

▸▸ Question 6

A patient with imaging showing lytic/isthmic spondylolisthesis and a clinical history of progressive low back and bilateral leg pain undergoes a noncontrast MR lumbar spine. Where would you expect to find neural element compression (▸ Fig. 3.3)?

- A. You would not expect to find neural element compression in isthmic spondylolisthesis
- B. Central canal
- C. Lateral recess
- D. Neural foramen
- E. Central canal and neural foramina

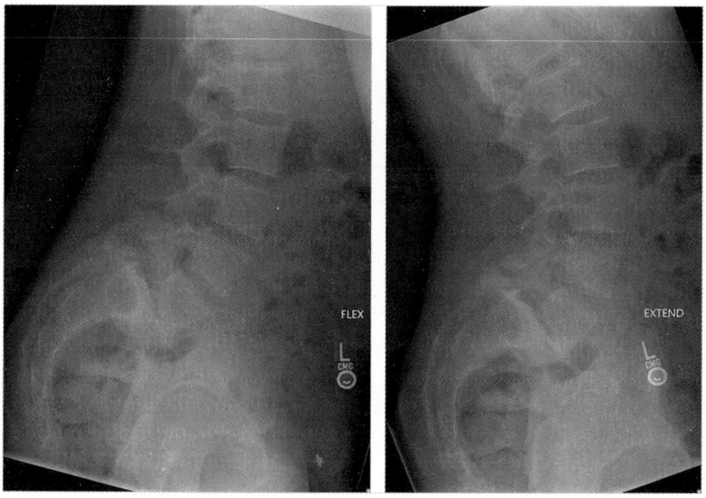

Fig. 3.2

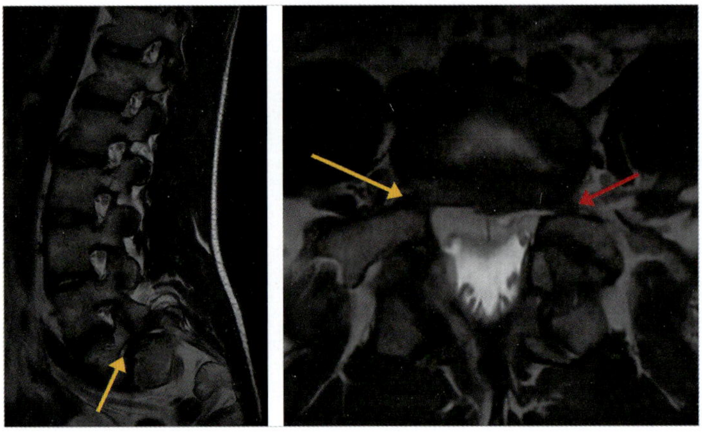

Fig. 3.3

Correct answer is D

In the most common type of spondylolisthesis—degenerative spondylolisthesis—there is a narrowing of the spinal canal, as the posterior elements of the cephalad vertebra translate anteriorly relative to the vertebral body of the caudal vertebra. Consequently, there is stenosis in the lateral recesses, commonly leading to a clinical picture of neurogenic claudication. However, in this patient's case, the bilateral pars defects mean that the L5 vertebral body is able to translate anteriorly while the posterior elements (the Gill body) remain stationary. Consequently, there is no significant narrowing of the spinal canal or lateral recesses; conversely, there is often an expansion of the anterior-posterior diameter of the canal. However, the fracture edge of the L5 body does translate with the vertebral body, bringing it closer to the L5/S1 disk and posterior edge of the S1 body. As the pars defines the posterior border of the foramen and the intervertebral disk and posterior vertebral body define the posterior and anterior borders of the neural foramen, respectively, there is a collapse of the AP dimension of the foramen. This resultant stenosis can compress the exiting L5 nerve roots as the spondylolisthesis progresses, causing radicular leg pain.

▸▸ Question 7

A 25-year-old male presents with bilateral radicular leg pain and imaging showing an L5/S1 isthmic spondylolisthesis. After trials of nonoperative therapy, he presents with new lower extremity weakness. Weakness in which of the following movements would be most consistent with his known pathology?

- A. Hip flexion.
- B. Knee extension
- C. Foot dorsiflexion
- D. Great toe extension
- E. Foot plantarflexion

Correct answer is D

As discussed in the previous question, the point of compression in isthmic spondylolisthesis is at the neural foramen, which leads to compression of the exiting nerve roots—L5 in this case. There is often multilevel innervation for the major muscle groups, but in general for the lower extremity, hip flexion is considered the L2 myotome, knee extension the L4 myotome, foot dorsiflexion the L4 and L5 myotome, great toe extension (extensor hallucis longus) the L5 myotome, and foot plantarflexion the S1 myotome. Patients may not complain of toe extensor weakness in the clinic but may instead note that they are more frequently tripping on curbs or having their feet catch on stairs. Those with significant dorsiflexor weakness will also commonly show a high-steppage gait, where the leg is lifted inordinately high in order to avoid the toes dragging on the ground. Patients may also employ an ankle-foot orthosis to help maintain the dorsiflexed position.

▸▸ Question 8

A young male with L5/S1 isthmic spondylolisthesis presents with bilateral leg and back pain that has progressed with nonoperative therapy. Which of the following surgical plans is most likely to offer long-term relief of his underlying symptoms?

- A. L5 laminectomy
- B. L5/S1 bilateral foraminotomy
- C. L5–pelvis fusion and gill laminectomy
- D. L5–S1 anterior lumbar interbody fusion
- E. L5/S1 interlaminar device placement

Correct answer is C

The patient's major presenting symptom was mechanical low-back pain resulting from his isthmic spondylolisthesis with a high slip angle. He subsequently developed bilateral EHL weakness due to compression of the exiting L5 nerve roots. As the compression is in the foramina, a laminectomy alone will not ameliorate his symptoms—there is no significant central or lateral recess stenosis. Similarly, while a bilateral L5/S1 foraminotomy may temporarily decompress the exiting L5 roots, he will likely experience a recurrence of his symptoms, as the high slip angle means his spondylolisthesis is likely to progress. An L5–S1 anterior lumbar interbody fusion is unlikely to allow for significant reduction of his spondylolisthesis; it is biomechanically inferior to a posterolateral fusion, and while it offers good segmental lordosis, sagittal misalignment is not this patient's main issue. L5–pelvis fusion is the best option, as it will arrest further progression of his spondylolisthesis and potentially also allow for reduction of the spondylolisthesis intraoperatively. The gill laminectomy/gill body resection will also help decompress the L5 roots. An interbody fusion is also reasonable in this case (e.g., an L5–S1 transforaminal lumbar interbody fusion), as it will provide an additional fusion surface and indirect decompression of the neural foramina, which have become elongated with the progressive slippage. Interlaminar devices are a poor option in this case, as they are less effective than decompression alone for central and lateral recess stenosis. Additionally, they are biomechanically inferior to fusion and will not offer the stability likely to address this patient's back pain.

▸▸ Question 9

Following an L5–S1 instrumented fusion and gill laminectomy for isthmic spondylolisthesis, a patient awakens with new right lower extremity dorsiflexor weakness and numbness on the top of his foot; neuromonitoring with free-running EMG was stable throughout the case. Which of the following examination findings would suggest that his injury was not a result of nerve root injury during surgery?

- A. Numbness in the first interspace
- B. Foot inversion weakness
- C. Foot eversion weakness
- D. Lateral shin numbness
- E. Extensor hallucis longus weakness

Correct answer is C

Concurrent foot eversion weakness (mediated by the peroneus longus and brevis, innervated by the superficial peroneal nerve) and dorsiflexion weakness (mediated primarily by the tibialis anterior, innervated by the deep peroneal nerve) would be suggestive of either a deep peroneal nerve palsy or a common peroneal nerve palsy. In this patient's case, the presence of numbness on the dorsum of the foot supports a common peroneal nerve palsy, which may occur due to compression at the fibular neck—though this is less likely in a prone-positioned spine case.

Importantly, foot inversion is mediated by the tibialis posterior, which receives innervation from the L5 nerve root via the tibial nerve, and is not affected by a common peroneal nerve injury. Therefore, preserved inversion with weakness of dorsiflexion and eversion may suggest a peripheral nerve lesion, whereas weakness of all three (inversion, eversion, and dorsiflexion) would be more consistent with an L5 radiculopathy.

The first dorsal webspace is innervated by the deep peroneal nerve, and while sensory loss might suggest a deep or common peroneal nerve injury, it cannot reliably distinguish between a peroneal neuropathy and an L5 radiculopathy, as both share this territory within the L5 dermatome. Similarly, numbness over the lateral shin, also in the L5 dermatome, could be due to injury to the superficial peroneal nerve or reflect a more proximal L5 nerve root lesion.[9]

▸▸ Question 10

A 31-year-old male presents to the local emergency department via ambulance after being involved in a single-vehicle collision as an unrestrained passenger. The patient is able to recall the circumstances of the event. On admission, his systolic blood pressure is in the 100 s, he has a normal heart rate, and his SpO_2 is in the mid-90 s. After stabilizing the patient's spine with sandbags or a cervical orthosis, which of the following is the next best step in the evaluation of this patient?

- A. Bedside ultrasound or CT of the abdomen/pelvis
- B. Vasopressin infusion for blood pressure support
- C. Noncontrast head CT
- D. Intubation
- E. Toxicology screening

Correct answer is A

The patient presents following a motor vehicle accident and may have unknown intracranial or spinal injuries. However, all trauma evaluation begins with the evaluation of the "ABCs." As the patient is able to recall the circumstances of his injury and is protecting his airway, no emergent intubation is merited. Additionally, his blood oxygenation percentage is in the mid-90 s, indicating that he is oxygenating appropriately. However, he is hypotensive and has a normal heart rate, which would be unusual in the case of high-energy trauma, where there is commonly increased sympathetic outflow, which manifests as tachycardia, often with hypertension. There are several reasons a patient posttrauma may have a normal or reduced blood pressure, the worsening of which may lead to shock. The first to rule out is hypovolemic shock, which requires urgent fluid resuscitation and often blood transfusion (replace blood with blood). A bedside ultrasound (FAST scan) or CT of the abdomen/pelvis can help rule out intra-abdominal bleed that would require emergent exploratory laparotomy. The patient should also undergo head CT and CT of the pan-spine for evaluation of intracranial and spinal injuries, but ruling out intra-abdominal injury takes precedence. If the patient does require vasopressors, norepinephrine is the agent of choice for cardiogenic, neurogenic, and spinal shock.[10]

▸▸ Question 11

A young male with multiple injuries following a motor vehicle accident has CT imaging of his cervical spine (▸ Fig. 3.4). Which of the following physical examination findings is most consistent with the injury seen below?

- A. Left elbow extensor weakness
- B. Right shoulder abductor weakness
- C. No motor abnormalities
- D. Bilateral hand intrinsic weakness
- E. Left elbow flexor weakness.

Correct answer is A

The imaging demonstrates a fracture through the left lateral mass of C6 with likely compression of the C6/C7 foramen. As the cervical nerve roots exit above their like-numbered vertebra, compression at the C6/C7 nerve root will result in C7 nerve root weakness, which on physical examination is most likely to manifest as elbow extensor weakness. The C5 root is conventionally held to be

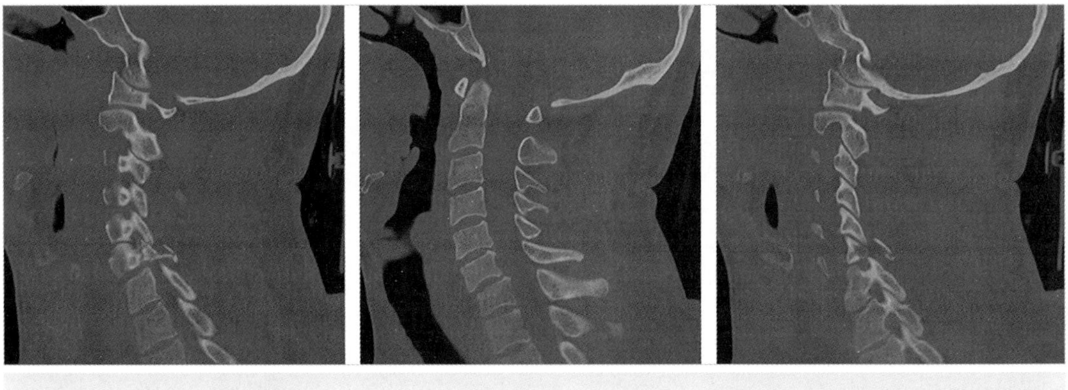

Fig. 3.4

responsible for shoulder abduction, C6 for wrist extension or elbow flexion, C8 for finger flexion, and T1 for hand intrinsics. Also note on the second image that there is an anterolisthesis of C6 on C7 with < 50% slippage. This is a classic finding for separating unilateral facet joint injury or unilateral jumped facet from bilateral facet joint injury/ bilateral jumped facets. Bilateral injury generally presents with ≥ 50% slippage.

▸▸ Question 12

A patient presents with moderate distal bilateral upper extremity weakness and flaccid lower extremity paraplegia with priapism. CT of the cervical spine shows bilateral C6/C7 jumped facets. His proximal arm musculature is full strength on examination. Which of the following is the next best step in management (▸ Fig. 3.5)?

- A. Emergent operating room for C6–C7 anterior cervical diskectomy and fusion
- B. Emergent operating room for C5–T1 fusion, C6–C7 laminectomy
- C. MR of the cervical spine
- D. IV methylprednisolone
- E. Awake cervical traction with fluoroscopy.

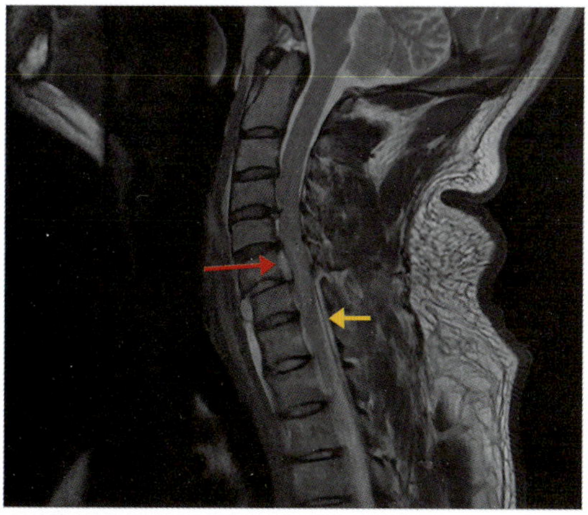

Fig. 3.5

Correct answer is C

The examination findings are out of proportion to the bony injury seen on his CT of the cervical spine; his physical examination shows diffuse flaccid paraplegia/atonia and priapism (loss of sympathetic tone), which is most consistent with a combination of neurogenic shock (high cervical or thoracic cord injury [above T5] resulting in loss of sympathetic outflow) and spinal shock (areflexia and flaccidity below the level of injury. It is therefore highly likely that the patient has sustained a severe spinal cord injury; further imaging in the form of an urgent/emergent MR is merited to evaluate this injury. There may be an unrecognized epidural hematoma requiring evacuation. Alternatively, there may be cord transection, which would result in irreversible injury. Consequently, the best next step in management is to rule out the presence of ongoing spinal cord compression. MR of the cervical spine is the best next step for this, and in the case of this patient, there was circumferential hematoma from the level of C4–T3 with focal compression at the C6 level. The intervertebral disk was also noted to be compromised, indicating the patient's injury affected all three columns, rendering it highly unstable.

Additionally, from this examination, one can assign the patient an American Spinal Injury Association (ASIA) grade, which evaluates a patient's neurological status on a scale from A to E based on the last normal spinal cord level, and the sensory and motor function distal to the injured level. A—patient has no preserved sensorimotor function distal to the injury and perianal wink is absent; B—patient has no motor function distal to the injury but some sensation is preserved (at minimum in S4–S5 segments); C—patient has preserved motor function but > 50% of motor groups distal to the injury have < 3/5 strength; D—patient has preserved motor function distal to the injury with > 50% of motor groups being ≥ 3/5 strength; E—the patient's sensorimotor examination is intact. Patients with more severe injuries (poorer ASIA score) have a lower likelihood of recovery. In this case, the patient has signs of spinal shock (flaccidity and loss of tone in the lower extremity), and so his true injury severity cannot be assessed. Rather, several days may be required to determine the true severity of injury. Regardless, the injury is severe and merits intervention.

Proceeding directly to surgery prior to obtaining additional imaging is incorrect in this case, as the patient has examination findings that cannot be explained by his current workup. The exact nature of the injury should be appreciated prior to proceeding to operative intervention. Last, while IV corticosteroids gained favor in the 1990s to improve neurological function following acute cervical spinal cord injury, the NASCIS trials failed to provide evidence supporting their efficacy, though they did show that patients treated with corticosteroids had higher risks of pneumonia and other complications. Based on this, the 2013 CNS/AANS cervical spine trauma guidelines recommend against giving IV corticosteroids following acute spinal cord injury. Cervical traction may be a reasonable option to reduce the jumped facets *if* MR demonstrates no ongoing compression, and the patient is able to comply with the examination. However, it is important to rule out a ventrally situated disk herniation/fragment that could result in permanent paralysis if reduced into the cord during traction.

▸▸ Question 13

A patient with bilateral C7/T1 jumped facets and ongoing cord compression is taken for C4–T2 posterior segmental instrumented fusion and C4–T1 laminectomy/decompression. Intraoperative neuromonitoring is used throughout the case. During the course of the procedure, which of the following changes in monitoring signals would be considered most predictive of a new postoperative deficit?

- A. Decrease in left leg SSEP amplitudes of 60%.
- B. Decrease in abductor pollicis brevis MEP of 40%
- C. Increase in right arm SSEP latency of 5%.
- D. EMG firing from the right vastus lateralis
- E. Absent transcortical MEPS in the right leg prior to positioning

Correct answer is A

In general, significant changes in neuromonitoring signals are a 10% increase in SSEP latency, a 50 to 60% decrease in SSEP signal amplitude, a 50% decrease in MEP amplitude, or loss of EMG activity from a given nerve root. EMG activity increases with nerve root irritation and can result from compression, stretching, or pulling of the nerve root. Neuromuscular blocking agents interfere with the ability to follow transcortical MEPs and EMG activity; they are commonly used for exposure in spine cases, but must wear off or be reversed with sugammadex (which reverses rocuronium and vecuronium) prior to resumption of neuromonitoring. Of note, repeat rounds of neuromuscular paralysis followed by reversal are usually not possible; so, this must be taken into account during exposure. For spinal cord tumors, D wave monitoring, which monitors transmission of signal from the transcranial electrode to an epidural or subdural electrode, provides real-time feedback and likely offers the greatest specificity for true changes. It is not available at all centers and is not indicated in most cases. A 50% decrease in amplitude in MEP and SEP from baseline is predictive of a new severe neurological deficit. Poor baseline motor signals (e.g., absent signals from the leg) likely indicate a severe baseline injury but provide no information to suggest that surgery is no longer the best option for this patient (▸ Table 3.2).[11,12]

Table 3.2 Common EMG recording sites

Level	Muscle	Level	Muscle
C4	Supraspinatus	L1	Iliopsoas
C5	Deltoid and biceps	L2	Adductor longus
C6	Biceps and wrist extensors	L3	Adductor longus and vastus medialis
C7	Triceps, wrist flexors, and finger extensors	L4	Vastus medialis and vastus lateralis
C8	Hand intrinsics and finger flexors	L5	TA and extensor hallucis longus
T1	Hand intrinsics	S1	Medial gastrocnemius and peroneus longus
T6–12 (uncommon target)	Rectus abdominis	S2–5	Perianal musculature and urethral sphincter

▸▸ Question 14

A patient undergoes cervical decompression and fusion for traumatic cervical spinal cord injury. As the fascia is being closed at the end of the procedure, neuromonitoring reports a new 80% decrease in transcranial motor-evoked potential (TcMEP) signals from the bilateral abductor pollicis brevis. Which of the following is the best next step?

- A. No intervention required; loss of TcMEPs is typical with emergence from anesthesia.
- B. Reopen the fascia and interrogate the wound for ongoing compression.
- C. Close and transfer to the ICU for blood pressure augmentation
- D. No intervention required; the signal change is likely due to prolonged anesthetic
- E. Administration of 10 mg dexamethasone

Correct answer is B

The reported 80% decrease in abductor pollicis brevis TcMEPs represents a significant change in neuromonitoring signals. It may be a harbinger of new spinal cord or nerve root compression (though cord is more likely in the setting of bilateral changes). Such compression can happen due to a shift in bone graft material during closure. Continuing closure is the wrong answer, as this is the best opportunity to remove any new such compression. Should interrogation of the wound fail to demonstrate any obvious compression, the next consideration should be revision of any reduction maneuver done as part of the instrumentation procedure. Occasionally, significant changes in sagittal and/or coronal alignment can lead to spinal cord or nerve root compression. Removing this reduction and reinspecting for areas of potential correction is the best choice. Should no inspection be appreciated, then the rods (longitudinal elements) can be replaced, and closure can proceed. However, if there is no rebound in neuromonitoring signals and no evidence of compression, blood pressure augmentation to a mean arterial pressure of > 80 to 85 mm Hg is considered standard of care. The administration of IV corticosteroids is not supported in the treatment of spinal cord injury. While neuromonitoring signals may be lost at the end of a surgical case with the switch from intravenous to inhaled anesthesia, the question does not mention a change in the anesthetic agent, and so the observed drop in TcMEPs likely represents a real change.

▸▸ Question 15

During a long posterior thoracolumbar fusion for correction of adolescent idiopathic scoliosis, there is an 80% decrease in the transcranial motor-evoked potentials (TcMEPs) for the lower extremities. The decrease remains despite reversal of correct maneuvers and interrogation of all implants. The decision is made to close the case and extubate the patient. Which of the following interventions is the best next step for improving the patient's odds of recovery?

- A. Administer a 5-day course of intravenous corticosteroids
- B. Mean arterial pressure (MAP) augmentation with norepinephrine to a target of 85 mm Hg
- C. MAP augmentation with phenylephrine to a target of 85 mm Hg
- D. MAP augmentation with norepinephrine to a target of 70 mm Hg
- E. Transfusion to a hemoglobin target of ≥ 10 g/dL

Correct answer is B

In this patient's case, the bilaterally decreased abductor pollicis brevis TcMEPs appear most consistent with spinal cord injury. For these patients, MAP augmentation to a target MAP > 85 to 90 mm Hg is considered standard of care. Norepinephrine is the preferred agent for cervical and upper thoracic injuries, with phenylephrine another option. In the case of concurrent spinal shock, a sympathomimetic agent, such as norepinephrine, is preferred. Ensuring that the patient has adequate oxygen delivery may help maximize recovery, but it does not have strong evidence to support it, and a hemoglobin goal of ≥ 10 g/dL is likely to increase the risk of adverse effects, such as transfusion-associated lung injury and transfusion-associated cardiac overload, without clear benefit.[13,14]

▸▸ Question 16

A 45-year-old female with no significant medical comorbidities undergoes an uncomplicated C2–T2 posterior segmental instrumented fusion and C3–C7 laminectomy. The patient awakens at her apparent neurological baseline and begins mobilizing out of bed on postoperative day 1. On postoperative day 2, she endorses new weakness in her left shoulder abduction, which on examination is 4/5. Her weakness worsens on postoperative day 3 to the point that she is no longer able to abduct her right shoulder antigravity. Which of the following is the best explanation?

- A. The patient has delayed spinal cord ischemia/ a new spinal cord infarct
- B. The patient has an antalgic shoulder, and her weakness is pain-limited
- C. The patient has a new C5 palsy
- D. The patient has new radial nerve palsy from surgical positioning
- E. The patient has an upper trunk injury from surgical positioning

Correct answer is C

The patient's finding is unilateral and appears isolated to the deltoid (C5 myotome). Consequently, a spinal cord infarct is unlikely; this would usually be an intraoperative surgical complication manifesting with bilateral findings. Though the patient may have pain with movement of her arm, the fact that the onset is delayed (postoperative day 2) and worsens over the subsequent 24 hours makes it unlikely that her weakness is just a pain-limited examination finding. While arm positioning can cause pain and subjective weakness postoperatively, it is often bilateral and is usually present on postoperative day 1. Patients should also be able to overcome it with effort. Last, the radial nerve does not innervate the deltoid and so would not be expected to cause shoulder weakness. Innervation of the deltoid is via the C5 root → upper trunk → posterior division → posterior cord → axillary nerve.

C5 palsy is the best explanation for this examination finding and affects 8 to 12% of patients following posterior cervical fusion. It can also be seen following anterior cervical diskectomy and fusion, though this is less common. The exact pathogenesis is unknown, but nerve root traction from cord float back, intraoperative thermal injury, new foraminal stenosis due to sagittal plane correction, and cord ischemia have all been suggested. Median onset is day 3, and the weakness often worsens in the first 1 to 2 days after onset. It is self-limiting, but recovery is variable; it is worse for those with greater deficits at the injury nadir (i.e., more profound weakness at the period of maximum deficit) and those with bilateral deficits.

▸▸ Question 17

A patient undergoes posterior cervical decompression and fusion for cervical myelopathy. On postoperative day 2, she is noted to have new left shoulder abduction weakness. Which of the following is the best next step in management for this patient?

- A. Short course of IV corticosteroids
- B. Intense physical/occupational therapy
- C. Urgent nerve transfer
- D. Continue observation
- E. Return to the operating room for surgical exploration.

Correct answer is D

The patient's new deficit is most consistent with C5 palsy, which is a self-limiting process. At present, there is no good evidence to suggest that there is any intervention that can improve the overall outcome. While physical and occupational therapy are always valid interventions to enhance mobilization after surgery, there is no suggestion that this will improve the patient's long-term outcome. In some cases, significant correction of lordosis may result in compression of the foramina with resultant radiculopathy ± weakness; however, this is uncommon, and the question does not describe a significant correction or lordosis or compression across the C4–C5 lateral masses. The latter would cause stenosis at the C4/C5 foramina, in which case surgical exploration with foraminotomies may help facilitate recovery, though evidence for this is limited, at best.[15,16,17]

▸▸ Question 18

A 75-year-old male presents to the clinic with complaints of difficulty swallowing and difficulty walking. The patient is seen in the clinic and when sitting across from you, he adopts a notably slumped posture in the chair. He endorses chronic neck pain, but denies difficulty with fastening buttons or handwriting, denies urinary incontinence, and has no overt weakness on physical examination. He does endorse difficulty walking. Which of the following imaging modalities is the best next step in his evaluation?

- A. MR of the cervical spine
- B. CT of the cervical spine

- C. Cervical spine X-ray with flexion/extension view
- D. Full-length (36") scoliosis radiographs
- E. None; patient has no signs/symptoms that merit imaging

Correct answer is A

The patient endorses difficulty with walking, which could be due to hip pathologies, spinal deformity/sagittal imbalance, normal pressure hydrocephalus, inner ear dysfunction, cervical myelopathy, or any of a number of other pathologies. However, given his age and endorsement of neck pain, spondylotic myelopathy is a possible, surgically treatable explanation of his imbalance. MR provides the best means of evaluating cervical stenosis. Flexion-extension views may also provide clues of dynamic cord compression, but generally would only be indicated if the MR shows cord signal change consistent with myelopathy but without evidence of static compression. CT of the cervical spine may also be a part of his workup. It can demonstrate whether the compressive discoligamentous elements are ossified (e.g., as in ossified posterior longitudinal ligament [OPLL]). It can also help assess for motion segment autofusion, which is often seen in the facet joints of older patients. This can influence the decision of which levels to fuse and can help inform whether disk arthroplasty is a surgical option for the patient.[18]

▸▸ Question 19

A 54-year-old man presents with progressive difficulty walking and swallowing and an MR of the cervical spine is shown below. He also endorses difficulty holding his head up as his neck muscles become tired as the day wears on. He is sent for additional cervical spine radiographs (▸ Fig. 3.6). Which of the following is the best explanation of his walking difficulties?

- A. Parkinson disease
- B. Vitamin B12 deficiency
- C. Chin-on-chest deformity
- D. Myelopathy from dynamic spinal cord compression
- E. Hirayama disease

Correct answer is C

The images here demonstrate a patent spinal canal on supine MR and a kyphotic cervical spine. Though Parkinson disease can explain gait difficulties in the aging population and may be associated with swallowing difficulties, there is no mention of either bradykinesia (slowness of movement) or a resting tremor—two of the cardinal features of Parkinsonism. In this patient's case, he was trialed on carbidopa/levodopa to determine if early-stage Parkinson disease was contributing to his symptoms, but he experienced no benefit. Vitamin B12 deficiency is also a potential cause of myelopathy (subacute combined degeneration); however, this is uncommon even in patients with vitamin B12 deficiency (14.8% of cases). It also presents radiographically with a V-shaped hyperintensity of the posterior spinal cord on T2-weighted imaging. This patient's MR shows no T2-hyperintensity consistent with this pathology. For similar reasons, dynamic myelopathy is unlikely, as there are no T2 signal changes. However, the radiograph demonstrates significant

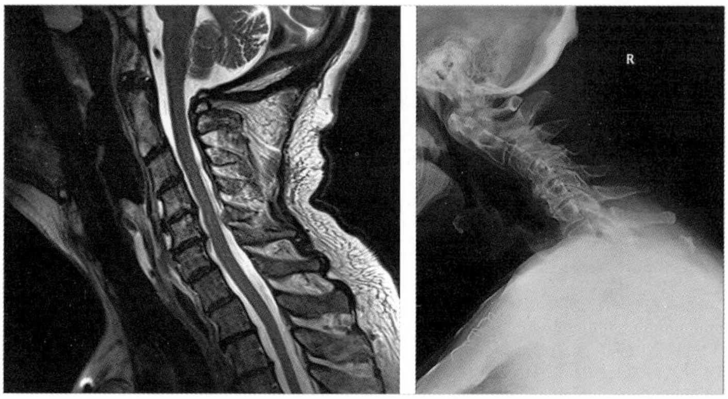

Fig. 3.6

kyphosis—a chin-on-chest or "swan neck" deformity with the occiput–C1 and C1–C2 joints in maximal extension. This suggests that the baseline alignment of the patient's spine precludes him from looking forward, which may be contributing to his altered gait. Additionally, he likely has suboccipital and paraspinal neck pain from constant, maximal retraction of his cervical paraspinal musculature as he attempts to maintain forward gaze. Hirayama disease—monomelic amyotrophy—is predominately a pathology of young, Asian males characterized by bilateral upper extremity weakness ± sensory changes. It is inconsistent with the patient's demographics and clinical history.[19]

▸▸ Question 20

A patient presents with difficulty walking and a stooped forward posture. He undergoes upright scoliosis radiographs and computed tomography (▶ Fig. 3.7) demonstrating cervical spine deformity and is offered surgical intervention. Which of the following is most likely to address his underlying pathology?

- A. C3–T1 anterior cervical diskectomy and fusion
- B. C2–C7 posterior cervical fusion
- C. C3–C7 anterior cervical diskectomy and fusion (ACDF); C2–T4 posterior fusion
- D. C2–T10 posterior fusion
- E. C3–C7 anterior fusion; C4–C6 corpectomy and reconstruction with expandable titanium cage

Correct answer is C

There is variability in surgical planning, but the best surgical plan to address the patient's deformity is option **C**. The scoliosis films show a high T1 slope and an apex near the cervicothoracic junction, indicating the deformity is a cervicothoracic deformity. A surgical plan involving only the cervical spine (option **B**) will therefore not treat the underlying deformity; the patient may, in fact, be at increased risk of distal junctional disease. The CT demonstrates large osteophytes in the subaxial spine, which will likely limit correction for a posterior-only correction (option **D**). Consequently, an anterior stage is merited to debulk and release these osteophyte complexes. Anterior interbodies will also allow for correction of the multilevel degenerative disk space collapse, physiologically correcting the subaxial kyphosis. Last, a multilevel ACDF, even one instrumenting C7/T1 (often difficult to access due to the manubrium) will create a long fusion mass that places significant forces on the cephalad and caudad motion segments. A posterior stage will improve the biomechanical stability of the construct and so improve the odds of successful fusion in the long term. An isolated anterior fusion with multilevel corpectomy is similarly a poor choice; a complementary posterior construct is merited to the stability of the construct.[20]

▸▸ Question 21

A patient is set to undergo cervical decompression and fusion for cervical spondylotic myelopathy. During his preoperative medical clearance appointment, the week before surgery, the patient reports a significant tobacco history and active tobacco use. He agrees to discontinue cigarettes at that time. How should this influence the timing of surgical intervention?

- A. The patient's surgery should be cancelled indefinitely.
- B. The patient's surgery should be delayed for 4 to 8 weeks
- C. The patient's surgery should be delayed for 2 weeks
- D. The patient's surgery can proceed next week without alteration
- E. The patient's surgery can proceed next week if a nicotine metabolite test on the day before surgery is negative

Correct answer is B

Smoking has been associated with a wide variety of complications following spine surgery, including nonunion, wound infection, and respiratory complications. However, a prior history of cigarette use is not an absolute contraindication to surgery (option **A**). Prior research has suggested that smoking cessation leads to an increase in respiratory secretions with a resultant increase in respiratory complications in the 4 to 8 weeks following surgery. The American College of Surgeons suggests cessation of smoking 4 to 6 weeks prior to surgery, and cessation of smoking preoperatively has been associated with a 25 to 50% reduction in respiratory complications, including bronchospasm, atelectasis, lung infection, pleural effusion, pneumothorax, pulmonary embolism,

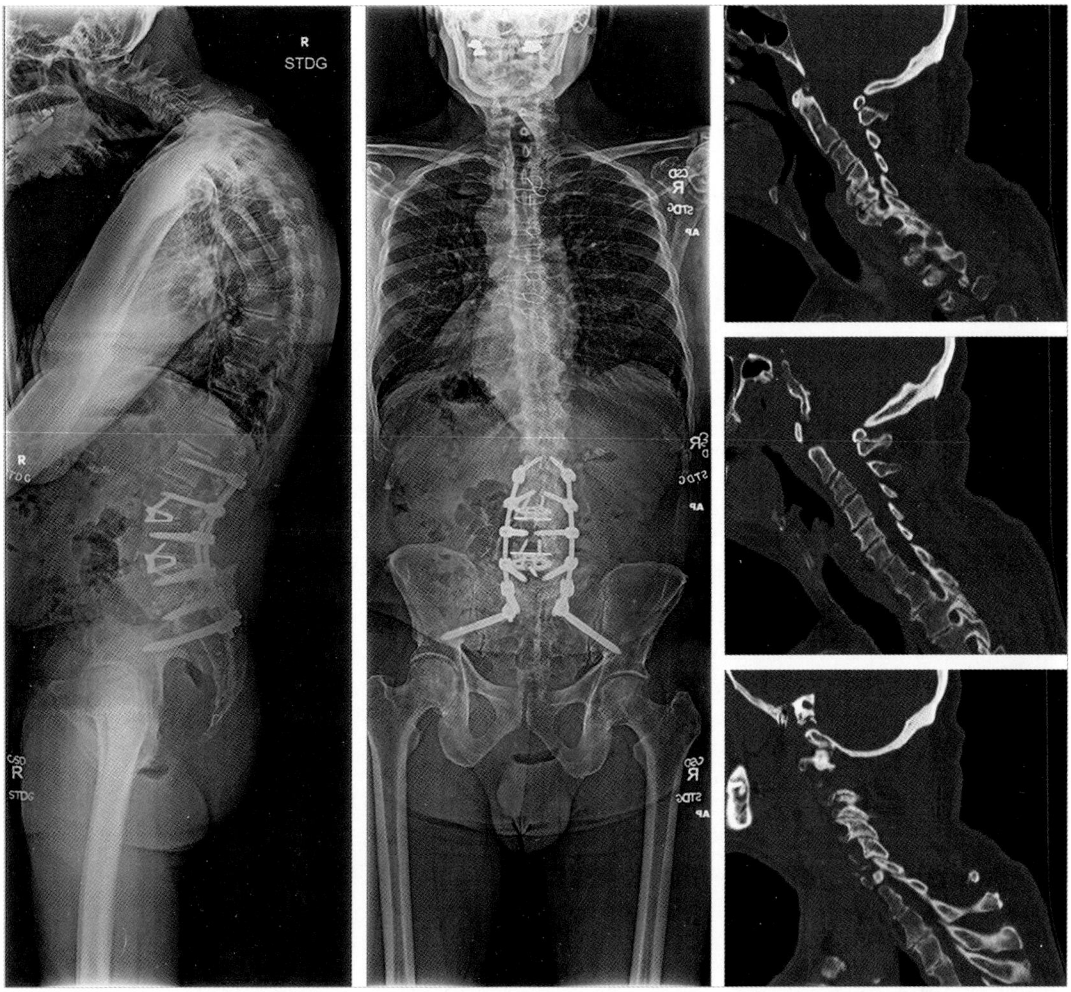

Fig. 3.7

reintubation, new postoperative oxygen requirement, and acute respiratory distress syndrome. If the patient is a smoker, it will be important to know that they have stopped smoking, which can be verified with a cotinine/nicotine metabolite test. Continued smoking places the patient at increased risk of wound infection/breakdown and nonunion and may be considered a contraindication to this elective surgery (option **D**). Delaying this patient's surgery for 4 to 8 weeks could significantly improve their perioperative risk profile. Additionally, given the patient's reported history of smoking, it is also advisable that they undergo a bone mineral density (BMD) evaluation, as tobacco use has been correlated with accelerated BMD loss. Poor BMD is a risk factor for mechanical complications following instrumented spine surgery (screw cutout/pull out, junctional failure, interbody subsidence). Dual-energy X-ray absorptiometry (DXA/DEXA) is considered the gold standard, but alternative techniques, including trabecular bone score and biomechanical CT, are now FDA-acceptable alternatives. Growing evidence now suggests that opportunistic bone quality evaluation using Hounsfield units on CT may provide superior risk stratification.[21,22]

►► Question 22

A 63-year-old female with past medical history of obesity and hyperlipidemia presents to the clinic with complaints of 10 years of progressive low-back pain and several years of progressive bilateral lower extremity pain that worsens with ambulation. Which of the following findings in the patient's history/clinical examination would suggest her symptoms are due to neurogenic pseudoclaudication as opposed to vascular claudication?

- A. The patient is limited to 1 block of ambulation before requiring rest
- B. The patient's feet are cold on examination
- C. The patient reports she is still able to use her bicycle without issue
- D. The patient reports pain that is equal in both extremities
- E. The patient endorses paresthesias in her toes bilaterally

Correct answer is C

Neurogenic pseudoclaudication from lumbar stenosis and vascular claudication can present with a number of shared features, including worsening of symptoms with ambulation and bilateral lower extremity pain. However, vascular claudication results from insufficient blood supply to the extremity muscles to meet the demands placed by exertion. The limb becomes hypoxic, leading to pain. This will be seen regardless of whether the activity is done in the upright or seated position. However, neurogenic pseudoclaudication is caused by compression of the cauda equina roots with upright posture. Symptoms will often worsen even with upright posture (e.g., standing) without exertion. Patients may note that pain is worsened when descending inclines (body adopts a more lordotic posture to maintain balance, worsening compression), and improves with forward posture (e.g., resting on a shopping cart/"shopping cart sign," exercising in seated posture, e.g., on the bike). Both vascular claudication and neurogenic pseudoclaudication can have pain that is equal bilaterally. With progression of both conditions, the patient's walking tolerance will worsen; so, a limitation of 1 block may be seen with either advanced peripheral artery disease (vascular claudication) or advanced stenosis (neurogenic pseudoclaudication), or lumbar radiculopathy.

►► Question 23

A 70-year-old woman with progressive lower extremity pain worsened with walking and upright posture. Her initial workup includes upright lumbar spine radiographs (► Fig. 3.8). The patient has multilevel degenerative disease, including a spondylolisthesis at L3/L4. Based on the Meyerding classification scale, what grade of spondylolisthesis does this patient have?

- A. Grade 1
- B. Grade 2

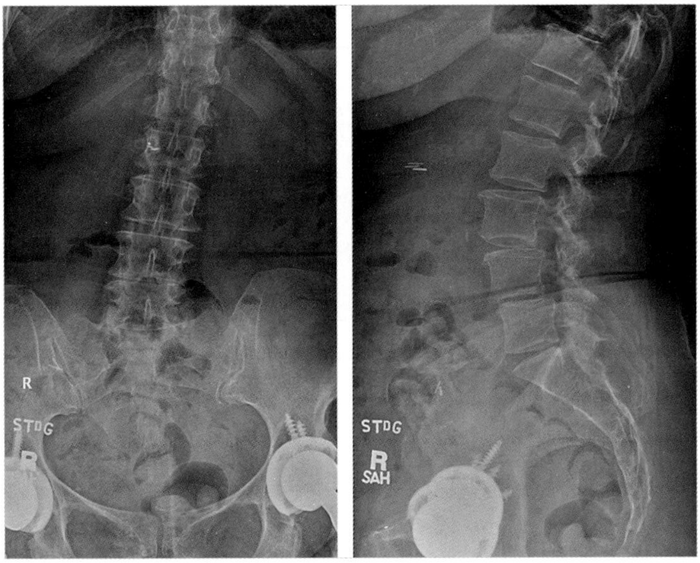

Fig. 3.8

- C. Grade 3
- D. Grade 4
- E. Grade 5

Correct answer is A

Although radiographs are unlikely to show the underlying pathology here (lumbar stenosis), for insurance purposes, patients often undergo radiographs before undergoing MR. Radiographs can also be helpful to demonstrate the patient's spinal alignment prior to surgery, to help develop the surgical plan. The radiographs here show multilevel degeneration with a slight leftward lean on the PA view, likely due to an antalgic hip (bilateral hip arthroplasty is noted). Additionally seen are significant collapse of the L4/L5 disk space and an anterolisthesis of L3 and L4, representing a Meyerding grade 1 spondylolisthesis.

Spondylolistheses can be categorized using two classification systems. The Meyerding system classifies the spondylolisthesis based on the degree of slippage on upright radiographs, where slippage is defined by the quotient given by dividing the anterior-posterior distance between the anterior-inferior edge of the cephalad vertebral body and the anterior-superior edge of the caudal vertebral body by the total anterior-posterior length of the caudal vertebral body. Grade 1 = 0 to 25% slippage; grade 2 = 25 to 50% slippage; grade 3 = 51 to 75% slippage; grade 4 = 76 to 100% slippage; and grade 5 ≥ 100% slippage (spondyloptosis).

Spondylolisthesis can also be classified by presumed etiology using the Wiltse classification as below:

- Type 1—dysplastic, congenital spondylolisthesis characterized by anterior and superior rounding of the S1 endplate.
- Type 2—isthmic; subtype A caused by stress fracture of pars interarticularis (spondylolysis), where type B is caused by repetitive fracture and healing with elongation of the pars; common at L5/S1 and less so at L4/5; thought due to extension and twisting motions, for example, rowing that place excess force on the pars.
- Type 3—degenerative; progressive weakening of the ligamentum flavum allows anterior slippage; most common subtype.
- Type 4—traumatic.
- Type 5—pathologic (e.g., tumor).
- Type 6—iatrogenic, for example, a patient having undergone prior laminectomy with resultant insufficiency fracture.

An additional point to study on the radiography is the slip angle of spondylolisthesis —the angle formed between the superior endplate of the caudal body and the horizon. Among degenerative cases (the most common spondylolisthesis type), high slip angle spondylolistheses are thought to be at higher risk for progression.[23,24]

▸▸ Question 24

A 54-year-old male presents with symptoms of neurogenic pseudoclaudication and an MR lumbar spine (▶ Fig. 3.9). On questioning, the patient reports that the majority of his pain runs down the lateral leg and into the dorsum of the foot. He additionally notes his right foot catching on steps when walking up stairs and on the curb, though he has no clear deficits on bedside examination. Which of the following points of compression best explains his symptoms?

- A. Central stenosis at the level of L4/L5
- B. Foraminal stenosis at the level of L5/S1
- C. Lateral recess stenosis at the level of L3/L4
- D. Lateral recess stenosis at the level of L4/L5
- E. Foraminal stenosis at L2/L3

Correct answer is D

The symptoms described by the patient are most consistent with a subtle dorsiflexor weakness (footdrop), although this may not be appreciated on bedside examination. Dorsiflexion is mediated by the tibialis anterior, itself innervated by the deep peroneal nerve, which derives innervation from the L4 and L5 roots. In the context of degenerative lumbar pathologies, the two most common points of compression are the lateral recess, which affects the descending root, and the neural foramen, which affects the exiting nerve root. For the L5 nerve roots, this is most commonly lateral recess stenosis at L4/L5. The imaging for this patient illustrates significant lateral recess stenosis at the L4/L5 level, which explains her findings. Though he may have L5/S1 foraminal stenosis, it is not seen on the images shown and is not the best explanation (option **B**). The imaging also shows his compression at L4/L5 is greater than at L3/L4, so while lateral recess stenosis can

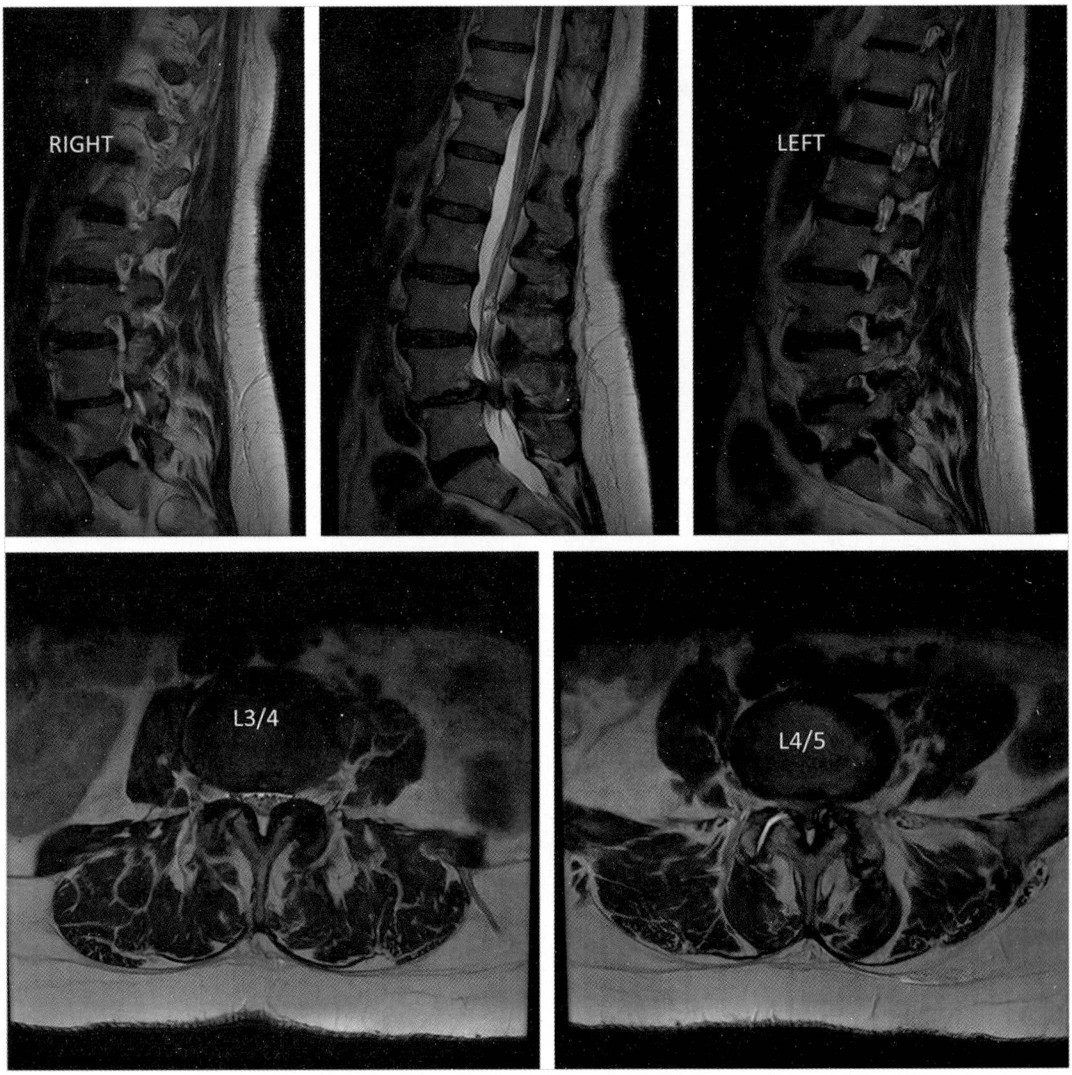

Fig. 3.9

cause compression of any of the descending roots, the space at L4/L5 is much more stenotic and consequently more likely to be driving her symptoms as compared to L3/L4.

▸▸ Question 25

A patient with symptoms of neurogenic pseudoclaudication and imaging showing lateral recess stenosis at L3/L4 and L4/L5, and large facet joint effusions at L4/L5 presents for surgical evaluation. The patient indicates that while her leg pain led her to evaluation, approximately 40% of her pain is localized to her back. Which of the following surgical options is most likely to address both her leg and back pain?

- A. L3/L4, L4/L5 anterior lumbar interbody fusion
- B. L3, L4, L5 laminectomy without fusion
- C. L3–L5 instrumented fusion with L3/L4, L4/L5 interlaminar decompression
- D. L3/L5 open laminectomy without fusion
- E. L3/L4, L4/L5 interspinous device placement

Correct answer is C

The patient's leg pain doubtlessly stems from the significant stenosis at the L3/L5 levels. This compression is due to predominately facet joint hypertrophy with lateral recess compression, though there is also a discogenic component at L4/L5. The best means of addressing this is through direct decompression, whether through traditional open laminectomy or minimally invasive hemilaminotomy with bilateral decompression. Her foraminal stenosis is mild at best, and not likely to cause symptoms and so a foraminotomy alone will not address her symptoms (option **D**). Similarly, an anterior approach can help address the diskogenic component of the compression and can create indirect decompression through restoration of disk space height, but it will not allow the lateral recess stenosis to be effectively addressed. As the patient says her back pain is also significant and her MR demonstrates fluid in the L4/L5 facet joints bilaterally, it is possible that she also has some instability at the L4/L5 motion segment. This can be addressed with an instrumented fusion. A comprehensive surgical plan aimed at addressing both the stenosis and instability could therefore include both a decompression and instrumented fusion (option **C**). Interbody fusion is frequently used but is not always necessary. The main advantages of the interbody fusion (e.g., transforaminal lumbar interbody fusion [TLIF]) are that it can allow for the induction of segmental lordosis in a person with flatback syndrome, can allow for indirect decompression through restoration of disk space height, and create an additional space for fusion. The downsides of TLIF include that it increases surgical invasiveness and operative time and requires resection of the facet joint on one side, eliminating the most important component of the posterolateral fusion surface. If this patient presented with complaints of neurogenic pseudoclaudication alone, decompression without fusion may be a reasonable option, as current evidence from randomized controlled trials suggests that the addition of fusion to decompression for Meyerding grade 1 to 2 spondylolistheses without evidence of instability offers no additional symptomatic benefit compared to decompression alone. Interlaminar and interspinous devices are an incorrect answer, as they are much less effective than decompression for symptoms of stenosis and fail to offer the biomechanical stabilization that would help address the instability evidenced by her facet joint effusions. A hemilaminectomy through a tubular retractor is able to preserve the spinous process and ligaments and able to decompress the bilateral lateral recess as well as the unilateral foramen, if needed, while still preserving stability to prevent the need for a fusion. In general, lumbar decompression procedures such as laminectomy or laminotomy tend to be for leg pain, whereas fusion tends to be better for back pain; however, patients frequently have improvements in their back pain since they are able to stand up straighter, which can help the back pain with laminectomy.[25,26,27,28,29]

▸▸ Question 26

In speaking with her surgeon, a patient undergoing evaluation for lumbar decompression and fusion mentions she uses ibuprofen to help manage the pain for her osteoarthritis. She asks if it would be okay to continue this medication through the perioperative period and to help reduce her opioid analgesic use postoperatively. For which of the following complications is she at greatest risk were she to continue using the celecoxib in the perioperative period?

- A. Wound infection
- B. Venous thromboembolic event
- C. Pseudoarthrosis
- D. Screw pullout
- E. Wound dehiscence

Correct answer is C

Ibuprofen is a nonselective nonsteroidal anti-inflammatory drug (NSAID) that inhibits both COX-1 and COX-2 enzymes, while celecoxib (Celebrex) is a selective COX-2 inhibitor. Both medications are commonly used for pain management in patients with osteoarthritis, and both have opioid-sparing effects in the postoperative period. However, NSAIDs as a class have been associated with impaired bone healing and increased rates of pseudoarthrosis following spinal fusion procedures, particularly when used for extended durations or at high doses.

Some studies suggest that short-term use of celecoxib may have a more favorable safety profile compared to nonselective NSAIDs like ibuprofen, particularly in terms of gastrointestinal side effects and bleeding risk. Additionally, because celecoxib is COX-2 selective, it may theoretically have less inhibitory effect on bone healing than traditional NSAIDs, though the data remain mixed. Despite these potential benefits, celecoxib still carries a dose- and duration-dependent risk of impairing fusion, and the greatest concern in the perioperative period remains pseudoarthrosis if celecoxib is continued around the time of spinal instrumentation and fusion.

Thus, while celecoxib may be considered in some perioperative pain management strategies due to its opioid-sparing benefits, it should still be used cautiously in patients undergoing spinal fusion due to the risk of nonunion.[30]

▸▸ Question 27

A 91-year-old male with past medical history of obstructive sleep apnea, atrial fibrillation (on warfarin), hyperlipidemia, and thoracic aortic aneurysm presents to the local emergency department following a ground-level fall at home. Immediately following the fall, he was noted to have jerking movements of the bilateral lower extremities along with paresthesias and weakness of the left lower extremity. On evaluation, he was noted to have 4-/5 left deltoid weakness, 4-/5 elbow flexor weakness, and 4/5 weakness in the remainder of the extremity. In the emergency department, he undergoes CT of the cervical spine, as illustrated in ▸ Fig. 3.10. Which of the following best describes his injury?

- A. Jefferson fracture
- B. Type I odontoid fracture
- C. Type II odontoid fracture
- D. Type III odontoid fracture
- E. None of the above

Correct answer is E

The imaging shows a complex fracture of the dens with at least two points of fracture and comminution. The major fracture line is oriented anterior-superior to posterior-inferior with approximately 8 mm of retrolisthesis of the odontoid peg relative to the C2 body, and 30 degrees of angulation. Jefferson fractures are a type of axial loading injury of the C1 ring, with a full Jefferson fracture involving the bilateral anterior and posterior arches. Odontoid fractures are the most common cervical spine injury in the elderly population, accounting for 10 to 20% of all cervical spine injuries in those older than 65 years. Odontoid fracture can be classified using the Anderson D'Alonzo classification system as type I, II, or III. Type I injures are avulsion fractures of the alar ligaments and comprise 1% of injuries. Type II injuries are the most common and occur through the neck of the odontoid; they comprise approximately 75% of odontoid fractures. The Grauer modification splits type II factures into type IIA (minimal displacement), type IIB (displaced fracture with anterosuperior to posteroinferior fracture line orientation), and type IIC (displaced fracture with anterosuperior to posteroinferior fracture line orientation). Type III fractures extend into the C2 body. The present fracture has both type 2 and 3 fracture lines with comminution and so does not fall cleanly into any of the predefined categories.[31]

▸▸ Question 28

A 93-year-old woman on warfarin presents to the emergency department following a ground-level fall. CT shows the fracture in ▸ Fig. 3.11. The patient's anticoagulation is reversed, and he has consented to surgery. Which of the following surgical options will best address his fracture?

- A. C1–C2 anterior cervical diskectomy and fusion
- B. Odontoid screw
- C. C1–C2 fusion
- D. Occiput–C3 instrumented fusion
- E. Transoral odontoidectomy

Correct answer is C

The patient's instability is at the C1–C2 level; fusion of the atlanto-occipital joint (O–C1) is not necessary and can be very morbid in this patient population (option **D**). It is responsible for the majority of head flexion-extension (approximately 50%) and its fixation and fusion, especially in older patients, restricts their ability to view their feet while walking, making them an extremely high fall risk. The atlas (C1) does not have a vertebral body and there is no C1/C2 intervertebral disk; so, a C1–C2 anterior cervical diskectomy and fusion is not a procedure that can be performed. This leaves an odontoid screw and C1–C2 fusion. The odontoid screw is considered an elegant surgical option, as it is a lag screw that can directly reduce the odontoid fracture and spare motion at the C1–C2 joint. However, only a select set of fractures are candidates for this procedure. Patients with

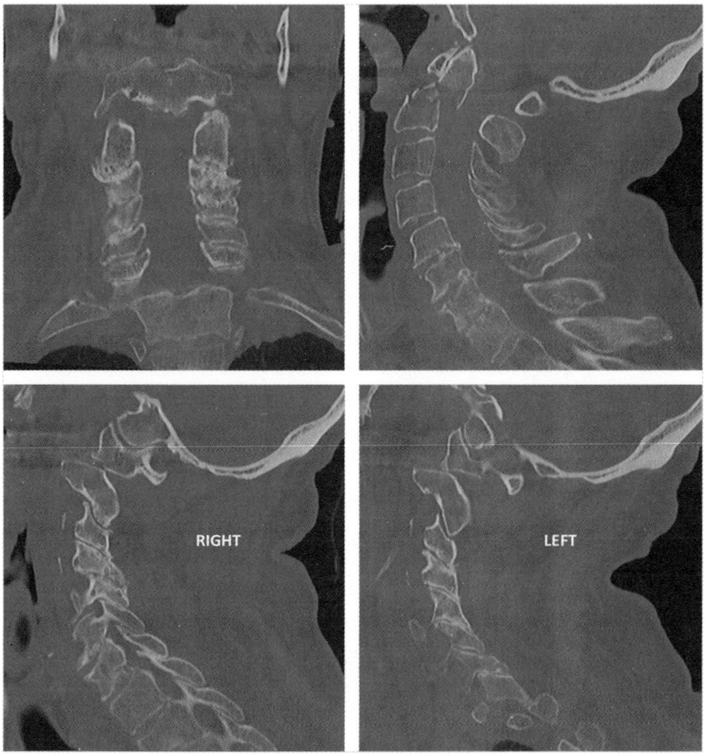

Fig. 3.10

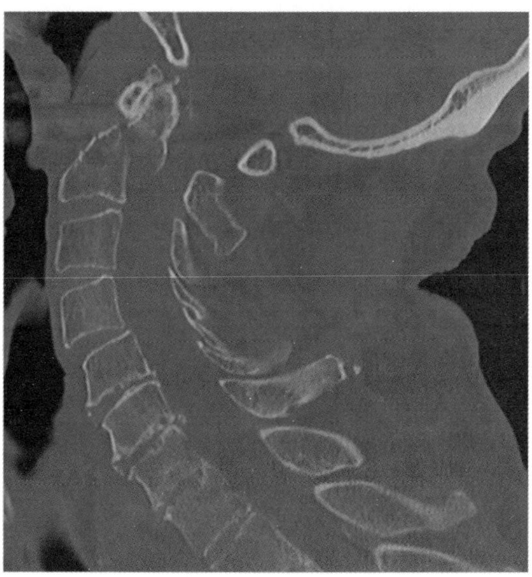

Fig. 3.11

highly angled fragments (> 11 degrees) or displaced fractures (> 2–3 mm) are unlikely to have their fragment reduced by the odontoid screw. Additionally, those with chronic nonunion (i.e., those without fresh fracture edges)—generally considered ≥ 6 months following the injury—have a more than threefold lower likelihood of successful fusion with an odontoid screw. The ideal candidate also has an anterosuperior to inferoposterior-oriented fracture line, which places the fracture line orthogonal to the long axis of the odontoid screw, maximizing screw capture. Those with poor underlying bone quality or with anteroinferior to posteroinferior fracture lines are unlikely to allow the odontoid screw sufficient purchase to reduce the fracture. Comminuted fractures are similarly not amenable to the odontoid screw, which cannot capture all of the fracture fragments. Last, advanced patient's age (increased risk of dysphagia with the procedure) and having a thick neck/barrel chest are considered relative contraindications, with the later making it difficult to achieve the correct angle for screw placement.

A C1–C2 posterior fusion is the ideal approach for this pathology. The most common approach employs lateral mass screws in the atlas (C1) and pedicle screws or pars screws in the axis (C2). Rib autograft, fibular autograft, or structural allograft can also be wired between the posterior C1 arch and C2 arch. Prior to instrumentation, it is advisable to look at the course of the vertebral artery, as a high-riding vertebral artery in the C2 neural foramen is associated with small pedicle diameter that can preclude placement of a C2 pedicle screw at this level. "Bail-out" options include translaminar screw and lateral mass screw. The major disadvantage of the C1–C2 fusion compared to the odontoid screw is a significant loss in rotational range of motion—approximately 50% of cervical spine rotation occurs at the atlantoaxial joint. Transoral odontoidectomy—historically used for retroodontoid pannus in the setting of rheumatoid arthritis—is at high risk for surgical site infection and will not address the instability suggested by the retrolisthesis of C1 on C2 seen in the CT.[31]

▸▸ Question 29

An elderly patient undergoes C1–C2 posterior fusion for a displaced type 2 odontoid fracture with concomitant central cord syndrome. The patient recovers well from the operation, but beginning on day 2 he begins to report numbness along his posterior scalp. What is the best explanation for this?

- A. Iatrogenic nerve injury
- B. Side effects of anesthesia
- C. Compression of the C2 roots by the bone graft
- D. Evolution of his central cord injury
- E. Expected of a malpositioned C2 screw

Correct answer is A

Though the onset of symptoms appears to be delayed, in all likelihood, the patient has had this deficit since surgery and is only now noticing it as the effects of anesthesia fully wear off. The numbness likely results from ligation of the C2 roots intraoperatively (iatrogenic injury, option **A**), which is commonly performed to expose the posterior aspect of C1 and facilitate placement of the C1 lateral mass screws. Bone graft for the C2 fusion is generally packed in the C1–C2 joints, where fusion is being targeted. Extrusion of bone graft from the joint could impinge upon the root, but nerve root irritation by graft or the screw head would be expected to present with pain or paresthesias as opposed to numbness. Central cord syndrome would not be expected to cause numbness on his posterior scalp. The effects of anesthesia should be diminishing 2 days after surgery, not worsening (option **B**). If the deficit was from a malpositioned screw, the deficit would be expected to be due to an inferiorly placed C1 screw as the sensory deficits are in the distribution of the greater occipital nerve, which runs between the C1 posterior arch and C2 laminae.[32]

▸▸ Question 30

To improve the probability of successful long-term fusion, collagen sponges with adsorbed recombinant bone morphogenetic protein-2 (BMP2, tradename Infuse, Medtronic) are placed in the atlanto-axial joint spaces in off-label fashion. Currently, there is only one FDA-approved indication for BMP2. For which of the following surgeries does this bone graft substitute have on-label indications?

- A. 1- or 2-level anterior cervical diskectomy and fusion
- B. 1- or 2-level transforaminal or posterior lumbar interbody fusion
- C. 5 + level posterolateral instrumented fusion
- D. 3- to 5-level thoracolumbar fusion for nonunion
- E. 1-level anterior lumbar interbody fusion

Correct answer is E

BMP2 adsorbed collagen sponges (INFUSE) were originally FDA-approved for a one-level L4–L5 or L5–S1 anterior lumbar interbody fusion (ALIF) in 2002, with subsequent approvals for tibial nonunion, and maxillofacial reconstruction. Its use in posterolateral cervical or thoracolumbar fusion is considered off-label, as is in XLIF/LLIF/DLIF, oblique lumbar interbody fusion, posterior lumbar interbody fusion, and transforaminal lumbar interbody fusion. However, it is often used in off-label fashion for patients deemed to be at increased risk of nonunion, such as those with significant smoking history, long-segment fusion, and revision fusion operations. BMP2 has been associated with seroma formation, nerve root irritation (BMP-associated radiculitis), ectopic bone formation, and retrograde ejaculation (when used in ALIF). Though there were originally fears that BMP2 could increase the risk of bone malignancy, this has not born out in the literature. Its use in anterior cervical operations is contraindicated and in 2009 the FDA put out a patient warning.[33,34]

►► Question 31

A 63-year-old female with a past medical history of obesity presents for evaluation of years of chronic low back and leg pain, predominantly in the anterior thighs and buttocks, which worsens throughout the day. She describes the pain as achy and notes that it is somewhat improved when she wakes up in the morning. The patient brings with her a set of standing radiographs, which are shown in ► Fig. 3.12. Which of the following best explains her leg pain?

- A. Neurogenic pseudoclaudication
- B. Vascular claudication
- C. Sagittal imbalance
- D. Bilateral hip osteoarthritis
- E. Sacroiliac joint dysfunction

Correct answer is C

The patient's pain localizes to the buttocks and thighs and worsens throughout the day, consistent with a fatigue-type picture. Neurogenic claudication generally worsens over the course of minutes to hours, though it also worsens with sustained upright posture. It is also generally described as sharp and commonly radiates distal to the knees. Vascular claudication similarly evolves over the course of minutes with exertion/muscle activation, creating a mismatch between oxygen supply and muscle demand. Though it is more difficult to appreciate in these films, the patient's left hip does not show bone-on-bone contact as might be expected from end-stage osteoarthritic changes of the left hip. Consequently, option **C** is the best answer.

In patients with adult spinal deformity, which affects 32 to 68% of those over 65 years of age, chronic sagittal imbalance can lead to leg (anterior thigh), buttock, and low-back pain as the patient subconsciously attempts to maintain upright posture. This involves initially extension of the back (decrease in or reversal of thoracic kyphosis with resultant back pain from paraspinal muscle activation), followed by pelvic retroversion (gluteal muscle activation and resultant buttock pain), and bending of the knees (anterior thigh pain from quadriceps activation to maintain a constant degree of knee flexion). These changes are best described under the paradigm of Dubousset's "cone of economy," whereby the body adopts changes in position to maintain the head and trunk over the patient's center of balance.[35,36,37]

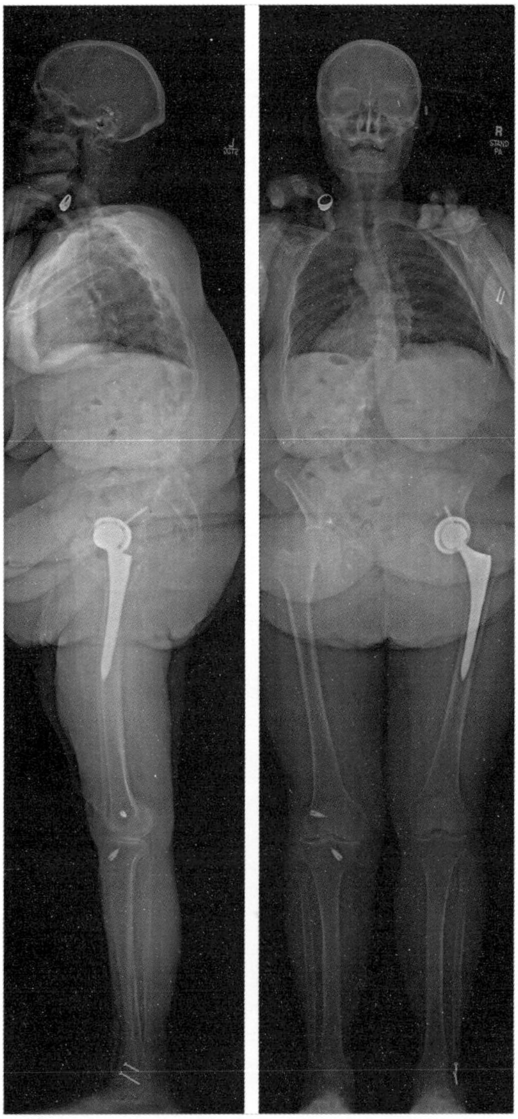

Fig. 3.12

▸▸ Question 32

A 91-year-old male presents to the emergency department with imaging showing a type 2 odontoid fracture with 40 degrees of posterior angulation. On meeting the patient, you explain his imaging but find that he is neurologically intact on examination. His first question is whether he needs to have surgery. He is currently independent in his activities of daily living and says that his main priority is returning to his current quality of life. Which of the following is the best response?

- A. Yes, he should have surgery because he has ongoing spinal cord compression and needs surgery to relieve this compression
- B. Yes, he should have surgery because his fracture is unlikely to heal without surgery
- C. No, he does not need to have surgery; his fracture will heal with bracing alone
- D. No, he is too old for surgery
- E. No, his history of thoracic aortic aneurysm makes him too high risk for surgery

Correct answer is B

The patient's imaging shows a fracture with comminution, significant displacement (> 3 mm), and significant angulation. All three features suggest a fracture that is unlikely to heal on its own (option **C**). Across all comers, surgical intervention for type II odontoid fractures has been associated with reduced mortality and superior functional outcomes, even among geriatric patients (option **D**). Type I and type III odontoid fractures are generally nonsurgical. They should undergo close radiographic follow-up to ensure successful bony union though. Declining the patient surgical intervention because of his aortic aneurysm is not reasonable, though it should be discussed with the anesthesiologist supporting the surgical case.[38,39]

▸▸ Question 33

A patient undergoing preoperative evaluation for thoracolumbar fusion for adult spinal deformity reports a history of prior Roux-en-Y gastric bypass. Nutritional optimization before surgery is requested by the consulting surgeon. Which of the following levels is most important for the patient to have tested prior to being scheduled for instrumented fusion to correct her deformity?

- A. Zinc
- B. Copper
- C. Cholecalciferol (vitamin D2)
- D. Vitamin B12
- E. Vitamin B3

Correct answer is C

Patients with a previous history of Roux-en-Y gastric bypass are at risk for multiple dietary insufficiencies. The most common include vitamin B12 and iron. However, neither of these has been linked to poorer fusion outcomes in patients undergoing instrumented fusion (option **C**). Vitamin D deficiency is increasingly recognized as a modifiable risk factor for improving successful fusion. Low zinc levels are associated with poorer wound healing outcomes and are occasionally seen only in the context of prior Roux-en-Y surgery.[40,41]

▸▸ Question 34

A patient with prior left total hip arthroplasty is being considered for long-segment thoracolumbar fusion. The patient undergoes preoperative bone health testing, including a dual-energy X-ray absorptiometry (DXA/DEXA), which shows a total hip bone mineral density of 0.728 g/cm^2 (T score: -2.2; Z score: -1.5). Which of the following best describes her underlying bone quality?

- A. Normal bone density
- B. Osteopenia
- C. Osteoporosis
- D. DXA cannot be used for patients with adult spinal deformity
- E. DXA cannot be used for patients with prior hip arthroplasty

Correct answer is C

Patient's bone mineral density (BMD) is classified currently based on the results of DXA. Areas measured include the femoral neck, total hip, distal radius, and L1–L4 spine. Degenerative changes in the lumbar spine make this a suboptimal location for assessing BMD. Total hip and femoral neck are preferred, though increasingly other metrics, such as HU of the lumbar spine, are being investigated. Classification is made by T-score, which compares the patient's measured BMD to that of a young sex-matched adult with peak bone mass. A DXA T-score ≥ -1.0 corresponds to normal bone density, scores -1.0 to -2.4 correspond to osteopenia (low bone mass), and a score of -2.5 or lower diagnoses osteoporosis. While DXA of the hip is considered nondiagnostic for patients with bilateral hip arthroplasty, this patient has only a unilateral implant and so imaging of the contralateral hip is valid.

▸▸ Question 35

Surgical correction with long-segment thoracolumbar fusion is recommended for a patient with significant degenerative kyphoscoliosis. However, the patient's preoperative bone health testing shows osteopenia. To optimize the patient's odds of a good outcome from surgery, it is decided that she should undergo preoperative therapy with teriparatide (Forteo). Which of the following is the target of teriparatide?

- A. The parathyroid hormone receptor
- B. Sclerostin
- C. The RANKL ligand
- D. Pyrophosphate mimic in osteoclasts
- E. Vitamin D transporters in the small intestine

Correct answer is A

Teriparatide (Forteo) and abaloparatide (Tymlos) are parathyroid hormone-related peptide analogs that bind to the PTH1 receptor, resulting in the stimulation of osteoblast function. Denosumab (Prolia) binds to the RANKL ligand on osteoclasts. Romosozumab (Evenity) binds to and inhibits sclerostin, a negative regulator of the Wnt/β-catenin pathway. Bisphosphonates (zoledronic acid, alendronate, risedronate, ibandronate) act as pyrophosphate analogs that prevent bone resorption. PTH-related peptide analogs (abaloparatide, teriparatide), denosumab, and romosozumab are all anabolic agents—they can build bone mass, whereas bisphosphonates are antiresorptive agents, aimed at preventing further bone loss. Oftentimes, patients will be started on antiresorptive therapies upon discontinuing anabolic agents, as withdrawal of these agents can lead to accelerated bone loss.

▸▸ Question 36

A patient with progressive degenerative kyphoscoliotic deformity is noted to have an L1–S1 lumbar lordosis of 28 degrees and a pelvic incidence of 70 degrees. It is determined that as part of her surgical operation she should undergo significant sagittal plane correction in the inferior lumbar spine. Which of the following options will offer the greatest correction?

- A. Smith-Peterson osteotomy/partial facet resection
- B. Ponte osteotomy/complete facet resection
- C. Pedicle subtraction osteotomy (PSO)
- D. Transforaminal lumbar interbody fusion with lordotic cage
- E. Sacral dome osteotomy

Correct answer is C

Sagittal plane correction is achieved through a combination of interbody device placement/anterior column lengthening and osteotomy/posterior column shortening. Schwab and colleagues published a classification system for spinal osteotomies in 2014. Of the options listed, PSO is the most aggressive posterior column shortening and can offer up to 25 degrees of segmental lordosis. An extended PSO can offer up to 40 degrees of correction. However, it is an extremely morbid procedure with blood loss often exceeding a liter and prolonged hospitalization as compared to similar procedures without PSO. The associated blood loss may also require a short stay in the ICU for closer monitoring of hemodynamic status. Complications are also common, with a large multicenter series published by Smith and colleagues noting complications in more than 75% of patients. While sacral dome osteotomy can also provide correction, it is an uncommonly employed technique and is technically more complex than a PSO. It is generally used only for the correction of high-grade spondylolisthesis versus spondyloptosis in patients with high pelvic incidence.[42,43,44,45,46,47,48]

▸▸ Question 37

A 72-year-old female presents with chronic low-back pain worsened with upright posture and prolonged activity. Preoperative imaging shows a flat back deformity. It is decided to try and achieve sagittal correction with multilevel interbody placement, including interbody fusion at L4/L5 and L5/S1. Which of the following strategies will be most effective at correcting her lumbar lordosis–pelvic incidence (PI-LL) mismatch?

- A. L5/S1 anterior lumbar interbody fusion (ALIF)
- B. L5/S1 XLIF
- C. L5/S1 TLIF
- D. L5/S1 PLIF
- E. L5/S1 TLIF with bilateral facetectomies

Correct answer is A

The ALIF allows for the greatest segmental lordosis of any of the interbody techniques, though some groups have suggested that an oblique lumbar interbody fusion or extreme lateral (XLIF)/direct lateral (DLIF) approach can offer similar correction with the new hyperlordotic cages. However, the XLIF/DLIF technique cannot be performed at the L5/S1 level, as the pelvic wing/iliac crest blocks a lateral approach to the disk space (option **B**). TLIF/PLIF, when performed properly with a lordotic cage, can offer 10 degrees of correction; however, the cage must be positioned at the front of the disk space and generally there should be compression on the screws posteriorly. By comparison, an ALIF offers 15 degrees or more. In a recent publication by the International Spine Study Group, a multicenter collaboration of spinal deformity surgeons found that deformity correction including L5/S1 ALIF (vs. TLIF) was associated with 70% increased odds of achieved ideal sagittal balance as well as a substantial clinical benefit in patient-reported outcomes at 2-year follow-up. In another recent comparison by this group directly comparing results in patients treated with ALIF or TLIF at L4–L5 and/or L5–S1 as part of their surgical correction, the authors noted that ALIF at L5/S1 afforded nearly double the segmental lordosis of TLIF. Additionally, the large footprint of ALIF cages means they exert lower von Mises stresses on the adjoining endplates, reducing the risk of implant subsidence. The addition of bilateral facetectomies to the TLIF will help increase lordosis. However, in the hands of most surgeons, it would not be expected to provide as great of a sagittal plane correction as an ALIF with a hyperlordotic implant.

▸▸ Question 38

A patient undergoing evaluation for correction of her degenerative scoliosis mentions to the surgeon that she has a friend who also underwent spinal fusion recently with a procedure called an "extreme lateral interbody fusion (XLIF)." The patient says she heard this procedure is minimally invasive and wants to know if she would be a candidate. In discussing the possibility of XLIF/direct lateral interbody fusion (DLIF) as part of her surgical plan, which of the following complications is most important to discuss?

- A. Aorta/great vessel injury
- B. Durotomy
- C. Femoral nerve palsy
- D. Retrograde ejaculation
- E. Durotomy

Correct answer is C

The transpsoas/direct lateral approach (XLIF/DLIF/LLIF) is a minimally invasive, "muscle-splitting" approach for lumbar interbody fusion that uses a transpsoas corridor to access the lumbar disk space. Advantages are that it avoids dissection of the paraspinal musculature, minimizes risk to the nerve roots and thecal sac (as it uses an approach that is purely ventral to these structures), and minimizes risk posed to the great vessels. However, the lumbar plexus traverses the psoas muscle, and consequently the transpsoas approach places the lumbar plexus at risk for injury. It is estimated that up to one-third of patients will have transient hip flexor weakness up to 6 weeks postoperatively; however, the prevalence of femoral nerve injury is 1 to 2% (highest risk at L4/L5 interspace as the femoral nerve is most anteriorly positioned at this level). The biggest risk factor for this injury is thought to be prolonged retractor time, though this has not been consistently borne out by the literature. "Breaking the table"—a maneuver used to increase the ease of accessing the disk space by inducing a convexity at the target level—can also increase the risk of postoperative motor deficits. Intraoperative neuromonitoring with EMG is considered a standard part of the transpsoas approach and is aimed at reducing intraoperative lumbar plexus injury. A threshold of

8 mA is used by many surgeons; triggering EMG potentials with ≤ 8 mA is thought to highlight a lumbar plexus that is too close to the retractor, and which is at risk for injury. However, EMG is imperfect, and other modalities, notably saphenous nerve somatosensory evoked potentials, are currently being explored to reduce the odds of intraoperative nerve injury.[49,50,51,52]

▸▸ Question 39

A patient undergoes L2–L5 posterior fusion and L2/L3, L3/L4 lateral interbody fusion for degenerative lumbar scoliosis. The patient was discharged from the hospital uneventfully but returned to the clinic for her 6-week follow-up with a painless bulge on the side of surgery that has persisted since surgery, but which reduces with palpation. What is this bulge and what is the best explanation for it?

- A. Approach-related hernia due to improper wound closure
- B. Pseudohernia from injury to the nerve in the abdominal wall musculature
- C. Genitofemoral nerve injury during passage of the retractor through the psoas muscle
- D. Stunning of the lumbar plexus during triggered EMG
- E. Wound site hematoma

Correct answer is B

The pathology described is abdominal pseudohernia, which is reported to occur in approximately 2% of patients. It results from injury to the motor branches of the subcostal (T12), iliohypogastric (T12–L1), and/or ilioinguinal (predominantly L1; some T12 fibers) nerves. The subcostal nerve innervates the external oblique and rectus abdominis, while the iliohypogastric and ilioinguinal nerves innervate the internal oblique and transversus abdominis muscles. Injury to the motor branches results in paralysis of these muscles with resultant weakening of the abdominal wall and pseudohernia. Abdominal pseudohernia is thoroughly documented in the abdominal and gynecological surgery literature and is now recognized as an uncommon complication of direct lateral/transpsoas surgery. In one large multicenter series by Dakwar and colleagues, 10 of 568 patients experienced abdominal pseudohernia. Eight experienced recovery by 6-month follow-up. A hematoma would be noted in the first several days postoperatively and would be appreciated as a palpable mass. By 6-week follow-up, it should be appreciably smaller in size.[53]

▸▸ Question 40

A 66-year-old male with past medical comorbidities including type 2 diabetes mellitus complicated by nephropathy and neuropathy, paroxysmal atrial fibrillation, chronic osteomyelitis, and chronic kidney disease presented to the local emergency department after a fall at home. Patient complains of back pain, urinary incontinence, and bilateral lower extremity weakness. The patient's white cell counts and inflammatory markers are elevated. During the bedside examination, the patient showed weakness in the bilateral lower extremities with noticeable drift. What is the next step in evaluation?

- A. CT of the cervical/thoracic/lumbar spine
- B. MR of the cervical/thoracic/lumbar spine
- C. PET/CT scan
- D. Upright scoliosis radiographs
- E. CT of the head

Correct answer is B

The patient with a known history of osteomyelitis presents with new bilateral lower extremity weakness. This is concerning for the development of an epidural abscess with resultant spinal cord compression, or cauda equina, which is reported to occur in 17% of cases. The best test for evaluating this is an MRI of the spine with and without gadolinium contrast. The weakness in the lower extremities could be explained by compression present at any level at or above the lumbar spine. Imaging should include cuts through the thoracic and cervical spine and the lumbar spine. CT can be used to evaluate the extent of bony destruction caused by the underlying osteomyelitis; however, it will not provide information about spinal cord compression. PET/CT may show increased uptake at the site of osteomyelitis, but it will not be instructive as part of surgical evaluation. Upright scoliosis radiographs will not provide useful information about the need for surgical intervention. There is nothing on this patient's examination to suggest that intracranial pathology is the cause of his presentation, and he should undergo spinal imaging for initial evaluation.

▸▸ Question 41

A patient with new bilateral lower extremity paraparesis, urinary incontinence, and elevated inflammatory markers undergoes MR and CT of his thoracic spine (▶ Fig. 3.13). What is the next best step in his management?

- A. Intravenous antibiotics and admission to the general care floor
- B. Intravenous antibiotics and fine needle aspiration of the epidural abscess for organism identification
- C. T6–T7 laminectomy and evacuation of the epidural abscess

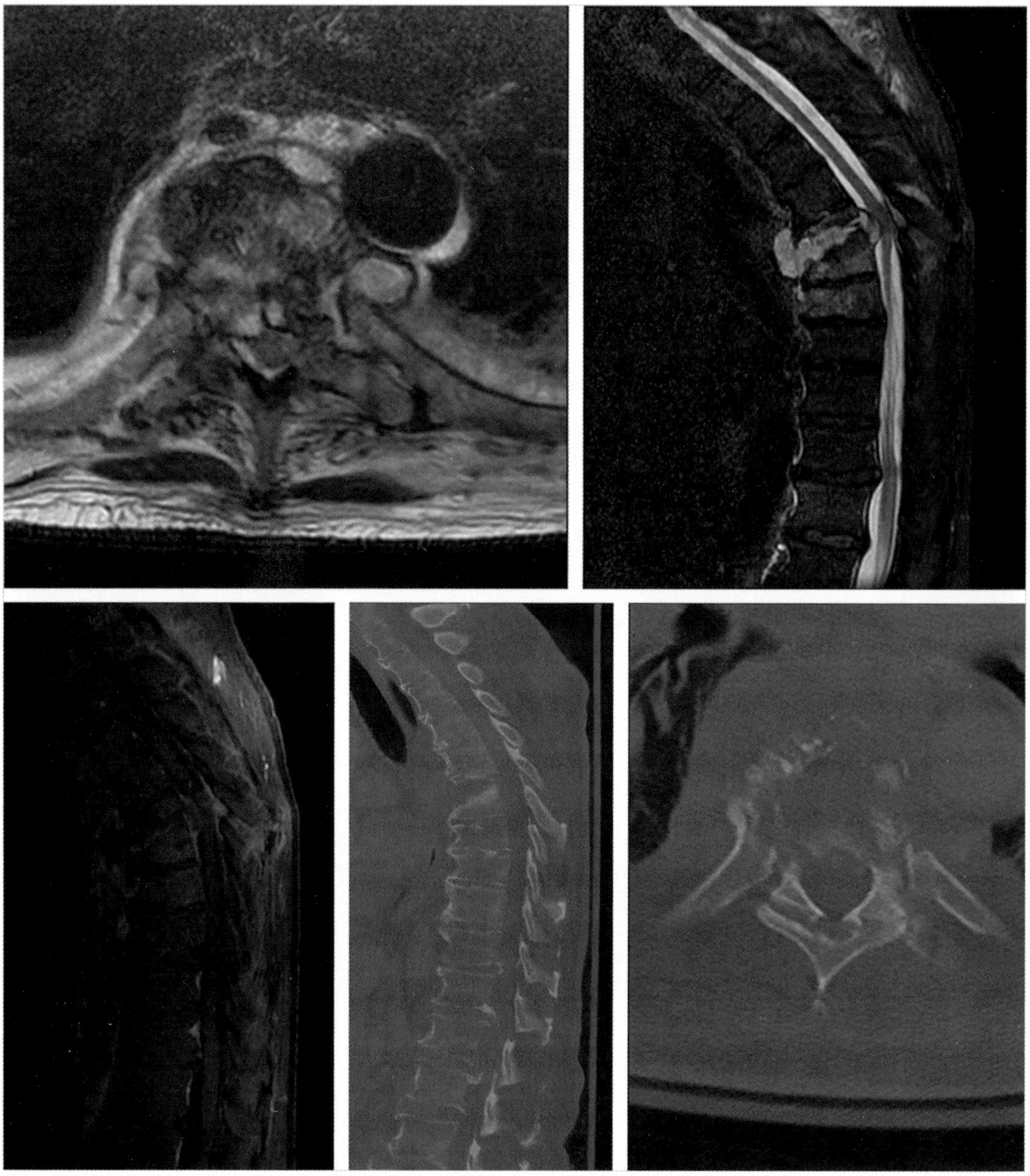

Fig. 3.13

- D. T4–T9 fusion; T6–T7 laminectomy; evacuation of the epidural abscess
- E. T5–T8 anterior fusion; T5–T6 corpectomy

Correct answer is C

The patient's MR and CT demonstrate osteomyelitis at the T6–T7 level with a circumferential epidural abscess causing compression of the mid-thoracic spinal cord. The CT demonstrates erosion of the T6/T7 disk space with focal kyphosis at this level, which will likely demonstrate worsened kyphosis on load-bearing films (upright X-rays). The chronic osteomyelitis has left the bony spine structurally incompetent and ultimately surgical intervention will require both spinal cord decompression and evacuation of the abscess, as well as stabilization of the spine. A decompression alone (option **C**) will not address the underlying instability; a staged decompression followed by fusion is plausible but carries with it an additional anesthesia event and the risks accordant with that. A T5–T8 standalone anterior fusion (option **E**) will not provide the same degree of stabilization as the T4–T9 posterior fusion, though the corpectomy will allow for anterior column support. Nevertheless, the anterior transthoracic approach is excessively morbid for this patient. Of note, a recent review by Boody et al recommended surgical intervention for patients with vertebral osteomyelitis if there is a new neurological deficit, > 50% spinal cord compression, involvement of 5 + contiguous vertebrae, radiological evidence of spinal instability, kyphosis > 60 degrees at the site of osteomyelitis, involvement of all three columns (anterior, middle, and posterior columns of Denis), or development of an epidural abscess.

▸▸ Question 42

A patient with a history of intravenous drug use presents to the emergency department with new lower extremity paraparesis and undergoes MR of the thoracic spine showing T6 osteomyelitis with an associated epidural abscess. He undergoes surgical evacuation of the abscess, during which bacterial cultures are drawn. Which of the following organisms is most likely to be identified from the culture data?

- A. *Staphylococcus epidermidis*
- B. *Staphylococcus aureus*
- C. *Aspergillus* species
- D. *Pseudomonas aeruginosa*
- E. No organisms identified (culture-negative osteomyelitis)

Correct answer is B

Although all of the above are possibilities, *Staphylococcus aureus* is the most common cause of vertebral osteomyelitis. Intravenous drug use is a risk factor for the development of osteomyelitis, as are a history of diabetes mellitus, coronary heart disease, an immunosuppressed state, active cancer, and renal failure. In one study of seven Cleveland area hospitals, the most common sources for the vertebral osteomyelitis were the skin or soft tissue infection, infection of a vascular access site, endocarditis, bursitis, and septic arthritis. Roughly 50% of cases of pyogenic vertebral osteomyelitis—the most common type of osteomyelitis—occur secondary to hematogenous spread (e.g., endocarditis), whereas 15 to 40% occur from direct inoculation of the bone or disk space. It is estimated that some 17% of cases of vertebral osteomyelitis are complicated by epidural abscess, and 38% of patients with vertebral osteomyelitis will develop neurological complications.

▸▸ Question 43

A patient with a history of intravenous drug use presents with low-back pain and undergoes an MRI showing diskitis. She is treated with 4 weeks of intravenous antibiotics, but repeat imaging shows persistent diskitis. Which of the following features of the intervertebral disks complicates the treatment of osteomyelitis/diskitis with intravenous antibiotics?

- A. The intervertebral disks are avascular
- B. The intervertebral disks are immunoprivileged
- C. The intervertebral disks are deep-seated tissues and so see lower doses of antibiotics
- D. Osteomyelitis/diskitis is characterized by higher rates of infection with resistant organisms
- E. Intravenous antibiotics is not the first-line treatment for diskitis

Correct answer is A

The intervertebral disks are avascular anatomic compartments and antibiotic penetration of the intervertebral disk tissue relies on diffusion from the capillary beds of the adjoining vertebral body endplates. Intravenous antibiotics are the first-line therapy for osteomyelitis/diskitis without epidural abscess.

▸▸ Question 44

A patient with a history of a prior kidney transplant on chronic immunosuppression presents with bilateral lower extremity paraparesis and imaging showing a lumbar epidural abscess with complete effacement of the thecal sac. The patient was being treated with broad-spectrum antibiotics for 6 weeks. Surgical decompression is recommended. Which of the following steps is most likely to improve his long-term neurological outcome?

- A. Administration of 10 mg dexamethasone intravenously
- B. Blood pressure augmentation to a mean arterial pressure > 85 mm Hg
- C. Decompression within 24 hours of symptom onset
- D. Early transition to broad-spectrum antibiotics
- E. Use of intraoperative vancomycin powder

Correct answer is C

The patient is already on intravenous antibiotics, and as evidenced by the radiographic and clinical progression, his current antibiotic regimen is unable to control the underlying osteomyelitis infection. Although a broader-spectrum agent may be useful in the ultimate clearance of the infection, it will not reverse the epidural abscess or neurological deficits (option **D**). Blood pressure augmentation is recommended to improve outcomes in patients with acute spinal cord injury, but it is not the best option for spinal epidural abscess. Dexamethasone is often given in the context of metastatic epidural spinal cord compression, but as an immunosuppressant, it is the wrong option here and will likely be ineffective, especially if the epidural phlegmon has become organized. Emergent decompression (< 24 hours after symptom onset) will offer this patient the best chance at long-term neurological recovery. One study by Rigamonti and colleagues considering 75 patients with spinal epidural abscess found that poor outcomes—defined as paraplegia or incontinence of bowel/bladder—were fivefold less common in those decompressed within 24 hours of presentation. Intraoperative vancomycin powder use has not been shown to improve infection clearance in osteomyelitis/diskitis.[54,55,56,57]

▸▸ Question 45

A 62-year-old woman with a past medical history of hyperlipidemia presented to the clinic with lower-back pain progressive over a 1-year period, localizing predominantly to the tailbone. She also endorsed occasional pain at night and pain with sitting. She denied pain or sensory changes in her legs. After initial management with conservative therapies, she underwent imaging that showed the mass (▸ Fig. 3.14). What is the next best step in management?

- A. Bladder scan for post-void residual
- B. Core needle biopsy
- C. Transrectal fine needle aspiration

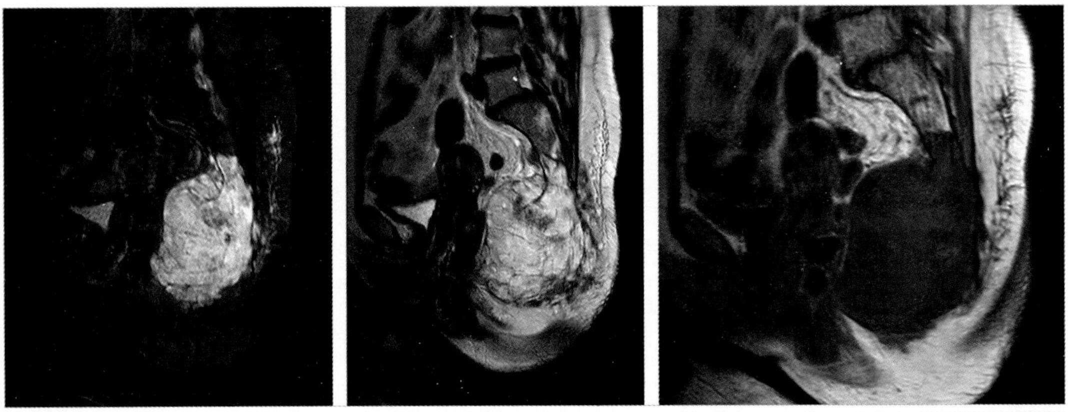

Fig. 3.14

- D. Resection of the mass
- E. Serial imaging

Correct answer is B

The imaging demonstrates a T1 hypointense, T2 hyperintense sacral lesion involving the S2–S5 sacrum and coccyx, likely with the involvement of the sacral nerve roots. These imaging findings are concerning for a primary vertebral column malignancy, such as chordoma, chondrosarcoma, or osteosarcoma. While the best oncologic treatment for these lesions hinges on *en bloc* resection with negative margins where possible, it is important to first verify that the mass is a primary malignancy. The surgical approach will vary significantly if the mass is found to be a schwannoma (which can have intrasacral extension and erosion of the sacral bone) or a metastatic lesion; in both of these cases, piecemeal resection is a reasonable option and would afford significantly reduced morbidity. Therefore, a biopsy to determine the pathology is imperative to guide treatment. Given that prior studies have suggested the tumor cells are capable of seeding the biopsy tract site, the biopsy should be performed through the planned surgical incision. A transrectal biopsy is not recommended, given the potential to seed the tumor into the rectum. Serial imaging is not appropriate, as the mass appears consistent with a primary spinal column neoplasm, for which treatment, often in the form of surgical resection, is merited.[58,59]

▸▸ Question 46

A 55-year-old woman presents with progressive low-back pain and MR imaging showing a large sacral mass. She undergoes a biopsy of the mass, which stains positive for brachyury. From which of the following embryological tissues did this mass arise?

- A. Somitic mesoderm
- B. Notochord
- C. Neural crest cells
- D. Lateral plate mesoderm
- E. Prechordal mesoderm

Correct answer is B

The mass stains positively for *brachyury*, which identifies it as a chordoma. Chordoma arises from the notochord—a rod of mesoderm running along the cephalocaudal axis that is essential for dorsal-ventral patterning through the formation of a sonic hedgehog gradient. The only remnants of the notochord in the adult body are the nuclei pulposi of the intervertebral disks.[58,60]

▸▸ Question 47

A patient presents with low-back pain and imaging demonstrating a large sacral mass shown to be biopsy-proven chordoma. Given the rarity of the lesion, the patient is referred to a tertiary care center and her case is presented in front of a multidisciplinary tumor board consisting of multiple medical specialists. Her staging imaging shows disease isolated to the sacrum, with no other sites of disease noted along the spine or on CT of the chest/abdomen/pelvis. Which of the following surgical approaches is the board most likely to recommend as the best approach to treat her disease?

- A. Subtotal resection
- B. Gross total piecemeal resection
- C. No resection; chemoradiation therapy alone
- D. *En bloc* resection
- E. Hemicorporectomy

Correct answer is D

Primary vertebral column tumors are extremely resistant to both radiotherapy and chemotherapy. Surgical resection is considered the core of definitive management, where possible. In this patient's case, an *en bloc* sacrectomy is likely to be recommended. *En bloc* resection encompasses surgical resection of the mass with a surrounding cuff of healthy, noninvolved tissue. Violation of the capsule is thought to allow seeding of the resection cavity with tumor, raising the risk of recurrence. Studies such as that of Akiyama et al have suggested that even resection *en bloc* with negative margins may not remove all disease, as "micro-skip" metastases are present in over 40% of cases.[61] These lesions represent local tissue invasion up to 2 cm outside of the macroscopic tumor margin.

▸▸ Question 48

A patient with biopsy-proven, isolated sacral chordoma is recommended for surgical resection by the tumor board at her treating hospital. The tumor board also makes recommendations on adjuvant therapies. Which of the following adjuvant therapies is the tumor board most likely to recommend?

- A. Adjuvant chemotherapy with doxorubicin
- B. Adjuvant immunotherapy with nivolumab and ipilimumab

- C. Adjuvant radiotherapy with 7040 cGyE proton radiotherapy to the tumor bed
- D. Adjuvant chemotherapy with etoposide and 7040 cGyE stereotactic photon radiotherapy to the tumor bed
- E. Neoadjuvant chemotherapy with doxorubicin and adjuvant radiotherapy in the case of lesion progression on serial imaging

Correct answer is C

Due to the rarity of primary vertebral column malignancies, prospective data are limited and so most recommendations are based on level III evidence from retrospective cohorts. Nevertheless, these data suggest that the addition of adjuvant radiotherapy improves local control and recurrence-free survival. There is no evidence to suggest the superiority of proton/charged particle therapy over focused photon radiation (e.g., CyberKnife/linear accelerator-based therapy, intensity modulated radiotherapy), and the choice of modality is largely based on institutional availability and experience. Focused photon radiotherapy and charged particle therapy are preferred, as the more focused delivery of radiotherapy afforded by these modalities allows for delivery of therapeutic radiation doses to the operative bed while minimizing off-target toxicities.[62,63,64,65]

▸▸ Question 49

A patient with a newly diagnosed sacral chordoma is taken to the operating room for a staged surgery. The anterior stage creates a transverse osteotomy through the S1/S2 space, neurolyses the S1 roots, and neurectomizes the S2–S4 and coccygeal nerve roots. The second stage performs the remaining release and delivers the tumor. The patient spends a short time in the ICU before transferring to the floor and is successfully transferred to inpatient rehabilitation for post-hospitalization recovery. Which of the following deficits is the patient most likely to have on discharge?

- A. Urinary and stool incontinence
- B. Dorsal foot numbness
- C. Plantarflexor weakness
- D. Great toe extensor (extensor hallucis longus) weakness
- E. Foot dorsiflexor weakness

Correct answer is A

The procedure as described indicates that the patient underwent intraoperative sacrifice of the S2, S3, S4, S5, and coccygeal nerve roots. These nerve roots provide sensation on the perineum as well as the function of the bowel and bladder. In one review by Zoccali et al, all patients who underwent sacrifice of both S2 nerve roots and all nerve roots distal to this level had major bowel problems in 96.4% of cases and major bladder dysfunction in 97.8% of the cases.[66] For comparison, motor function was reported as normal in 56.3% of the cases. Sparing of at least one S2 root was associated with significantly superior retention of urinary and bowel function, with major bladder dysfunction in only 75% of cases and major bowel dysfunction in only 37.5% of the cases.[67]

▸▸ Question 50

A 71-year-old male with a history of metastatic prostate cancer presented to the local emergency department with 2 days of progressive lower-extremity weakness and numbness, progressing to the point of non-ambulation. On examination, he has activation of all major muscle groups in the lower extremities but cannot lift his legs off the bed. He also endorses numbness in both legs. He undergoes imaging as demonstrated in ▸ Fig. 3.15. Which of the following is the next best step in management?

- A. Delayed thoracic laminectomy and resection of epidural disease
- B. Emergent thoracic laminectomy and resection of epidural disease
- C. Emergent transthoracic T6 corpectomy and resection of epidural disease
- D. Scheduled intravenous corticosteroids
- E. Radiotherapy with charged particle therapy or focused photon radiotherapy

Correct answer is B

The patient's CT demonstrates multifocal osteoblastic lesions consistent with multifocal metastatic prostate cancer. Additionally, MR demonstrates a heterogeneously gadolinium-enhancing mass of the T5 vertebral body with significant epidural disease burden causing spinal cord compression (Bilsky grade 3/epidural spinal cord compression grade 3). The patient's clinical

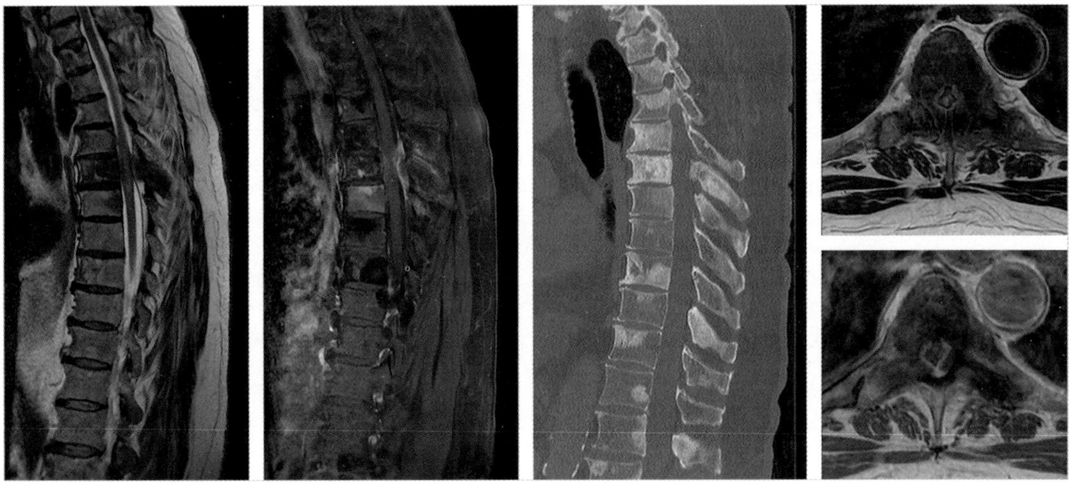

Fig. 3.15

and radiographic pictures are suggestive of symptomatic, high-grade epidural spinal cord compression. The gold standard of treatment for this pathology is spinal cord decompression, which in this case is best achieved through laminectomy and resection of the epidural disease component. Evidence for this strategy is derived from the randomized controlled trial by Patchell and colleagues in 2005, who compared treatment of epidural spinal cord compression with surgical decompression followed by adjuvant radiotherapy to radiotherapy alone. They found that the mean time retaining the ability to walk was significantly greater in patients treated with decompression and radiotherapy (122 vs. 13 days).

Conventionally, an expected prognosis of 3 to 6 months was used to divide patients who were surgical candidates from those who should be treated nonsurgically. However, with the increasing development of minimally invasive techniques, the proportion of patients who are surgical candidates has increased; prognoses in oncology are also increasing as a whole. Though the evidence from the Patchell trial still guides therapy, the increased availability of these minimally invasive techniques has led to a paradigm shift at many centers toward "separation surgery," where surgery is treated as a neoadjuvant to definitive radiotherapy. Decompression is performed at the points of high-grade compression to debulk the epidural disease and create a tumor-free margin around the spinal cord. The remaining tumor is then irradiated. In this patient with multifocal metastatic cancer, a transthoracic approach is likely to be a morbid procedure and affords no benefit for neurological recovery as compared to a posterior decompression.[68,69,70,71,72]

▸▸ Question 51

A patient with metastatic prostate cancer undergoes thoracic MRI and CT to evaluate new rapidly progressive bilateral lower extremity paresis, which shows multifocal osteoblastic metastases and epidural spinal cord compression at T5. Despite his malignancy, the patient was reportedly independent in all of his activities of daily living prior to his recent decline. He endorses nonspecific, "achy," mid-back pain, but is unable to identify any exacerbating factors. Based on this, which of the following surgical strategies will best address his symptoms?

- A. T2–T7 instrumented fusion, T4–T6 laminectomy, T5 partial corpectomy
- B. T4–T6 laminectomy; T3–T7 percutaneous fusion
- C. T4–T6 laminectomy; resection of epidural disease
- D. T4–T6 laminectomy followed by T5 percutaneous vertebroplasty
- E. T5–T6 interlaminar decompression

Correct answer is C

The formulation of a surgical plan for spinal metastasis is encapsulated in the NOMS framework, as articulated by Laufer et al at Memorial Sloan Kettering. This considers patients based on four factors—neurological status ("N"), oncology/the underlying pathology ("O"), mechanical assessment ("M"), and systemic assessment ("S"). The neurological assessment questions what the tumor is doing to the spinal cord and nerve roots; grading can be performed using the Bilsky grading scale (see references), where high-grade epidural spinal cord compression (grades 2–3) generally merits surgical decompression. In this patient's case, there is grade 3 compression of the spinal cord at T5 and so any surgical plan must include a T5 laminectomy for central decompression, though likely an inferior T4 partial laminectomy and superior T6 partial laminectomy should likely be included at a minimum to ensure complete decompression. Next, the patient's pathology is known. Prostate cancer is often considered to be relatively radioresponsive; so, radiation can be reasonably considered for the treatment of residual disease after a safe margin has been created around the spinal cord. Next, the mechanical assessment can be guided by the Spinal Instability Neoplastic Score (SINS), which evaluates the perceived mechanical stability of the affected spine segment. In this patient's case, he has a lesion of the semirigid spine (1 point), associated with nonmechanical pain (1 point), that is blastic (0 points), without deformity or vertebral body collapse (0 points), but which involves > 50% of the vertebral body (1 point) and both pedicles (3 points). This means the lesion has a SINS score of 6 and is likely a biomechanically "stable" lesion; so, internal fixation is not necessary. The final metric—systemic assessment—is used to assess the patient's suitability for/ability to tolerate surgery. Increasingly surgery is offered to sicker, more frail patients. Regardless, this patient was reportedly independent in all activities of daily living prior to presentation (Karnofsky performance status 90—only mild symptoms) and so is a reasonable surgical candidate. Based on this, his surgical plan should include decompression but does not require the addition of a stabilization procedure.[69,73,74,75,76]

▸▸ Question 52

The patient undergoes the surgical procedure above and successfully discharges from the acute care hospital on postoperative day 7 to home. The patient's home is a considerable distance from the hospital, and the decision is made to have him undergo hypofractionated radiotherapy with 24 Gy in three fractions on postoperative days 5, 6, and 7 prior to discharging home. The risk for which of the following complications is most likely increased by this early initiation of radiotherapy?

- A. Malignancy degeneration of the tumor
- B. Radiation-induced spinal cord injury/neurological decline
- C. Wound dehiscence
- D. Venous thromboembolism
- E. Atrial fibrillation

Correct answer is C

The evidence describing the relation of wound complications to the initiation of adjuvant radiotherapy is low quality; however, of the data available, there appears to be a suggestion that earlier initiation of radiotherapy may be associated with increased odds of wound complications. In a systematic review by Kumar et al, the authors noted mixed evidence with preoperative radiotherapy being cited as the most common risk factor for wound complications, though they found that the bulk of the evidence suggested irradiation within 7 days of surgery increases the risk of wound complications.[70,77,78]

▸▸ Question 53

A 49-year-old male presents to the clinic with 4 years of progressive back pain, now with several months of left lateral thigh paresthesias. Patient underwent MR of the lumbar spine with and without gadolinium contrast, which is shown below. Which of the following is the best explanation for these imaging findings (▶ Fig. 3.16)?

- A. Conus medullaris arteriovenous malformation
- B. Extramedullary spinal cord tumor
- C. Intrathecal disk herniation
- D. Epidural abscess
- E. Arachnoiditis

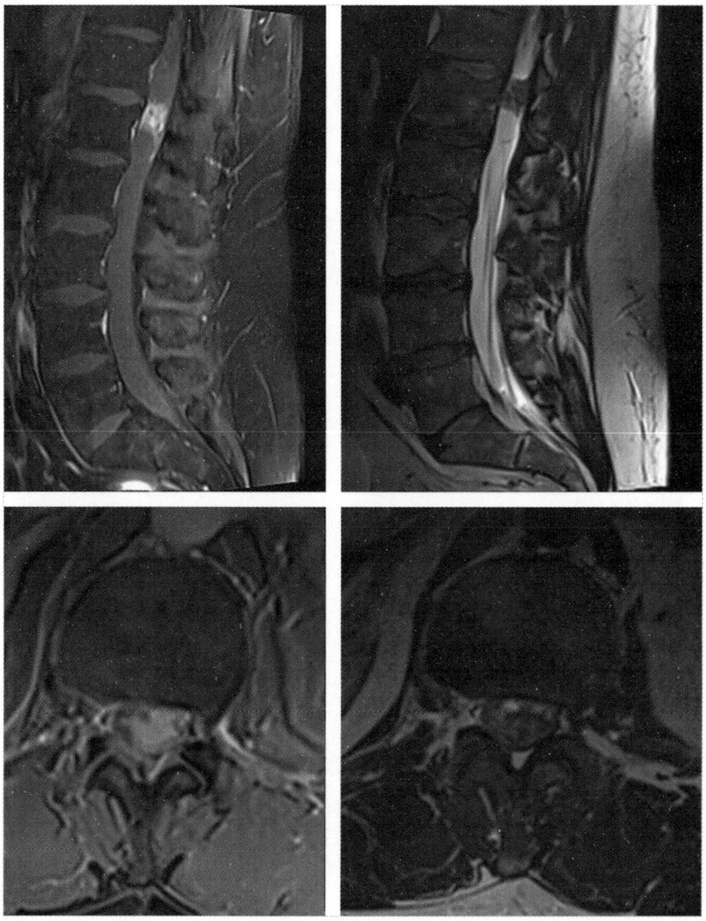

Fig. 3.16

Correct answer is B

The imaging demonstrates a heterogeneously enhancing 2.0 × 1.0 × 1.5 cm solid/cystic mass at the level of T12/L1 that is effacing the spinal canal. While disk herniations can become intrathecal, they would not be expected to show gadolinium enhancement, which is one means of differentiating recurrent disk herniations from postoperative inflammation in patients with recurrent symptoms following diskectomy. An abscess would not be expected to form a discrete intrathecal mass like the one demonstrated here, and it would additionally be uncommon in the absence of osteomyelitis or a clear risk factor, such as intravenous drug use, endocarditis, or an epidural injection that could directly inoculate bacteria into this space. Last, conus medullaris arteriovenous malformations will show contrast enhancement, but should also show extramedullary flow voids on T2-weighted imaging, which are not seen here.[79,80,81]

▸▸ Question 54

A patient presents with insidiously progressive low-back pain. MR of the lumbar spine shows a 3-cm intradural extramedullary lesion at the level of the conus medullaris with imaging features suggestive of an intradural primary spinal cord tumor. He is neurointact on evaluation and opts for serial observation; however, this demonstrates progressive enlargement on consecutive MR and surgical resection is recommended. Which of the following surgical strategies will best address the tumor?

- A. L1–L2 laminectomy; gross total resection of tumor
- B. T12–L1 laminectomy; gross total resection of tumor

- C. T12–L1 laminectomy; T11–L2 instrumented fusion; gross total resection of tumor
- D. T12–L1 laminectomy; subtotal resection of tumor
- E. T12/L1 interlaminar approach for piecemeal resection

Correct answer is B

The patient has an extramedullary mass localizing to the T12–L1 level; a T12–L1 laminectomy is necessary to provide sufficient craniocaudal exposure for resection of the tumor; however, laminoplasty or minimally invasive hemilaminectomy can also be considered. The patient is not reporting any mechanical back pain and the laminectomy itself would not be expected to cause iatrogenic instability so long as care is taken to preserve the facet joint capsules during exposure. Instrumented fusion is therefore not necessary for this patient's pathology (option **C**). Extramedullary tumors generally have a clearly defined plane with the spinal cord; schwannomas generally arise from sensory nerve rootlets, which can be sectioned at the points of entry and exit from the tumor to allow *en bloc* resection of the mass. Meningiomas similarly have a defined plane separating them from cord parenchyma; resection should include repairing the dural defect (with synthetic graft material). Likewise, myxopapillary ependymomas arise from the filum terminale and can be resected *en bloc* by dividing the filum cephalad and caudad to the tumor. The interlaminar window at T12/L1 is too small to allow for an interlaminar approach to this pathology.[82,83]

▸▸ Question 55

A 54-year-old male is taken to surgery for resection of an intradural extramedullary tumor. Upon opening the arachnoid, the tumor is identified. A thin, white fibrous band is seen exiting the cranial and caudal poles of the tumor. Which of the following pathologies is most likely to be identified on pathologic examination?

- A. Meningioma
- B. Schwannoma
- C. Neurofibroma
- D. Myxopapillary ependymoma
- E. Angiolipoma

Correct answer is D

Myxopapillary papillary ependymomas arise from the ependymal cells of the filum terminale; they can be found at other spinal levels, but classically localize to the lumbar spine. Resection of these lesions involves separating them from the surrounding nerve roots of the cauda equina, identifying the cranial and caudal points of attachment to the filum, and sectioning these attachments to allow for delivery of the tumor. The cranial attachment should be sectioned first to prevent retraction of the lesion out of the surgical field. Meningiomas will show adherence to the spinal dura, as they originate from arachnoid cap cells. Schwannomas and neurofibromas arise from the nerve roots, which generally have a slightly yellowish appearance due to the myelination of the nerve roots. The nerve roots can additionally be distinguished from the filum terminale using a nerve stimulator, which will be negative if the filum is being stimulated.

▸▸ Question 56

During surgery for a myxopapillary ependymoma at the level of the conus medullaris, the attending surgeon discusses whether to approach the tumor with piecemeal or en bloc resection to achieve gross total resection. Which of the following complications is more likely with piecemeal resection?

- A. Intrathecal drop metastases
- B. Postoperative urinary retention
- C. Malignant degeneration
- D. Persistent cerebrospinal fluid leak
- E. Postoperative foot/toe paresthesias

Correct answer is A

Though meningiomas and schwannomas can be resected in piecemeal fashion to reduce neural element manipulation, myxopapillary ependymomas are thought to have a high risk of local recurrence if the tumor capsule is violated. Consequently, for myxopapillary ependymomas, *en bloc* resection is recommended.

▸▸ Question 57

A 43-year-old male undergoes gross total resection of a myxopapillary ependymoma. He recovers well and is discharged home on postoperative day 3. He presents to neurooncology outpatient clinic for his 6-week follow-up visit and asks if any additional therapies are recommended. Which of the following adjuvant therapies is recommended?

- A. Radiotherapy with focused photon radiation (e.g., CyberKnife)
- B. Oral chemotherapy with temozolomide
- C. Single-dose intrathecal cytarabine for prevention of leptomeningeal spread
- D. Combined chemoradiation with focused photon radiation and chemotherapy with temozolomide
- E. Observation alone

Correct answer is E

In the 2021 WHO guidelines, myxopapillary ependymoma was classified as WHO grade 2 lesions. However, there is no consistent evidence to suggest that radiotherapy will improve local control or overall survival in patients who undergo gross total resection. Some centers will consider upfront radiotherapy in patients who are known to experience tumor morcellation intraoperatively. However, radiotherapy is not benign and carries with it the risk of radiation-induced dermatitis and new neurological deficits. At present, there are no chemotherapy regimens with documented efficacy for myxopapillary ependymoma. Consequently, observation is generally considered the standard of care following gross total resection of these lesions. There is no indication for intrathecal chemotherapy for myxopapillary ependymomas.

▸▸ Question 58

A 63-year-old female with past medical history of obesity, hypothyroidism, and chronic kidney disease presented with a 20-year history of right lower extremity paresthesias, 18 months of progressive left lower extremity paresthesias, and bilateral lower extremity weakness and urinary retention. She underwent MR that showed the following pathology (▸ Fig. 3.17). Which of the following imaging modalities is the next best step in management?

- A. CT of the thoracic spine
- B. Thoracic spine radiographs
- C. Upright scoliosis radiographs
- D. Cervical spine MR
- E. Bone scintigraphy

Correct answer is A

The MR demonstrates a large central T9/T10 disk herniation with significant compression of the spinal cord and associated intrinsic spinal cord signal changes. The best next step in evaluation is determining whether the patient's disk herniation is calcified or not, which is best evaluated with computed tomography. In this patient's case, the CT demonstrated calcification, which is noted in 40% of cases. The presence of calcification on preoperative imaging may suggest that the herniated component cannot be "rolled out" from its more ventrally located position, and therefore an anterior transthoracic approach may be preferable. Additionally, the presence of a large, calcified

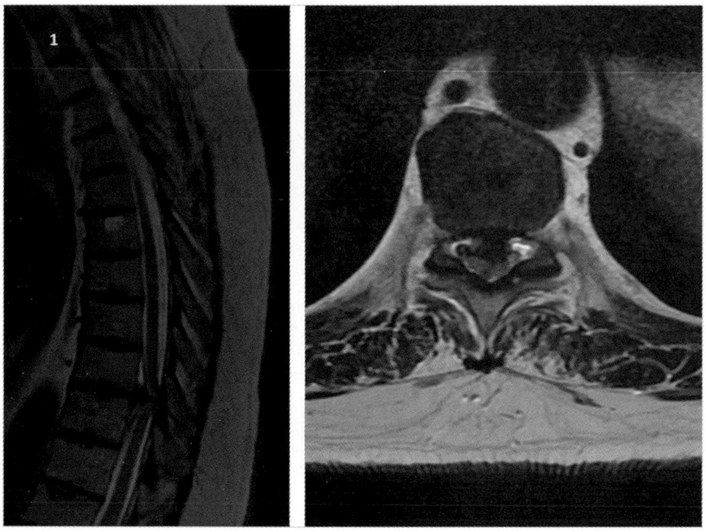

Fig. 3.17

disk herniation increases the odds that there is intradural extension of the disk herniation due to erosion and thinning of the dura. It has been suggested that as compared to all disk herniations, giant calcified thoracic disk herniations (as in the present case) are associated with intradural extension. This carries with it an elevated risk of ventral cerebrospinal fluid leak intraoperatively.[84,85,86]

▸▸ Question 59

A 53-year-old woman presents with gait difficulties with progressive imbalance and falls. Imaging shows a T9/10 central disk herniation. Surgical resection is recommended based on the patient's confluence of radiographic features and clinical symptoms. Which of the following surgical approaches will most safely address the patient's symptoms?

- A. T9–T10 laminectomy, T9/10 diskectomy
- B. T9/T10 medial facetectomy, right-sided T9–T10 hemilaminectomy; T9/T10 diskectomy
- C. T9–T10 right-sided hemilaminectomy; T9–T10 pediculectomy, T9/T10 diskectomy
- D. Thoracotomy, anterior T9/T10 partial corpectomy, T9/T10 diskectomy
- E. T8–T11 instrumented fusion; T9–T10 hemilaminectomy; T9–T10 pediculectomy; T9/T10 diskectomy

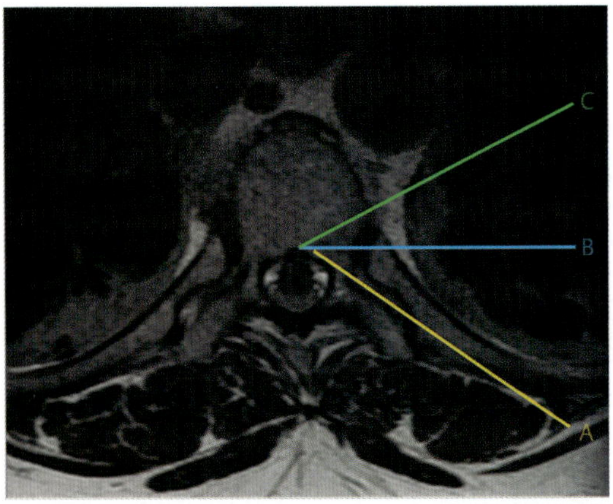

Fig. 3.18 (Source: Reproduced with permission from 14.6.2 Surgical Approaches. In: Baaj A, Kakaria U, Kim H, eds. Surgery of the thoracic spine: principles and techniques. 1st ed. New York: Thieme; 2019.)

Correct answer is D

Of these options, only **D** will most safely allow for resection of the disk. A costotransversectomy (**D**, below) or lateral extracavitary approach (**E**, below) will allow for a successful approach to the centrally located disk fragment; however, it will likely require resection of significant bone at the T9/T10 segment and an instrumented fusion. The transthoracic approach (likely thoracotomy, though a thoracoscopic approach is reasonable for soft/noncalcified disk herniations) is the best option as it approaches from the side of the disk herniation. The adjacent vertebral bodies are partially corpectomized to create a small cavity into which the disk fragment can be delivered. A direct posterior approach will not address this patient's symptoms, and the actual case of this patient was associated with permanent bilateral lower extremity paraplegia. A transfacet approach and even a pediculectomy (options **B, C, and E**) are also unlikely to afford sufficient access to the ventral epidural space to allow for safe resection of this calcified disk fragment. If a transthoracic approach is to be performed, the patient should undergo preoperative pulmonary function tests. Additionally, the anesthesia team must be prepared for intubation with a dual-lumen endotracheal tube, as single-lung ventilation will be required to allow for the surgical approach. Preoperatively, regardless of whether a transthoracic or lateral extra-cavitary approach is selected, the patient should be considered for placement of a gold seed at the target level under fluoroscopic guidance so as to prevent wrong-level surgery. For anterior approaches, instrumentation is merited when ≥ 50% of the vertebral body is resected.[87,88,98] ▸ Fig. 3.18 and ▸ Table 3.3 show surgical corridors to midline thoracic disk herniation. Axial MRI of a giant calcified thoracic disk herniation is shown—large hypointensity in the central canal. Line A demonstrates a costotransversectomy approach. There is a limitation of medial access and the contralateral side cannot be reached. Line B is the trajectory in a mini-open or minimally invasive surgery lateral transthoracic/retropleural approach. Line C is the anterior transthoracic approach. There is no retraction of the spinal cord required to reach the midline, ventral dura, and the contralateral disk in both the lateral (B) and anterior (C) approaches.

Table 3.3 Advantages and disadvantages of the surgical approach to midline thoracic disk herniations

Approach	Advantage	Disadvantage
Laminectomy	For lesions dorsal to the spinal cord	No midline exposure No ventral dura exposure High risk of neurological deficits
Costotransversectomy	Fair midline disk exposure Good for lateral or paracentral disk Intact pleura	No access to contralateral disk Limited ventral dura exposure Rhizotomy required
Lateral extracavitary	More midline exposure Intact pleura can access multiple levels	No access to contralateral disk Limited ventral dura exposure Rhizotomy required More boney resection needed
Minimally invasive lateral transthoracic/retropleural	Good midline disk exposure Good ventral dura exposure Can have intact pleura—may not require chest tube Can access contralateral dis Can access multiple levels	Limited view working through retractors Steep learning curve
Anterior transthoracic and thoracoscopic	Best midline disk exposure Best ventral dura exposure Can access contralateral disk	Requires cardiothoracic surgeon Steep learning curve Painful Requires chest tube Pulmonary complications

▸▸ Question 60

A 63-year-old female with a history of hyperlipidemia and hypothyroidism (on replacement) presented to clinical attention with diffuse paresthesias of the bilateral upper extremities. She also endorsed the sensation of an electrical shock traveling up and down her spine with flexion of her head. She had previously undergone C5/C6 foraminotomy for these symptoms with transient benefit, but during follow-up was found to have the imaging below. Which of the following is the most likely explanation for these imaging findings (▸ Fig. 3.19)?

- A. Multiple sclerosis
- B. Intramedullary spinal cord tumor
- C. Neuromyelitis optica
- D. Myelomalacia from chronic compression
- E. Spinal cord contusion

Correct answer is B

The imaging demonstrates a heterogeneously contrast-enhancing, T2-hypointense lesion located centrally within and expanding the spinal cord. This is characteristic of an intramedullary spinal cord tumor. Neuromyelitis optica and multiple sclerosis can both show gadolinium enhancement on imaging; however, they do not expand the cord. Multiple sclerosis also requires the disease to show dissemination in either space or time (the McDonald criteria). Spinal cord contusion is also unlikely to cause spinal cord expansion, and this patient has no reported history of trauma. Lastly, myelomalacia is associated with spinal cord atrophy as opposed to spinal cord expansion.

▸▸ Question 61

A patient with complaints of bilateral upper extremity paresthesias undergoes MR of the cervical spine showing a T2-heterogeneous mass with heterogenous contrast enhancement. The patient's lesion is initially worked up as neuromyelitis optica. Which of the following antibodies was most likely tested for to help rule out this diagnosis?

- A. Anti-NMDAR
- B. Anti-Hu
- C. Anti-aquaporin 4
- D. Anti-nicotinic acetylcholine receptor
- E. Anti-L-type calcium channel

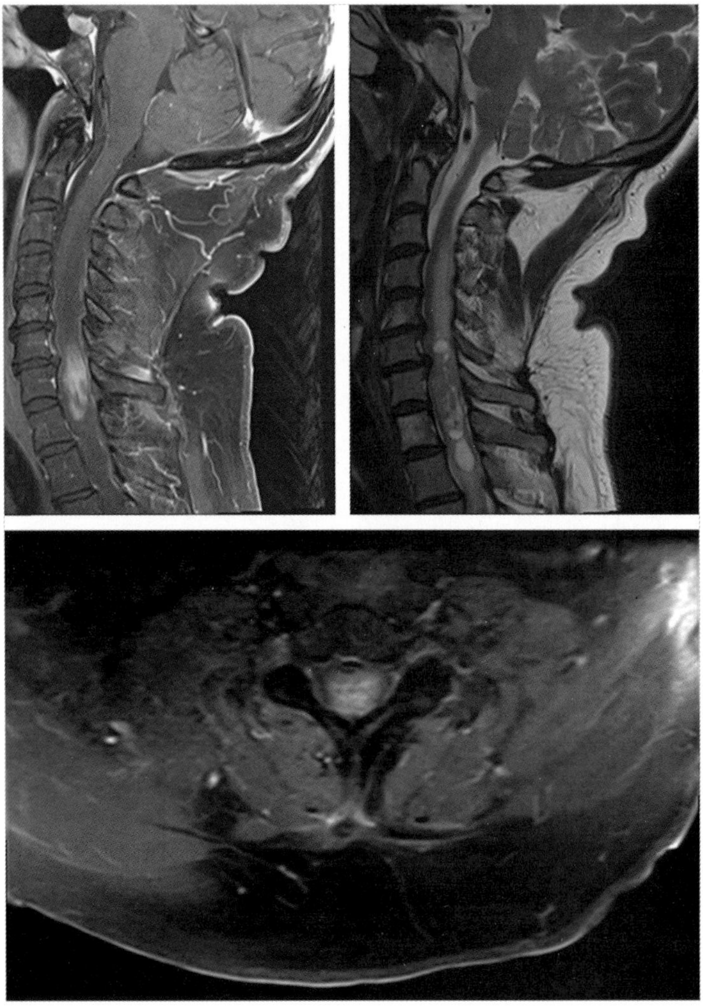

Fig. 3.19

Correct answer is C

In more than 80% of NMO cases, patients test positive for anti-aquaporin 4 antibodies. In 10 to 40% of the remaining individuals, tests for anti-myelin oligodendrocyte glycoprotein (anti-MOG) are positive. Anti-NMDAR antibodies are often seen in autoimmune encephalitis, characterized radiographically by mesial temporal lobe hyperintensities in 30% of cases and clinically by auditory and visual hallucinations, behavioral changes, seizures, dyskinesias, and delusions. Anti-Hu antibodies are seen in paraneoplastic disorders, most commonly in patients with small cell lung cancer. Anti-nicotinic acetylcholine receptor antibodies are seen in myasthenia gravis and anti-L-type calcium channel antibodies are seen in Lambert-Eaton myasthenic syndrome. These latter two are disorders of the neuromuscular junction and do not affect the spinal cord.[90,91]

▸▸ Question 62

A patient presents with progressive bilateral upper extremity, numbness, and paresthesias. Imaging demonstrates a solid-cystic mass of the cervicothoracic junction. She is diagnosed with an intramedullary spinal cord tumor. Which of the following pathologies is most likely based on her imaging findings?

- A. High-grade astrocytoma
- B. Low-grade astrocytoma
- C. Ependymoma
- D. Hemangioblastoma
- E. Neurocytoma

Correct answer is C

The imaging (▶ Fig. 3.20) demonstrates a heterogeneously contrast-enhancing mass arising centrally within and expanding the cervical spinal cord with cephalad and caudad T2-hyperintense collections. These are features suggestive of ependymoma, which is the most common intramedullary spinal cord tumor in adults. The lesion also has relatively well-defined borders, which are again suggestive of ependymoma as compared to astrocytoma, which generally have poorly defined borders. It is also centrally located as compared to astrocytomas, which are more commonly eccentrically located. Hemangioblastomas are far less common and generally show syrinxes that are much larger. They also show homogeneous enhancement. In the pediatric population, astrocytomas are the most common pathology, though in most cases these are low grade (WHO grade 1/2). Low-grade astrocytomas are also more common in adults; however, high-grade astrocytomas disproportionately affect adult patients.

▸▸ Question 63

A patient presents to the clinic with outside imaging showing a cervicothoracic intramedullary lesion consistent with a primary intramedullary spinal cord tumor. The patient has a nonfocal sensorimotor examination. She endorses mild neck

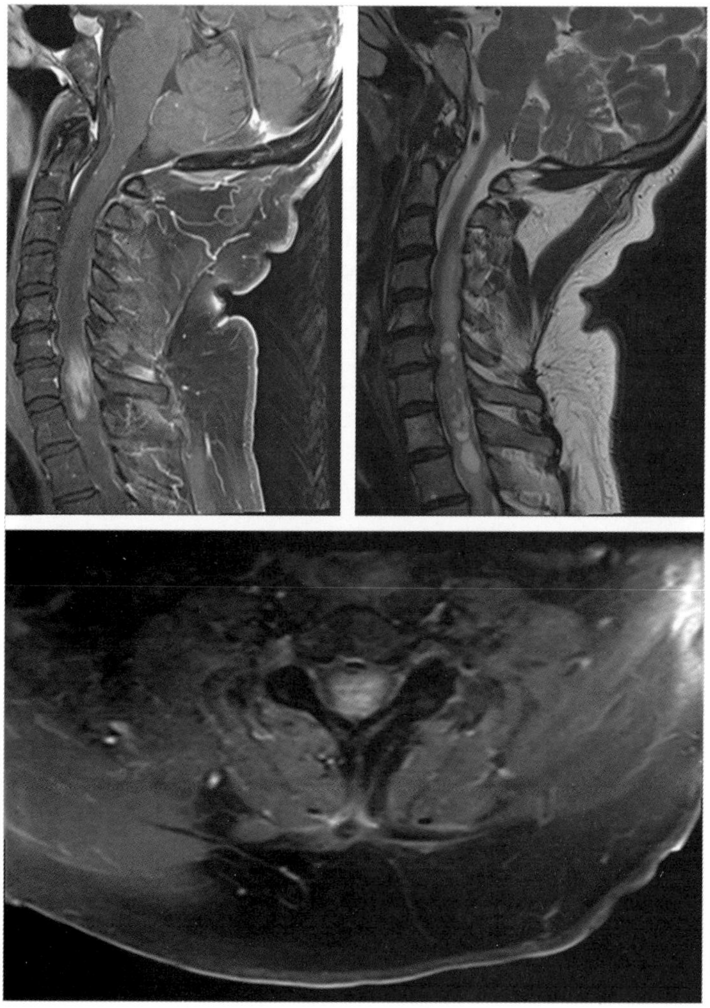

Fig. 3.20

pain with movement and subjective paresthesias in her fingers bilaterally. She has no hyperreflexia or pathological reflexes (e.g., Hoffman reflex, Babinski reflex). Which of the following is the best approach to the management of this patient?

- A. C6–T1 laminectomy; en bloc resection of the tumor
- B. C6–T1 laminectomy; subtotal resection of tumor
- C. Observation with repeat MR of the cervical spine in 6 months
- D. Chemoradiation with proton radiotherapy
- E. Focused photon radiotherapy with 12 Gy to 80% isodose line

Correct answer is C

While some surgeons may recommend or offer resection of the lesion at this stage, the scenario indicates that this patient is minimally symptomatic with no signs of myelopathy on examination. Surgical resection of these lesions is associated with new proprioceptive deficits in the majority of cases, as surgical resection requires splitting and retraction of the dorsal columns, which contain the ascending proprioceptive inputs (gracile and cuneate fasciculi). *En bloc* resection, that is, gross total resection of the lesion as one piece with a surrounding cuff of normal tissue, is never indicated for spinal cord tumors (option **A**), as this will needlessly resect healthy cord parenchyma. If there is a clear dissection plan, then gross total resection may be pursued, and is generally considered the gold standard of treatment for ependymomas. But this does not include resection of any healthy surrounding cord parenchyma. Additionally, a recent consensus statement by the spinal oncology working group of the North American Spine Society recommended observation for patients with IMSCTs who are asymptomatic or minimally symptomatic. For lesions without clear margins intraoperatively, then subtotal resection is reasonable; however, the goal for subtotal resection is symptom relief as compared to oncologic cure.[92,93]

▸▸ Question 64

A 27-year-old woman presents with imaging suggestive of a primary intramedullary spinal cord tumor. After serial observation, the patient returns to the clinic with complaints of increased difficulty walking, culminating in one recent fall, and difficulty with fine motor movements of her hands, including handwriting and fastening buttons. Surgical intervention is offered. The patient asks if there are any potential neurological complications of surgery. Which of the following new deficits should the patient be informed is most likely to present following surgical resection, assuming that there are no intraoperative complications?

- A. Weakness of the bilateral hands
- B. Radicular pain radiating into both arms
- C. Urinary and/or stool incontinence
- D. Worsening balance difficulties
- E. Dysesthetic pain of bilateral upper extremities

Correct answer is D

The surgical approach for resection of IMSCTs employs either a midline myelotomy dividing and retracting the bilateral dorsal columns, if the tumor is centrally located, or a dorsal root entry zone approach, if the tumor is eccentrically located. In both cases, the dorsal columns will be retracted, which carry the ascending fibers of the gracile fasciculus and cuneate fasciculus (above the level of T7). These carry the proprioceptive inputs for the lower and upper body, respectively. Retraction can cause palsy or damage to these fibers and resultant balance difficulties, which are seen in many patients. Radicular pain is most consistent with a nerve root injury and would not be expected in an uncomplicated surgery. Similarly, the corticospinal tracts are located eccentrically in the lateral funiculi, and the cell bodies of the α motor neurons innervating the hands are located in the lateral aspect of the ventral horn. Weakness in the hands would therefore not be expected in an uncomplicated surgery. Last, bowel/bladder symptoms can be seen in the context of chronic myelopathy, but new bowel/bladder symptoms would be far less likely than new proprioceptive/joint position sense symptoms.[92,93]

▸▸ Question 65

A patient presents for surgical resection of a primary intramedullary spinal cord tumor with imaging features suggestive of ependymoma. Which of the following surgical approaches is most likely to allow for the successful excision of the tumor and to minimize complications associated with resection?

- A. C5–T1 anterior fusion; C6 corpectomy; ventral median myelotomy; and resection of tumor
- B. C7 laminectomy; gross total resection of tumor
- C. C6–T1 laminectomy; gross total resection of tumor
- D. C5–T2 instrumented fusion; C5–T1 laminectomy; gross total resection of tumor
- E. C3–T5 instrumented fusion; C4–T2 laminectomy; gross total resection of tumor

Correct answer is D

Anterior approaches are never indicated for intramedullary spinal cord tumors, as the anterior spinal artery lies in the anterior median sulcus and would almost invariably be injured with such an approach. Injury of this vessel renders ischemic the anterior two-thirds of the spinal cord, including the ventral horns and corticospinal tracts with resultant paralysis. Based on the imaging, it can be seen that the tumor extends from the C6/C7 interspace to the mid-T1 body. A C7 laminectomy (option **B**) will therefore not afford enough exposure to allow a durotomy to be made that can expose the full craniocaudal extent of the lesion. The decision between the latter two options relies on the knowledge that multilevel laminectomy, especially when performed at the cervicothoracic junction, increases the patient's risk for post-laminectomy kyphosis. The removal of the posterior elements weakens the posterior tension band that helps prevent such kyphosis. In one series of 32 adults who underwent cervical laminectomy without fusion for intradural tumor resection, Sciubba et al showed that those who underwent ≥ three-level laminectomy had a sixfold higher odds of post-laminectomy kyphosis requiring subsequent fusion. Given this patient's relatively young age, the location of the tumor at the cervicothoracic junction, and the need for at least a three-level laminectomy to full expose the tumor, she is at high risk for this complication. Including instrumented fusion in her surgical plan will help avoid this complication. A C3–T5 instrumented fusion will require a surgical exposure that is much larger than required; stabilization is indicated only to prevent post-laminectomy kyphosis. Reducing the length of the exposure/injury to the posterior tension band can help prevent this complication.[94]

▸▸ Question 66

An 82-year-old woman with a history of hypertension, type 2 diabetes mellitus, undifferentiated connective tissue disease, and vertebral artery stenosis presents to the emergency department with progressive numbness in her bilateral hands, gait difficulty with falls, and difficulty with fine motor movements. She has recently undergone an MR of her cervical spine (▸ Fig. 3.21). Which of the following is the best initial management for this patient?

- A. C3/C4, C4/C5 cervical diskectomy and fusion
- B. C3/C4, C4/C5 cervical disk arthroplasty
- C. Transforaminal epidural corticosteroid injection
- D. C3–C5 laminectomy and fusion
- E. C2–C7 laminectomy and fusion

Correct answer is A

The patient presents with clear clinical and radiographic signs of cervical spondylotic myelopathy. Nonoperative management (option **C**) is unlikely to provide any substantive improvement in her symptoms. In this patient, the imaging demonstrates clear compression from disk-osteophyte complexes at C3/C4 and C4/C5. A posterior approach (option **D**) is unlikely to relieve this compression. In a patient with advanced age (82 years old), there is little inherent motion in the subaxial spine. Additionally, the facet joints may be autoarthrodesed, though a CT would be needed to evaluate this. Consequently, if present, disk replacement/arthroplasty is not a good option. The best option is a two-level anterior cervical diskectomy and fusion. A C2–C7 laminectomy is overly aggressive for the pathology in question, as there is no evidence of significant stenosis at C2/C3, C5/C6, or C6/C7.

▸▸ Question 67

A 68-year-old man presents with clinical evidence of cervical spondylotic myelopathy. Both anterior and posterior decompression approaches are presented to the patient. Benefits and risks of each procedure are discussed with the patient, and ultimately an anterior approach is selected. Which of the following complications is less likely from an anterior as compared to a posterior approach?

- A. Dysphagia
- B. C5 palsy

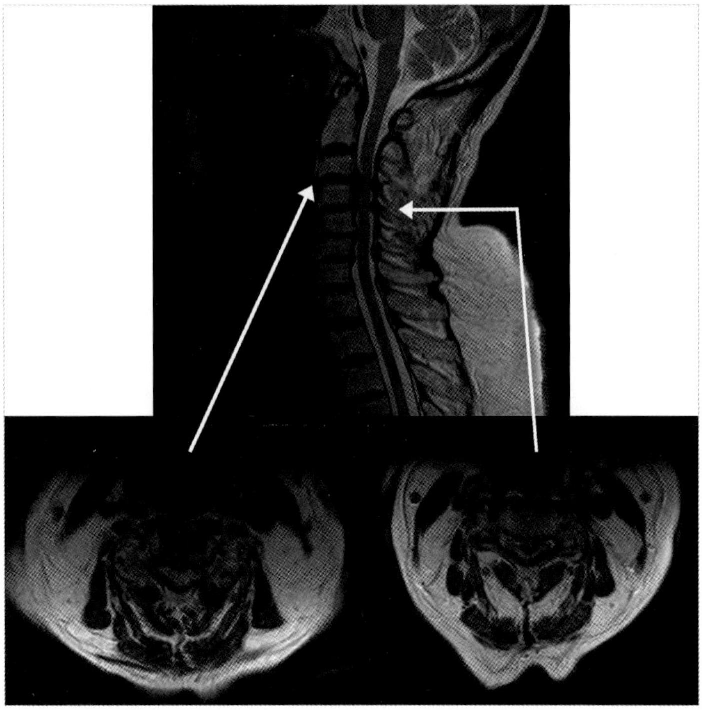

Fig. 3.21

- C. Hoarseness
- D. Horner syndrome
- E. Wound bed hematoma

Correct answer is B

The anterior cervical diskectomy and fusion is the workhorse approach to one and two-level diskogenic pathologies of the subaxial spine and can be employed for both cervical myelopathy and cervical radiculopathy. The anterior approach has, in general, a lower risk profile than the posterior approach, but is associated with an increased risk of swallowing difficulty (dysphagia), Horner syndrome (due to injury of the sympathetic chain that runs adjacent to the longus colli), and hoarseness (due to the manipulation of the trachea or injury to the recurrent laryngeal nerve—thought to be higher risk with right-sided approaches). Wound infection and C5 palsy are both more likely from a posterior approach. A wound bed hematoma is possible with either approach.[95,96,97]

▸▸ Question 68

A 75-year-old woman undergoes anterior cervical diskectomy and fusion for cervical spondylotic myelopathy. The Smith-Robinson anterolateral working corridor is used to expose the C3, C4, and C5 vertebral bodies. The longus colli muscles are elevated and a self-retaining retractor is placed. Which of the following interventions can best help reduce the risk of postoperative dysphagia?

- A. Use of an integrated fixation device versus a tension band plate
- B. Maintaining endotracheal cuff pressure ≤ 20 mm Hg
- C. Placing steroid-coated Gelfoam pledgets on the trachea prior to closure
- D. Thorough irrigation of the surgical bed prior to closure
- E. Use of non-toothed blades for the self-retaining retractor

Correct answer is B

Dysphagia following anterior cervical diskectomy and fusion is thought to result from a confluence of factors, including esophageal manipulation during the surgery, pharyngeal irritation by the endotracheal tube, elevated transmural esophageal pressure, and in some cases recurrent laryngeal nerve injury. Most cases of dysphagia are transient, but in a minority of cases, enteric feeding with a nasogastric tube or percutaneous endogastric tube may be required. A recent clinical trial of 98 patients by Sejkorová et al found that reducing endotracheal cuff pressure following retractor placement can lead to a significant reduction in postoperative hoarseness. Additionally, a systematic review published by Miller et al found endotracheal tube cuff pressure reduction was associated with 23% lower odds of postoperative dysphagia, though this difference did not prove significant. None of the other measures listed have been correlated with improved postoperative hoarseness or dysphagia outcomes.[98,99]

▸▸ Question 69

An 82-year-old woman undergoes a two-level anterior cervical diskectomy and fusion (ACDF) for degenerative cervical myelopathy. The procedure is uncomplicated, and she is transferred to the perioperative recovery area. In the recovery area, she begins to experience difficulty breathing, which does not improve with supplemental oxygen. On bedside examination, her breathing is rapid and oxygen saturation is 98% on a 6 L simple facemask. She moves her upper and lower extremities with full strength, and her neck appears firm. What is the next best step in management?

- A. Emergent endotracheal intubation
- B. Reopening of the surgical wound at the bedside
- C. Inhaled racemic epinephrine
- D. Intravenous hydrocortisone
- E. Inhaled albuterol/ipratropium nebulizer with positive pressure ventilation (CPAP or BiPAP)

Correct answer is A

The patient's recent anterior cervical operation with a tense surgical site and worsening respiratory status are concerning for a wound bed hemorrhage. The first step is securing the patient's airway, which can become rapidly compressed by the expanding hematoma, resulting in airway compromise and potential mortality. After the airway has been secured, the patient should be emergently returned to the operating room for wound reopening and exploration. The images below show CT angiograms of a patient who experienced a postoperative wound bed hemorrhage with progressive neck discomfort, swelling, and difficulty with swallowing and subjective dyspnea. Note the images show an endotracheal tube in place with leftward displacement of the trachea by the right-sided hematoma (▸ Fig. 3.22). This patient underwent interval hematoma evacuation prior to the image, but residual clot is present.[97]

▸▸ Question 70

A 77-year-old woman undergoes a two-level anterior cervical diskectomy and fusion for cervical radiculopathy. The patient is taken to recovery and is cleared for transfer to the floor. During the first day following surgery, she notes difficulty handling secretions and requires repeat suctioning by the nursing staff. She becomes increasingly agitated and is ultimately intubated. She undergoes cervical spine CT, which is shown in ▸ Fig. 3.23. Which of the following best explains her postoperative secretions difficulty?

- A. Esophageal perforation
- B. Inadequate resection of anterior osteophytes leading to postoperative dysphagia
- C. Intraoperative recurrent laryngeal nerve injury
- D. Aspiration pneumonia
- E. Gastroesophageal reflux disease

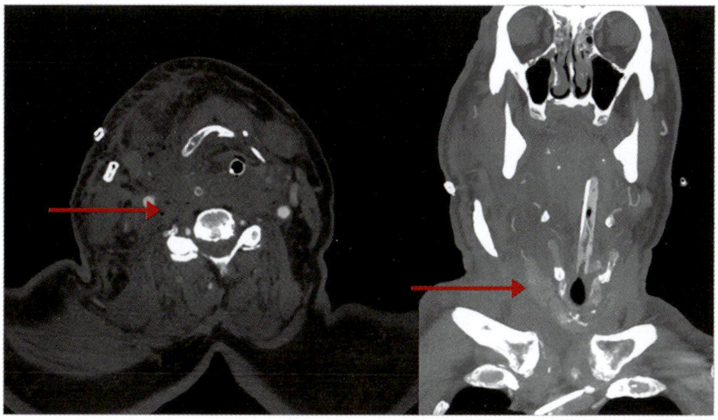

Fig. 3.22

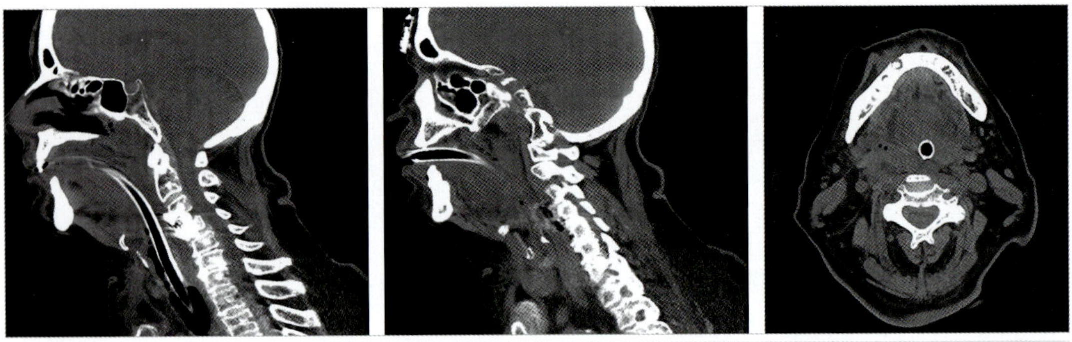

Fig. 3.23

Correct answer is A

The CT demonstrates multiple pockets of air along the surgical tract in the right anterior neck. While these are potentially compatible with surgery, they may also be indicative of esophageal injury. While anterior plate/anterior osteophyte prominence can lead to postoperative dysphagia, secretion burden significant enough to require intubation would be unlikely. Recurrent laryngeal nerve palsy occurs in 3 to 9% of cases, but is characterized by hoarseness, not dysphagia, as it innervates the vocalis/thyroarytenoid vocalis muscle (intrinsic laryngeal muscle responsible for vocal cord abduction). This patient underwent upper endoscopy to further evaluate her difficulty handling secretions, which showed an esophageal perforation (▶ Fig. 3.24). Otorhinolaryngology was consulted and took the patient to the operating room for primary repair. Her anterior cervical plate was also removed at that time to help facilitate healing of the posterior pharyngeal wall injury. Post-repair the patient must be made NPO to allow for healing of the repair. This patient underwent gastric tube placement after undergoing enteral feeds with a nasogastric tube.[97]

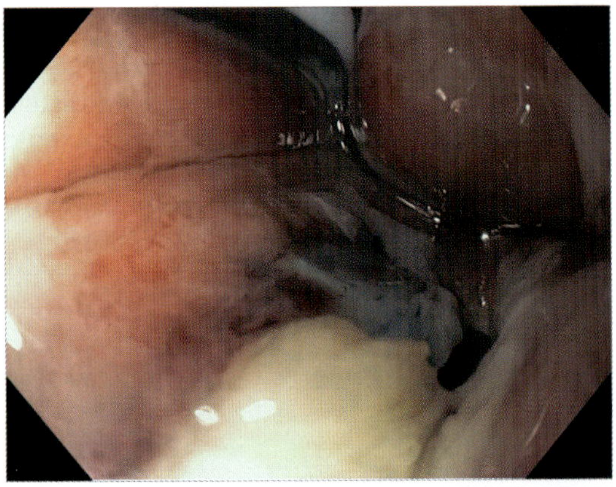

Fig. 3.24

▸▸ Question 71

An 80-year-old woman undergoes two-level anterior cervical diskectomy and fusion for cervical spondylotic myelopathy that is complicated by intraoperative esophageal injury. After a protracted hospital course, the patient was discharged with a PEG tube. She returns to the emergency room 6 months later with confusion and endorsing neck pain. On examination, she is found to have new left upper extremity weakness relative to her prior postoperative baseline. She undergoes MR (▶ Fig. 3.25). What is the best next step in management?

- A. C2–C5 posterior fusion; C3–C4 laminectomy
- B. C3–C4 anterior cervical corpectomy
- C. Intravenous antibiotics alone
- D. Conservative management with serial observation
- E. C3–C4 laminectomy

Correct answer is A

The imaging above shows a contrast-enhancing prevertebral mass with erosion of the C3 and C4 bodies with C3 and C4 vertebral body, consistent with osteomyelitis. This is likely related to the patient's known history of esophageal perforation, which likely seeded the interbody grafts with alimentary tract bacteria. Additionally, there is a ventral contrast-enhancing mass consistent with

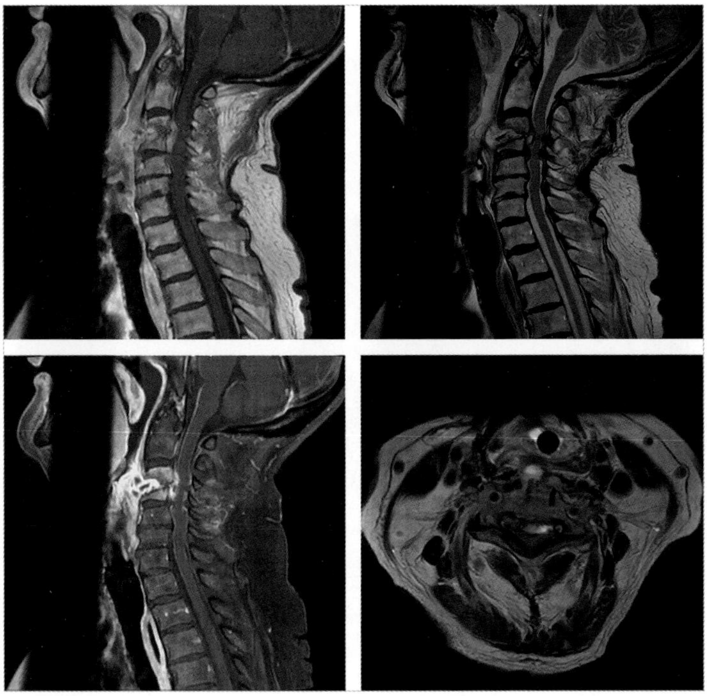

Fig. 3.25

an epidural abscess, which can be seen on MR to be causing significant spinal cord compression. The patient's neck pain is likely from a combination of the osteomyelitis-associated inflammation and instability from the bony erosion. Initial management of osteomyelitis is antibiotic therapy (4–6-week trial prior to operative management per 2015 position paper by the Infectious Diseases Society of America). However, in this case, there is a concurrent epidural abscess with spinal cord compression, which may explain the worsened left arm weakness on bedside examination. This merits operative intervention. Given the patient's prior esophageal perforation, a repeat anterior cervical operation is high risk and is likely to have an extremely high risk for recurrent perforation. Consequently, while an anterior approach would likely be preferred *ceteris paribus*, the patient's prior surgical history makes a posterior option preferable. Here, decompression will rely on the spinal cord floating back. As the patient is undergoing surgery, the underlying instability may also be addressed with instrumented fusion. Laminectomy alone in the setting of her osteomyelitis will likely result in kyphosis of the cervical spine as the imaging demonstrates erosion of the C3 and C4 bodies, with likely structural incompetence of the anterior column.[100,101]

▸▸ Question 72

A patient with a T12 burst fracture undergoes spinal stabilization surgery. Postoperatively, he is diagnosed with deep vein thrombosis. Which of the following is the most effective method to prevent deep vein thrombosis (DVT) in spinal cord injury patients?

- A. Early mobilization
- B. Mechanical compression devices
- C. Low-dose aspirin
- D. Low-molecular-weight heparin
- E. Inferior vena cava filter placement

Correct answer is D

In patients with spinal cord injuries, low-molecular-weight heparin is the most effective prophylactic agent against DVT. It reduces the incidence of thromboembolic events more effectively than mechanical methods or aspirin.

References

[1] 2013 CNS C spine guidelines. Accessed June 12, 2025 at: https://www.cns.org/guidelines/browse-guidelines-detail/guidelines-management-of-acute-cervical-spine-spin-2

[2] 2013 CNS C spine guidelines. Accessed June 12, 2025 at: https://www.cns.org/guidelines/browse-guidelines-detail/guidelines-management-of-acute-cervical-spine-spin-2

[3] 2013 CNS C spine guidelines. Accessed June 12, 2025 at: https://www.cns.org/guidelines/browse-guidelines-detail/guidelines-management-of-acute-cervical-spine-spin-2

[4] 2018 CNS TL spine guidelines. Accessed June 12, 2025 at: https://www.cns.org/guidelines/browse-guidelines-detail/guidelines-on-evaluation-treatment-of-patients-wit

[5] Liu K, Zhang Z. Reduction of lower cervical facet dislocation: a review of all techniques. Neurospine 2023;20(1):181–204

[6] McDonald CL, Daniels AH, Anderson GA, Alsoof D, Kuris EO. Traumatic cervical facet fractures and dislocation. JBJS Reviews 2022;10(5). Doi: 10.2106/JBJS.RVW.22.00023

[7] Wiltse LL, Newman PH, Macnab I. Classification of spondylolysis and spondylolisthesis. Clin Orthop Relat Res 1976:(117):23–29

[8] Meyerding H. Low backache and sciatic pain associated with spondylolisthesis and protruded intervertebral disk: incidence, significance, and treatment. JBJS 1941;23(2):461–470

[9] Gagnet P, Kern K, Andrews K, Elgafy H, Ebraheim N. Spondylolysis and spondylolisthesis: a review of the literature. J Orthop 2018;15(2):404–407

[10] 2013 CNS C spine guidelines. Accessed June 12, 2025 at: https://www.cns.org/guidelines/browse-guidelines-detail/guidelines-management-of-acute-cervical-spine-spin-2.

[11] Park JH, Hyun SJ. Intraoperative neurophysiological monitoring in spinal surgery. World J Clin Cases 2015;3(9):765–773

[12] Gonzalez AA, Jeyanandarajan D, Hansen C, Zada G, Hsieh PC. Intraoperative neurophysiological monitoring during spine surgery: a review. Neurosurg Foc 2009;27(4):E6

[13] Saadeh YS, Smith BW, Joseph JR, et al. The impact of blood pressure management after spinal cord injury: a systematic review of the literature. Neurosurg Foc 2017;43(5):E20

[14] Yang J, Skaggs DL, Chan P, et al. Raising mean arterial pressure alone restores 20% of intraoperative neuromonitoring losses. Spine (Phila Pa 1976). 2018;43(13):890–894

[15] Pennington Z, Lubelski D, Westbroek EM, et al. Time to recovery predicted by the severity of postoperative C5 palsy. J Neurosurg Spine 2019;32(2):191–199

[16] Pennington Z, Lubelski D, Westbroek EM, et al. Spinal cord float back is not an independent predictor of postoperative C5 palsy in patients undergoing posterior cervical decompression. Spine J 2020;20(2):266–275

[17] Lubelski D, Pennington Z, Planchard RF, et al. Use of electromyography to predict likelihood of recovery following C5 palsy after posterior cervical spine surgery. Spine J 2021;21(3):387–396

[18] Theodore N. Degenerative cervical spondylosis. N Engl J Med 2020;383(2):159–168

[19] Nouri A, Matur A, Pennington Z, et al. Prevalence of anemia and its relationship with neurological status in patients undergoing surgery for degenerative cervical myelopathy and radiculopathy: A retrospective study of 2 spine centers. J Clin Neurosci 2020;72:252–257

[20] Scheer JK, Lau D, Smith JS, et al. Alignment, classification, clinical evaluation, and surgical treatment for adult cervical deformity: a complete guide. Neurosurgery 2021;88(4):864–883

[21] Carrick MA, Robson JM, Thomas C. Smoking and anaesthesia. BJA Educ 2019;19(1):1–6

[22] Al-Bashaireh, Haddad LG, Weaver M, Chengguo X, Kelly DL, Yoon S. The effect of tobacco smoking on bone mass: an overview of pathophysiologic mechanisms. J Osteoporos 2018:2018:1206235

[23] Wiltse LL, Newman PH, Macnab I. Classification of spondylolisis and spondylolisthesis. Clin Orthop Relat Res 1976;(117):23–29

[24] Wiltse LL, Winter RB. Terminology and measurement of spondylolisthesis. J Bone Joint Surg Am 1983;65:768–772

[25] Gagnet P, Kern K, Andrews K, Elgafy H, Ebraheim N. Spondylolysis and spondylolisthesis: a review of the literature. J Orthop 2018;15(2):404–407

[26] Meyerding HW. Low backache and sciatic pain associated with spondylolisthesis and protruded intervertebral disc: incidence, significant, and treatment. J Bone Jt Surg 1941;23:461–470

[27] Huang RP, Bohlman HH, Thompson GH, Poe-Kochert C. Predictive value of pelvic incidence in progression of spondylolisthesis. Spine (Phila Pa 1976) 2003;28:2381–2385

[28] Kaiser R, Kantorová L, Langaufová A, et al. Decompression alone versus decompression with instrumented fusion in the treatment of lumbar degenerative spondylolisthesis: a systematic review and meta-analysis of randomised trials. J Neurol Neurosurg Psychiatry 2023;94:657–666

[29] Shukla GG, Chilakapati SS, Matur AV, et al. Laminectomy with fusion is associated with greater functional improvement compared with laminectomy alone for the treatment of degenerative lumbar spondylolisthesis. Spine (Phila Pa 1976) 2023;48:874–884

[30] Sivaganesan A, Chotai S, White-Dzuro G, McGirt MJ, Devin CJ. The effect of NSAIDs on spinal fusion: a cross-disciplinary review of biochemical, animal, and human studies. Eur Spine J 2017;26:2719–2728

[31] Nourbakhsh A, Hanson ZC. Odontoid fractures: a standard review of current concepts and treatment recommendations. J Am Acad Orthop Surg 2022;30:e561–572

[32] Kang MM, Anderer EG, Elliott RE, Kalhorn SP, Frempong-Boadu A. C2 nerve root sectioning in posterior C1–2 instrumented fusions. World Neurosurg 2012;78:170–177

[33] Gillman CE, Jayasuriya AC. FDA-approved bone grafts and bone graft substitute devices in bone regeneration. Mater Sci Eng C 2021;130:112466

[34] Food and Drug Administration. Life-threatening complications associated with recombinant human bone morphogenetic protein in cervical spine fusion. 2009.

[35] Smith JS, Shaffrey CI, Ames CP, Lenke LG. Treatment of adult thoracolumbar spinal deformity: past, present, and future. J Neurosurg Spine 2019;30:551–567

[36] Diebo BG, Shah NV, Boachie-Adjei O, et al. Adult spinal deformity. Lancet 2019;394:160–172

[37] Hasegawa K, Dubousset JF. Cone of economy with the chain of balance-historical perspective and proof of concept. Spine Surg Relat Res 2022;6:2022–2038

[38] Iyer S, Hurlbert RJ, Albert TJ. Management of odontoid fractures in the elderly: a review of the literature and an evidence-based treatment algorithm. Neurosurgery 2018;82:419–430

[39] Chapman J, Smith JS, Kopjar B, et al. The AOSpine North America Geriatric Odontoid Fracture Mortality Study. Spine (Phila Pa 1976) 2013;38:1098–1104
[40] Andari Sawaya R, Jaffe J, Friedenberg L, Friedenberg FK. Vitamin, mineral, and drug absorption following bariatric surgery. Curr Drug Metab 2012;13:1345–1355
[41] Mayo BC, Massel DH, Yacob A, et al. A review of vitamin d in spinal surgery: deficiency screening, treatment, and outcomes. Int J Spine Surg 2020;14:447–454
[42] Uribe JS, Schwab F, Mundis GM, et al. The comprehensive anatomical spinal osteotomy and anterior column realignment classification. J Neurosurg Spine 2018;29:565–575
[43] Schwab F, Blondel B, Chay E, et al. The comprehensive anatomical spinal osteotomy classification. Neurosurgery 2014;74:112–120
[44] Gupta MC, Gupta S, Kelly MP, Bridwell KH. Pedicle subtraction osteotomy. JBJS Essent Surg Tech 2020;10:e0028
[45] Smith JS, Shaffrey CI, Klineberg E, et al. Complication rates associated with 3-column osteotomy in 82 adult spinal deformity patients: retrospective review of a prospectively collected multicenter consecutive series with 2-year follow-up. J Neurosurg Spine 2017;27:444–457
[46] Mikula AL, Lakomkin N, Pennington Z, et al. Lumbar lordosis correction with transforaminal lumbar interbody fusion in adult spinal deformity patients with minimum 2-year follow-up. World Neurosurg 2022;167:e295–e302
[47] Passias PG, Ahmad W, Williamson TK, et al. Efficacy of varying surgical approaches on achieving optimal alignment in adult spinal deformity surgery. Spine (Phila Pa 1976) 2024;49(1):22–28
[48] Buell T, Shaffrey CI, Bess S, et al. Segmental lordosis restoration using ALIF vs TLIF in adults with flatback deformity. Spine J 2021;21(9):S69–S70
[49] Morgan CD, Katsevman GA, Godzik J, et al. Outpatient outcomes of patients with femoral nerve neurapraxia after prone lateral lumbar interbody fusion at L4–5. J Neurosurg Spine 2022;37(1):92–95
[50] Hijji FY, Narain AS, Bohl DD, et al. Lateral lumbar interbody fusion: a systematic review of complication rates. Spine J 2017;17(10):1412–1419
[51] Nie JW, Hartman TJ, Zheng E, MacGregor KR, Oyetayo OO, Singh K. Neuromonitoring in lateral approaches for lumbar interbody fusion: a systematic review. World Neurosurg 2022;168:268–277.e1
[52] Uribe JS, Isaacs RE, Youssef JA, et al. Can triggered electromyography monitoring throughout retraction predict postoperative symptomatic neuropraxia after XLIF? Results from a prospective multicenter trial. Eur Spine J 2015;24(S3):378–385
[53] Dakwar E, Le TV, Baaj AA, et al. Abdominal wall paresis as a complication of minimally invasive lateral transpsoas interbody fusion. Neurosurg Focus 2011;31(4):E18
[54] Sharfman ZT, Gelfand Y, Shah P, et al. Spinal epidural abscess: a review of presentation, management, and medicolegal implications. Asian Spine J 2020;14:742–759
[55] Nickerson EK, Sinha R. Vertebral osteomyelitis in adults: an update. Br Med Bull 2016;117:121–138
[56] Zimmerli W. Vertebral osteomyelitis. N Engl J Med 2010;362:1022–1029
[57] Boody BS, Jenkins TJ, Maslak J, Hsu WK, Patel AA. Vertebral osteomyelitis and spinal epidural abscess. J Spinal Disord Tech 2015;28:E316–E327
[58] Pennington Z, Ehresman J, McCarthy EF, et al. Chordoma of the sacrum and mobile spine: a narrative review. Spine J 2021;21:500–517
[59] Feghali J, Pennington Z, Hung B, et al. Sacrectomy for sacral tumors: perioperative outcomes in a large-volume comprehensive cancer center. Spine J 2021;21:1908–1919
[60] Pennington Z, Ehresman J, Pittman PD, et al. Chondrosarcoma of the spine: a narrative review. Spine J 2021;21:2078–2096
[61] Akiyama T, Ogura K, Gokita T, et al. Analysis of the infiltrative features of chordoma: the relationship between micro-skip metastasis and postoperative outcomes. Ann Surg Oncol. 2018;25(4):912–919
[62] Pennington Z, Ehresman J, Elsamadicy AA, et al. Systematic review of charged-particle therapy for chordomas and sarcomas of the mobile spine and sacrum. Neurosurg Focus 2021;50:E17
[63] Dea N, Fisher CG, Reynolds JJ, et al. Current treatment strategy for newly diagnosed chordoma of the mobile spine and sacrum: results of an international survey. J Neurosurg Spine 2019;30:119–125
[64] Gokaslan ZL, Zadnik PL, Sciubba DM, et al. Mobile spine chordoma: results of 166 patients from the AOSpine Knowledge Forum Tumor database. J Neurosurg Spine 2016;24:644–651
[65] Varga PP, Szövérfi Z, Fisher CG, et al. Surgical treatment of sacral chordoma: prognostic variables for local recurrence and overall survival. Eur Spine J 2015;24:1092–1101
[66] Zoccali C, Skoch J, Patel AS, Walter CM, Maykowski P, Baaj AA. Residual neurological function after sacral root resection during en-bloc sacrectomy: a systematic review. Eur Spine J. 2016; 25(12):3925–3931
[67] Zoccali C, Skoch J, Patel AS, Walter CM, Maykowski P, Baaj AA. Residual neurological function after sacral root resection during en-bloc sacrectomy: a systematic review. Eur Spine J 2016;25:3925–3931
[68] Patchell RA, Tibbs PA, Regine WF, et al. Direct decompressive surgical resection in the treatment of spinal cord compression caused by metastatic cancer: a randomised trial. Lancet 2005;366:643–648
[69] Bilsky MH, Laufer I, Fourney DR, et al. Reliability analysis of the epidural spinal cord compression scale. J Neurosurg Spine 2010;13:324–328
[70] Sciubba DM, Pennington Z, Colman MW, et al. Spinal metastases 2021: a review of the current state of the art and future directions. Spine J 2021;21:1414–1429
[71] Quraishi NA, Rajagopal TS, Manoharan SR, Elsayed S, Edwards KL, Boszczyk BM. Effect of timing of surgery on neurological outcome and survival in metastatic spinal cord compression. Eur Spine J 2013;22:1383–1388
[72] Park S, Park JW, Park JH, et al. Factors affecting the prognosis of recovery of motor power and ambulatory function after surgery for metastatic epidural spinal cord compression. Neurosurg Focus 2022;53:E11
[73] Laufer I, Rubin DG, Lis E, et al. The NOMS framework: approach to the treatment of spinal metastatic tumors. Oncologist 2013;18:744–751
[74] Fisher CG, DiPaola CP, Ryken TC, et al. A novel classification system for spinal instability in neoplastic disease: an evidence-based approach and expert consensus form the Spine Oncology Study Group. Spine (Phila Pa 1976) 2010;35:E1221–1229
[75] Pennington Z, Ehresman J, Cottrill E, et al. To operate, or not to operate? Narrative review of the role of survival

predictors in patient selection for operative management of patients with metastatic spine disease. J Neurosurg Spine 2021;34:135–149
[76] Dea N, Versteeg AL, Sahgal A, et al. Metastatic spine disease: Should patients with short life expectancy be denied surgical care? An international retrospective cohort study. Neurosurgery 2020;87(2):303–311
[77] Rothrock RJ, Barzilai O, Reiner AS, et al. Survival trends after surgery for spinal metastatic tumors: 20-year cancer center experience. Neurosurgery 2020;88:402–412
[78] Kumar N, Madhu S, Bohra H, et al. Is there an optimal timing between radiotherapy and surgery to reduce wound complications in metastatic spine disease? A systematic review. Eur Spine J 2020;29:3080–3115
[79] Kim LJ, Spetzler RF. Classification and surgical management of spinal arteriovenous lesions: arteriovenous fistulae and arteriovenous malformations. Neurosurgery 2006;59:S3–195–S3–201
[80] Spetzler RF, Detwiler PW, Riina HA, Porter RW. Modified classification of spinal cord vascular lesions. J Neurosurg Spine 2002;96:145–156
[81] Koeller KK, Shih RY. Intradural extramedullary spinal neoplasms: radiologic-pathologic correlation. RadioGraphics 2019;39:468–490
[82] Pesce A, Palmieri M, Armocida D, Frati A, Miscusi M, Raco A. Spinal myxopapillary ependymoma: the Sapienza University experience and comprehensive literature review concerning the clinical course of 1602 patients. World Neurosurg 2019;129:245–253
[83] Moses ZB, Barzilai O, O'Toole JE. Benign intradural and paraspinal nerve sheath tumors: advanced surgical techniques. Neurosurg Clin N Am 2020;31:221–229
[84] Court C, Mansour E, Bouthors C. Thoracic disc herniation: surgical treatment. Orthop Traumatol Surg Res 2018;104: S31–S40
[85] Yuan L, Chen Z, Li W, et al. Radiographic and clinical features of thoracic disk disease associated with myelopathy: a retrospective analysis of 257 cases. Eur Spine J 2021;30:2211–2220
[86] Quint U, Bordon G, Preissl I, Sanner C, Rosenthal D. Thoracoscopic treatment for single level symptomatic thoracic disc herniation: a prospective followed cohort study in a group of 167 consecutive cases. Eur Spine J 2012;21:637–645
[87] Gong M, Liu G, Guan Q, Li L, Xing F, Xiang Z. Surgery for giant calcified herniated thoracic discs: a systematic review. World Neurosurg 2018;118:109–117
[88] Malcolm JG, Moore MK, Refai D. Anterior/Anterolateral thoracic access and stabilization from posterior approach: transpedicular, costotransversectomy, lateral extracavitary approaches: standard intralesional resection. In: Sciubba DM, ed. Spinal Tumor Surg. 1st ed. Cham: Springer International Publishing; 2019:141–153
[89] Kshettry VR, Healy AT, Jones NG, Mroz TE, Benzel EC. A quantitative analysis of posterolateral approaches to the ventral thoracic spinal canal. Spine J 2015;15:2228–2238
[90] Filippi M, Bar-Or A, Piehl F, et al. Multiple sclerosis. Nat Rev Dis Prim 2018;4:43
[91] Jarius S, Paul F, Weinshenker BG, Levy M, Kim HJ, Wildemann B. Neuromyelitis optica. Nat Rev Dis Prim 2020;6:85
[92] Hussain I, Parker WE, Barzilai O, Bilsky MH. Surgical management of intramedullary spinal cord tumors. Neurosurg Clin N Am 2020;31:237–249
[93] Hersh AM, Pennington Z, Lubelski D, et al. Treatment of intramedullary spinal cord tumors: a modified Delphi technique of the North American Spine Society Section of Spine Oncology. J Neurosurg Spine 2023:40(1):1–10
[94] Sciubba DM, Chaichana KL, Woodworth GF, McGirt MJ, Gokaslan ZL, Jallo GI. Factors associated with cervical instability requiring fusion after cervical laminectomy for intradural tumor resection. J Neurosurg Spine 2008;8:413–419
[95] Huschbeck A, Knoop M, Gahleitner A, et al. Recurrent laryngeal nerve palsy after anterior cervical discectomy and fusion - prevalence and risk factors. J Neurol Surg A Cent Eur Neurosurg 2020;81(6):508–512
[96] Johnson MD, Matur AV, Asghar F, Nasser R, Cheng JS, Prestigiacomo CJ. Right versus left approach to anterior cervical discectomy and fusion: an anatomic versus historic debate. World Neurosurg 2020:135:135–140
[97] Fountas KN, Kapsalaki EZ, Nikolakakos LG, et al. Anterior cervical discectomy and fusion associated complications. Spine (Phila Pa 1976) 2007;32(21):2310–2317
[98] Sejkorová A, Bolcha M, Beneš J, Kalhous J, Sameš M, Vachata P. Intraoperative measurement of endotracheal tube cuff pressure and its change during surgery in correlation with recurrent laryngeal nerve palsies, hoarseness, and dysphagia after anterior cervical discectomy and fusion: a prospective randomized controlled trial. Global Spine J 2023;13(6):1635–1640
[99] Miller A, Griepp DW, Miller C, Hamad M, Ramos RDlG, Murthy SG. The effectiveness of reducing endotracheal cuff pressure after retractor placement to decrease postoperative laryngeal dysfunction in anterior cervical surgery: a meta-analysis. J Neurosurg Spine 2022:37(1):21–30
[100] Berbari EF, Kanj SS, Kowalski TJ, et al. 2015 Infectious Diseases Society of America (IDSA) Clinical Practice Guidelines for the diagnosis and treatment of native vertebral osteomyelitis in adults. Clin Infect Dis 2015;61(6):e26–e46
[101] Longo M, Pennington Z, Gelfand Y, et al. Readmission after spinal epidural abscess management in urban populations: a bi-institutional study. J Neurosurg Spine 2019;32 (3):465–472

4 Pediatric Neurosurgery

Syed I. Khalid, Jonathan Scoville, Sandi Lam

▸▸ Question 1

A 12-year-old patient presents with a tectal glioma resulting in hydrocephalus. You decide to proceed with an endoscopic third ventriculostomy (ETV; ▸ Fig. 4.1). The structure indicated by the arrow in the third ventricle is most likely:

- A. Foramen of Monro
- B. Mammillary bodies
- C. Hypothalamus
- D. Pineal gland
- E. Tuber cinereum

Correct answer is B

In an ETV, accurately identifying the anatomical landmarks within the third ventricle is crucial. The mammillary bodies are prominent structures located on the floor of the third ventricle, just posterior to the tuber cinereum and infundibulum. These structures are essential landmarks during the procedure to ensure accurate fenestration of the floor of the third ventricle, typically performed anterior to the mammillary bodies, to create communication with the interpeduncular cistern. ▸ Fig. 4.2 shows an explicative case.

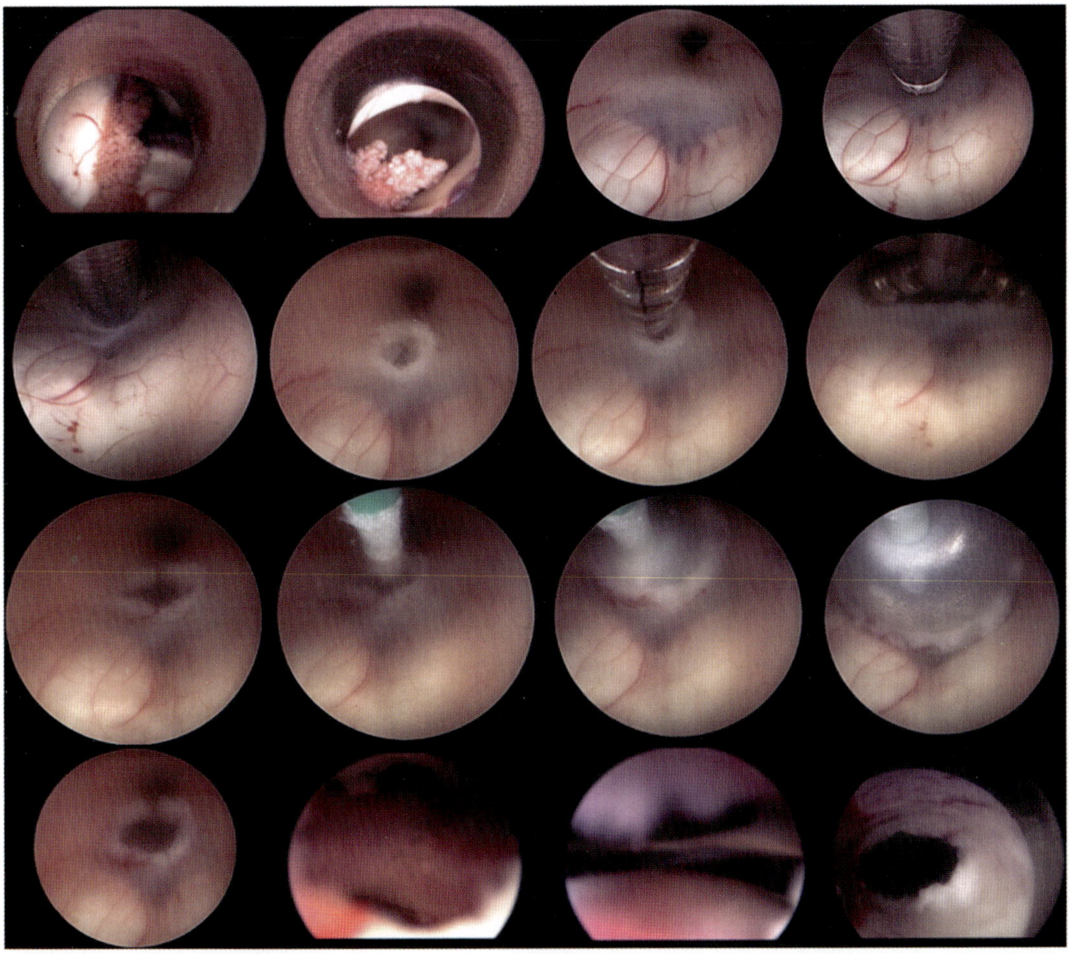

Fig. 4.1 (Source: Reproduced from Endoscopic third ventriculostomy. In: Torres-Corzo J, Rangel-Castilla L, Nakaji P, eds. Neuroendoscopic Surgery. 1st ed. New York: Thieme; 2016.)

(**A**) View from the endoscope after cannulation of the right lateral ventricle. (**B**) View of the floor of the third ventricle through the right foramen of Monro. (**C**) Fenestration of the floor of the third ventricle using a Fogarty balloon. (**D**) Floor of the third ventricle after the fenestration.

Abbreviations: BA, basilar artery; CP, choroid plexus; F, fornix; FC, Fogarty catheter; FE, fenestration; IR, infundibular recess; MB, mammillary body; MF, Monro foramen; OR, optic recess; PCA, posterior cerebral artery; SP, septum pellucidum; T, thalamus; TC, tuber cinereum; TSV, thalamostriate vein.

▸▸ Question 2

A 16-year-old male with a tectal glioma presents with new-onset headaches and is diagnosed with hydrocephalus. What is his endoscopic third ventriculostomy (ETV) success score?

- A. 40
- B. 60
- C. 70
- D. 80
- E. 90

Correct answer is E

The ETV success score (ETVSS) is a predictive tool used to estimate the likelihood of success for endoscopic third ventriculostomy based on patient age, hydrocephalus etiology, and prior shunt history. For a 16-year-old with a tectal glioma (typically non-communicating hydrocephalus), the ETVSS is calculated as follows (▶ Table 4.1).[1]

ETVSS = Age score + etiology score + previous shunt score

Calculation Example:

For a 16-year-old patient with a tectal glioma and no previous shunt:

- Age score: 50
- Etiology score: 30 (tectal tumor)
- Previous shunt score: 10 (no previous shunt)

Total ETVSS: 50 + 30 + 10 = 90

Table 4.1 Treatment of hydrocephalus

Category	Description	Value
Age	< 1 mo	0%
	1 to < 6 mo	10%
	6 mo to < 1 y	30%
	1 to > 10 y	40%
	≥ 10 y	50%
Etiology	Postinfectious	0%
	Myelomeningocele post-IVH	20%
	Non-tectal brain tumor	
	Aqueductal stenosis tectal tumor other	30%
Shunt history	Previous shunt	0%
	No previous shunt	10%
		Total (range: 0–90%)

Source: Reproduced from Treatment of hydrocephalus. In: Greenberg M, ed. Greenberg's Handbook of Neurosurgery. 10th ed. New York: Thieme; 2023.

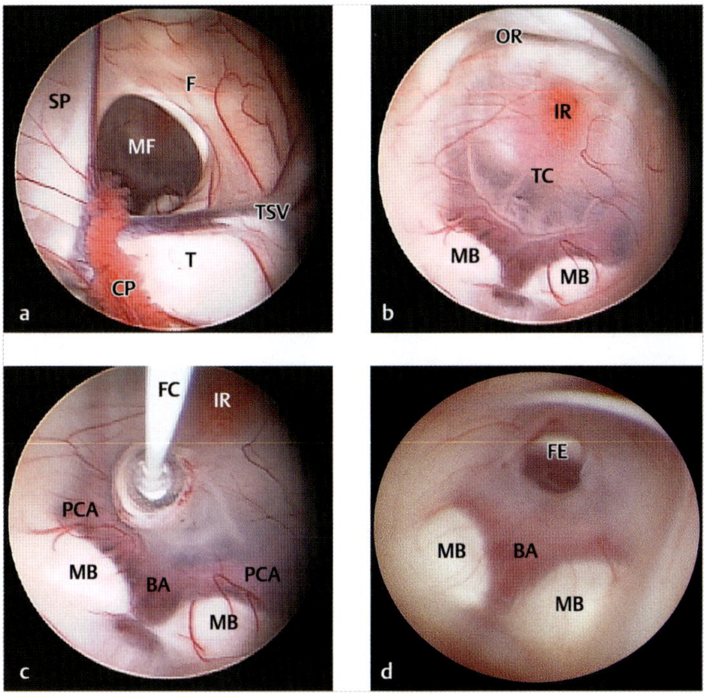

Fig. 4.2 (Source: Reproduced from Pearls. In: Gagliardi F, Gragnaniello C, Mortini P, Caputy A, eds. Operative Cranial Neurosurgical Anatomy. 1st ed. New York: Thieme; 2018.)

▸▸ Question 3

A 2-year-old male presents with a cerebellopontine angle mass and hydrocephalus. Tumor resection is undertaken, and pathology shows small blue cells with molecular marking of INI. What is the diagnosis?

- A. Medulloblastoma
- B. Ependymoma
- C. Atypical teratoid/rhabdoid tumor
- D. Choroid plexus carcinoma
- E. Pilocytic astrocytoma

Correct answer is C

Atypical teratoid/rhabdoid tumor (ATRT) is a rare and highly aggressive tumor primarily affecting young children. It is characterized histologically by small blue cells and genetically by the loss of the INI1 protein encoded by the *SMARCB1* gene. ATRT commonly presents in the posterior fossa or supratentorial regions and requires prompt and aggressive treatment, including surgery, chemotherapy, and often radiation (▸ Fig. 4.3).[2]

▸▸ Question 4

You admit a 7-year-old girl for surgery the next day. She weighs 27 kg. What is the appropriate maintenance fluid rate?

- A. 40 mL/h
- B. 50 mL/h
- C. 70 mL/h
- D. 80 mL/h
- E. 90 mL/h

Correct answer is D

The maintenance fluid rate for children can be calculated using the 4–2-1 rule[3]:

- 4 mL/kg/h for the first 10 kg
- 2 mL/kg/h for the next 10 kg
- 1 mL/kg/h for any additional kg

For a 27-kg child:

- First 10 kg: 10 kg × 4 mL/kg/h = 40 mL/h
- Next 10 kg: 10 kg × 2 mL/kg/h = 20 mL/h
- Remaining 7 kg: 7 kg × 1 mL/kg/h = 7 mL/h

Total = 40 + 20 + 7 = 67 mL/h, rounded to 70 mL/h.

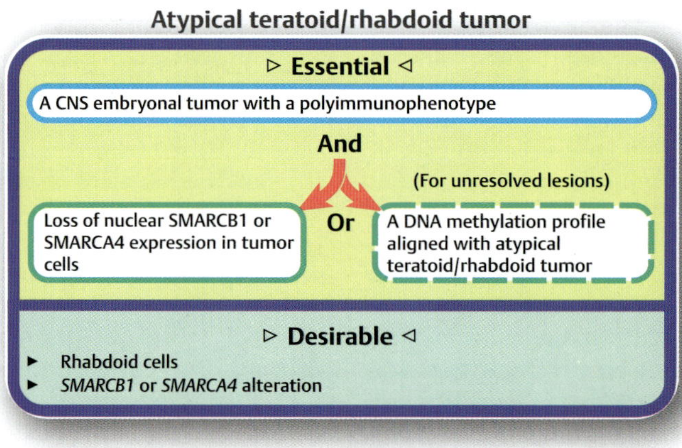

Fig. 4.3 (Source: Reproduced from Diagnostic criteria for atypical teratoid/rhabdoid tumor. In: Greenberg M, ed. Greenberg's Handbook of Neurosurgery. 10th ed. New York: Thieme; 2023.)

▸▸ Question 5

A newborn weighs 3.3 kg and has a cyst resulting in hydrocephalus. You plan to undertake surgery. What is the patient's circulating blood volume?

- A.150 mL
- B. 200 mL
- C. 250 mL
- D. 300 mL
- E. 350 mL

Correct answer is B

The circulating blood volume in neonates is approximately 80 to 100 mL/kg. For a newborn weighing 3.3 kg, the circulating blood volume can be estimated as follows:

- 3.3 kg × 60 mL/kg = 198 mL, rounded to 200 mL.

▸▸ Question 6

Which characteristics are most commonly associated with Apert syndrome but not Crouzon syndrome?

- A. Craniosynostosis
- B. Midface hypoplasia
- C. Syndactyly
- D. Hydrocephalus
- E. Proptosis

Correct answer is C

Apert syndrome and Crouzon syndrome are craniosynostosis syndromes with overlapping features such as craniosynostosis, midface hypoplasia, and proptosis. However, Apert syndrome is uniquely characterized by syndactyly, where the fingers and toes are fused. This feature is a distinguishing characteristic and is not typically seen in Crouzon syndrome.[4,5]

▸▸ Question 7

A 7-year-old boy is diagnosed with medulloblastoma. Molecular analysis reveals the tumor belongs to the WNT subgroup. Which of the following best describes the prognosis for this patient?

- A. Poor overall survival despite aggressive treatment
- B. Moderate survival with frequent recurrence
- C. Excellent prognosis with high survival rates
- D. Variable prognosis depending on resection extent
- E. Poor prognosis with limited treatment options

Correct answer is C

Medulloblastoma is categorized into four molecular subgroups: WNT, SHH, Group 3, and Group 4. Each subgroup has distinct genetic, clinical, and prognostic characteristics:

- **WNT subgroup:** This subgroup has the best prognosis, with overall survival rates exceeding

90% at 5 years. These tumors often have a good response to current therapies.

- **SHH (Sonic Hedgehog) subgroup:** The prognosis for this subgroup is intermediate and can vary significantly based on age and genetic mutations. Infants and patients with TP53 mutations within this subgroup tend to have poorer outcomes.
- **Group 3:** This subgroup is associated with the poorest prognosis, especially those with MYC amplification. The 5-year survival rate is significantly lower, often around 50% or less.
- **Group 4:** The prognosis for Group 4 medulloblastomas is intermediate, better than Group 3 but not as favorable as the WNT subgroup. The survival rate is typically around 75%.

The stratification of survival rates emphasizes the importance of molecular classification in guiding treatment and prognosis for medulloblastoma patients. ▶ Fig. 4.4 shows the prognosis and distribution of histologic variants among molecular

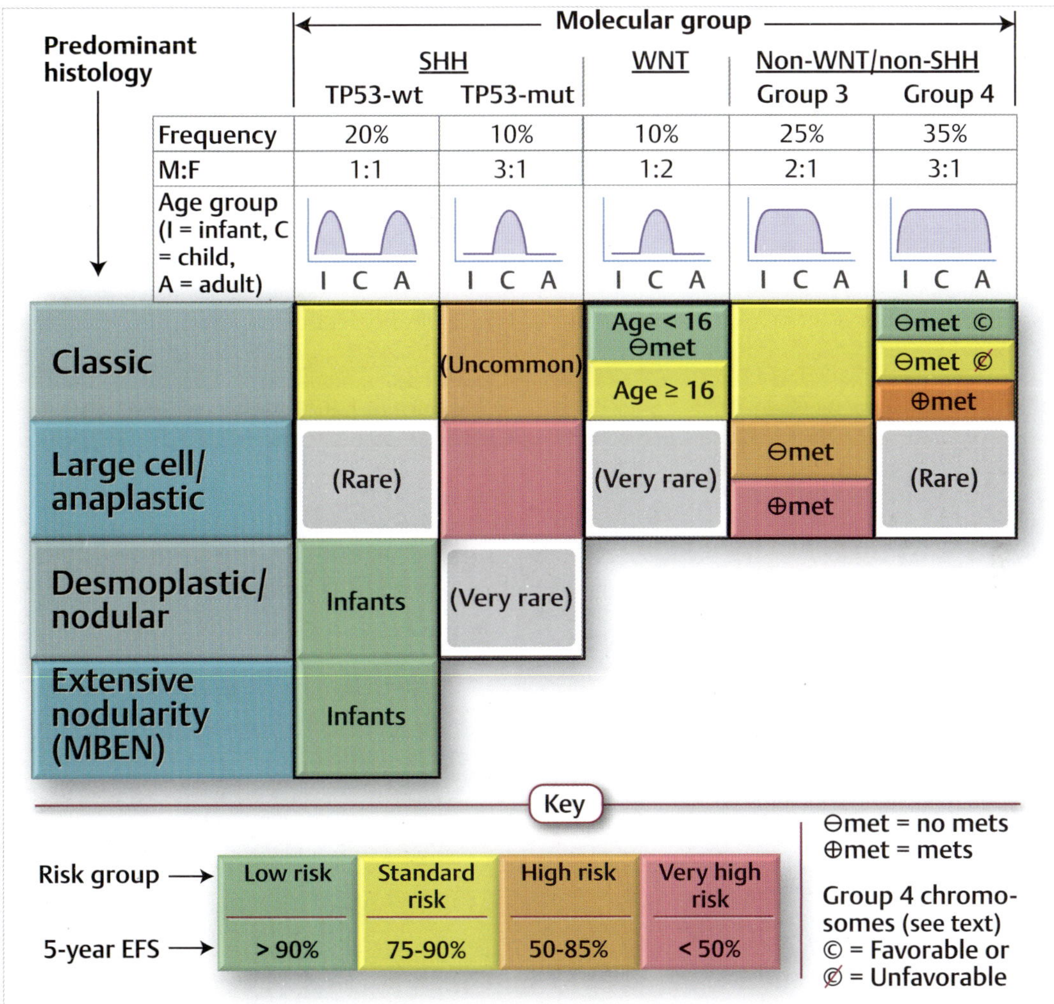

Fig. 4.4 (Source: Reproduced from Classification. In: Greenberg M, ed. Greenberg's Handbook of Neurosurgery. 10th ed. New York: Thieme; 2023.)

types of medulloblastoma. Box color indicates prognosis as follows:

5-year EFS rates: **low risk** > 90%, **standard risk** 75 to 90%, **high risk** 50 to 75%, **very high risk** < 50%.

No risk is shown for tumors of uncertain clinicopathological significance.

Abbreviations: EFS, event-free survival; MDB, medulloblastoma; SHH, activated sonic hedgehog; TP53, tumor protein 53; mut, mutant; wt, wild type; WNT, activated wingless/integrated (signal transduction pathway), ©, favorable chromosomal findings for non-WNT/non-SHH group 4: chromosome 7 gain, chromosome 8 loss, chromosome 11 loss, chromosome 17 gain.[6,7]

▸▸ Question 8

A 4-year-old boy presents with ataxia. MRI reveals vermian agenesis and midbrain–hindbrain malformation which resembles a "molar tooth." Which of the following is the most likely diagnosis (▶ Fig. 4.5)?

- A. Medulloblastoma
- B. Ependymoma
- C. Diffuse intrinsic pontine glioma
- D. Joubert syndrome
- E. Pilomyxoid astrocytoma

Correct answer is D

Joubert syndrome is a rare genetic disorder characterized by the "molar tooth sign" on MRI due to the abnormal development of the cerebellar vermis and brainstem. This condition often presents with hypotonia, ataxia, and developmental delays. The other conditions listed, such as medulloblastoma, ependymoma, and diffuse intrinsic pontine glioma, typically present with different imaging and clinical features.[8]

▸▸ Question 9

Which gene mutation is most commonly associated with neurofibromatosis type 1 in children, leading to multiple café-au-lait spots and an increased risk of optic glioma?

- A. PTEN
- B. BRAF
- C. NF1
- D. TP53
- E. H3F3A

Correct answer is C

Mutations in the *NF1* gene cause neurofibromatosis type 1 (NF1). It is characterized by multiple café-au-lait spots, neurofibromas, and an increased risk of developing optic gliomas and other tumors. The other genes listed are associated with different conditions and cancers, such as PTEN with Cowden syndrome, BRAF with certain melanomas, TP53 with Li-Fraumeni syndrome, and H3F3A with certain brainstem gliomas (▶ Box 4.1).

▸▸ Question 10

A 2-month-old infant presents with a sacral dimple and tuft of hair. Ultrasound reveals a tethered

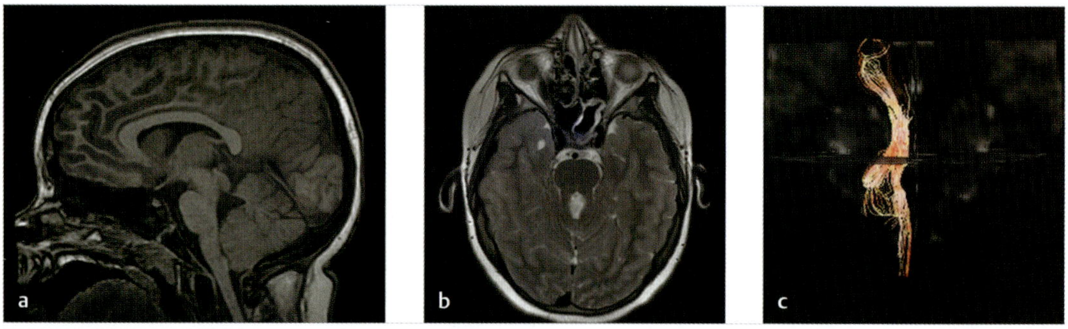

Fig. 4.5 (Source: Reproduced from Joubert syndrome. In: Choudhri A, ed. Pediatric Neuroradiology: Clinical Practice Essentials. 1st ed. New York: Thieme; 2016)

Box 4.1 Diagnostic criteria for NF1 according to NIH Consensus Conference

Diagnosis of NF1 requires **at least two** of the following (according to the **National Institutes of Health Consensus Conference**)
• Café au lait macules: ◦ In children: more than 5 macules of 0.5-cm diameter ◦ In adults: more than 5 macules of 1.5-cm diameter
• One plexiform neurofibroma or two or more neurofibromas of any type
• Multiple axillary or inguinal freckles
• Optic pathway gliomas (most commonly pilocytic astrocytoma)
• Distinctive bony abnormality (sphenoid wing dysplasia or congenital bowing or thinning of the long bone cortex with or without pseudoarthrosis)
• Two or more iris hamartomas (Lisch nodules)
• A first-degree relative with neurofibromatosis type 1

spinal cord. Which of the following embryonic stages is implicated in developing this condition?

- A. Gastrulation
- B. Neurulation
- C. Organogenesis
- D. Somitogenesis
- E. Neural crest migration

Correct answer is B

Tethered spinal cord syndrome is often associated with defects in the neurulation process, which involves the formation and closure of the neural tube during embryonic development. Other conditions, such as neural crest migration defects, can lead to different congenital abnormalities, but they do not typically result in tethered cord syndrome.[9]

▸▸ Question 11

A 10-year-old girl with a known diagnosis of tuberous sclerosis complex (TSC) presents with new-onset seizures. MRI of the brain shows multiple subependymal nodules and cortical tubers. Which pharmacologic agent is FDA-approved for the treatment of subependymal giant cell astrocytomas (SEGA) associated with TSC?

- A. Carbamazepine
- B. Levetiracetam
- C. Everolimus
- D. Vincristine
- E. Prednisone

Correct answer is C

Everolimus, a mammalian target of rapamycin inhibitor, is FDA-approved for the treatment of SEGA in patients with TSC. This medication helps reduce the size of these tumors. Other agents listed, such as carbamazepine and levetiracetam, are used for seizure control but are not specific treatments for SEGA.[10]

▸▸ Question 12

What is the primary difference in outcome for fetal myelomeningocele repair compared to postnatal repair?

- A. Improved leg function
- B. Decreased need for ventriculoperitoneal shunting
- C. Increased IQ
- D. Reduced incidence of hydrocephalus
- E. Lower risk of Chiari II malformation development

Correct answer is B

Fetal myelomeningocele repair has been shown to decrease the need for ventriculoperitoneal shunting postnatally, compared to repairs done after birth. This prenatal intervention does not necessarily improve leg function, increase IQ, or significantly reduce the incidence of hydrocephalus or Chiari II malformation, although it may have some impact on these outcomes.[11]

▸▸ **Question 13**

A 15-year-old boy presents with a rapidly growing mass in the cerebellum, headache, and vomiting. Biopsy reveals a highly malignant tumor with small blue cells. Which molecular marker would be most prognostically significant?

- A. WNT pathway activation
- B. MYC amplification
- C. IDH1 mutation
- D. H3 K27 M mutation
- E. 1p/19q co-deletion

Correct answer is A

Medulloblastomas are the most common malignant brain tumors in children and can be categorized into different molecular subgroups. WNT pathway activation is associated with the best prognosis among these subgroups. MYC amplification is linked with a poor prognosis. IDH1 mutations are more commonly seen in gliomas. H3 K27 M mutations are associated with diffuse intrinsic pontine gliomas, and 1p/19q co-deletion is characteristic of oligodendrogliomas.

▸▸ **Question 14**

Which of the following is the most common presenting symptom in children with an intracranial ganglioglioma?

- A. Headache
- B. Hemiparesis
- C. Seizures
- D. Visual disturbances
- E. Ataxia

Correct answer is C

Gangliogliomas are rare, usually benign brain tumors that often present with seizures, especially in children. They are commonly found in the temporal lobe, which is highly epileptogenic. Other symptoms, such as headache, hemiparesis, visual disturbances, and ataxia, can occur but are less common as initial presenting symptoms.[12]

▸▸ **Question 15**

For a child with craniosynostosis, which cranial suture is the most common site of premature fusion in nonsyndromic cases?

- A. Sagittal
- B. Coronal
- C. Metopic
- D. Lambdoid
- E. Squamosal

Correct answer is A

Sagittal synostosis is the most common type of nonsyndromic craniosynostosis. It results in a long, narrow head shape known as scaphocephaly. Coronal and metopic sutures are less commonly involved in isolated craniosynostosis, while lambdoid and squamosal synostoses are rare.[13]

▸▸ **Question 16**

Which of the following is the most appropriate initial step in managing a 3-month-old infant with plagiocephaly and right occipital skull flattening?

- A. Cranial orthotic therapy
- B. Surgical cranial vault remodeling
- C. Observation and reevaluation in 3 months
- D. Immediate MRI
- E. Physical therapy for torticollis

Correct answer is E

In cases of positional plagiocephaly, initial management often involves physiotherapy to address any associated torticollis, which is a common contributing factor. Cranial orthotic therapy can be considered if there is no improvement with conservative measures. Surgical interventions are generally reserved for craniosynostosis or severe cases that do not respond to less invasive treatments.

▸▸ **Question 17**

A 3-year-old boy has recently undergone gross total surgical resection of a fourth ventricular WHO grade II ependymoma. Molecular subgroup analysis is pending as is the decision whether he will undergo adjuvant treatment. What is the most accepted prognostic factor that will affect his overall survival?

- A. Tumor location
- B. Patient's age
- C. Tumor histology
- D. Extent of resection
- E. Presence of metastasis

Correct answer is D

The extent of resection is the most crucial prognostic factor in determining overall survival for patients with ependymoma. Gross total resection, confirmed by postoperative MRI, is associated with significantly improved progression-free and overall survival. Although molecular subgroups and histology can provide additional prognostic information, the completeness of the surgical resection remains paramount.

▸▸ Question 18

What medication reduces the risk of intraventricular hemorrhage (IVH) and improves outcomes in premature infants?

- A. Antibiotics
- B. Anticoagulants
- C. Corticosteroids
- D. Diuretics
- E. Antihypertensives

Correct answer is C

Antenatal corticosteroid administration is a well-established intervention that reduces the risk of IVH in premature infants. Corticosteroids help mature the fetal lungs and reduce the incidence of respiratory distress syndrome, which is associated with a decreased risk of IVH. The use of antibiotics, anticoagulants, diuretics, or antihypertensives does not have the same impact on IVH in this population.[14]

▸▸ Question 19

A 17-year-old male presented with a heterogeneously contrast-enhancing mass within the spinal cord, causing significant spinal cord expansion and compression. After laminectomy, an expansile intramedullary mass that appeared highly vascularized and infiltrative was found. A frozen section showed glioblastoma. What is the most appropriate next step in management?

- A. Complete resection
- B. Radiation therapy
- C. Chemotherapy
- D. Duraplasty without resection
- E. Steroid administration

Correct answer is D

Spinal cord glioblastoma is a rare and aggressive tumor. The extent of resection does not significantly improve survival, and aggressive resection can result in significant neurological deficits due to the infiltrative nature of the tumor. Duraplasty is performed to accommodate postprocedure edema and spinal cord decompression. Radiation therapy and chemotherapy can be considered as adjunctive treatments, but complete resection is generally not feasible or beneficial.

▸▸ Question 20

A 15-year-old girl with a history of epilepsy and learning disability presents with vomiting and somnolence. MRI shows obstructive hydrocephalus with a 3-cm calcified, contrast-enhancing intraventricular mass near the foramen of Monro, as well as several small subependymal nodules. Which cutaneous findings are most likely to be observed on physical examination?

- A. Café-au-lait spots
- B. Port-wine stain
- C. Hypopigmented macules
- D. Neurofibromas
- E. Hemangiomas

Correct answer is C

The clinical presentation suggests tuberous sclerosis complex (TSC), which is characterized by hypopigmented macules (ash leaf spots) among other features. Patients with TSC commonly have cortical tubers, subependymal nodules, and subependymal giant cell astrocytomas, which can cause obstructive hydrocephalus. Café-au-lait spots are associated with neurofibromatosis type 1, port-wine stains with Sturge-Weber syndrome, neurofibromas with neurofibromatosis, and hemangiomas are common vascular anomalies (▸ Box 4.2).

▸▸ Question 21

A 17-year-old cerebral palsy patient with spasticity undergoes intrathecal baclofen pump placement with significant objective improvement. Fifteen months later, he presents to the emergency department with recurrent spasticity. He is otherwise medically well, afebrile, and without signs or symptoms of infection. What is the next most appropriate step in management?

- A. Increase oral baclofen dosage
- B. MRI of the spine
- C. Shunt revision
- D. Refill the baclofen pump
- E. Pump interrogation and catheter assessment

Box 4.2 Clinical diagnostic criteria of tuberous sclerosis complex

Definitive diagnosis: 2 major criteria, or 1 major AND ≥ 2 minor
Possible diagnosis: 1 major or ≥ 2 minor
Major criteria
≥ 3 hypomelanotic macules ≥ 5 mm diameter
≥ 3 angiofibromas or fibrous cephalic plaque
≥ 2 ungual fibroma
Shagreen patch
Multiple retinal hamartomas
Cortical dysplasias (including tubers and cerebral white matter radial migration lines)
Subependymal nodules
Subependymal giant cell astrocytoma (SEGA)
Cardiac rhabdomyoma
Lymphangioleiomyomatosis
≥ 2 angiomyolipomas
Minor criteria
"Confetti" skin lesions
≥ 4 pits in dental enamel
≥ 2 intraoral fibromas
Achromic retinal patch
Multiple renal cysts
Nonrenal hamartomas

Source: Reproduced from Greenberg's Handbook of Neurosurgery. Greenberg M, ed. 10th ed. New York: Thieme; 2023.

Box 4.3 Assessing ITB infusion systems (adapted)

Interrogate the pump (with device programmer): alarm log for low reservoir, low battery, or end of service; check rotor log (rotor stops temporarily in MRI scanners)
Verify reservoir volume: aspirate the entire volume of drug and compare to the volume calculated by the programmer; discrepancies > 25% may signal mechanical faults. Refill the reservoir with the drug if empty (by an experienced ITB practitioner)
Obtain AP and lateral X-rays to assess the location of the catheter tip and to look for breaks,[a] kinks, or migration
Program the pump to administer a prescribed bolus, observe for decreased spasticity (takes up to 4 h)
Aspirate 3–4 mL through the catheter aspiration port (CAP). Difficulty aspirating or bubbles are abnormal
Contrast study (either of the following can miss a microleak): • If abrupt onset: aspirate the CAP (if unsuccessful, do *not* inject dye because of danger of overdose), then inject iodinated contrast into the CAP either under fluoroscopy or while the patient is in the CT scanner (do not move the patient between injecting and imaging). High rate of false negatives • Insidious onset: an indium study can be done; it takes ≈ 24 h to get the radio-isotope. DPTA radio-isotope is injected into the reservoir fill port—not into the CAP! (Okay for it to mix with baclofen). Image with nuclear medicine camera (length of study depends on programmed flow rate). This test is expensive, takes a long time to complete (2–3 days) from the time it is ordered, and has low sensitivity

[a]In 2012, Medtronic replaced the radiopaque catheter with a stronger Ascenda catheter, which is radiolucent except for a small spot on the distal tip.
Source: Reproduced from Intrathecal baclofen. In: Greenberg M, ed. Greenberg's Handbook of Neurosurgery. 10th ed. New York: Thieme; 2023.

Correct answer is E

In a patient with an intrathecal baclofen pump presenting with recurrent spasticity, the most appropriate initial step is to interrogate the pump and assess the catheter for potential issues. This approach can identify mechanical problems such as catheter kinks, disconnections, or pump malfunction. Increasing oral baclofen may provide temporary relief but does not address the underlying issue. MRI of the spine might be necessary if structural causes are suspected, but it is not the first step. Shunt revision is irrelevant in this context unless there is a shunt in place for hydrocephalus, which is not indicated here (▶ Box 4.3).

▸▸ Question 22

Following transsphenoidal resection of a large craniopharyngioma, what are the manifestations of a classic triphasic response?

- A. Hypothyroidism, hyperthyroidism, euthyroidism
- B. SIADH, diabetes insipidus, cerebral salt wasting
- C. Cerebral edema, meningitis, encephalitis
- D. Hypernatremia, hyponatremia, and return to normonatremia
- E. Hypovolemia, hypervolemia, normovolemia

Correct answer is D

The classic triphasic response following transsphenoidal resection of a large craniopharyngioma involves an initial phase of diabetes insipidus (leading to hypernatremia), followed by a phase of inappropriate antidiuretic hormone secretion (SIADH, leading to hyponatremia), and a subsequent return to normonatremia. This pattern is associated with the disruption and subsequent recovery of the hypothalamic–pituitary axis. Other options, such as thyroid disorders or cerebral salt wasting, are less relevant to this specific context.

▸▸ Question 23

What endocrinological complication is most common following radiotherapy for a posterior fossa tumor in childhood?

- A. Hyperthyroidism
- B. Hypothyroidism
- C. Diabetes mellitus
- D. Addison disease
- E. Hyperparathyroidism

Correct answer is B

Hypothyroidism is the most common endocrinological complication following radiotherapy for posterior fossa tumors in childhood. The thyroid gland is highly sensitive to radiation, and damage can lead to decreased thyroid hormone production. Monitoring thyroid function is crucial in children receiving radiotherapy to the head and neck region. Other endocrine complications, such as diabetes mellitus or Addison disease, are less commonly associated with this specific treatment.[15]

▸▸ Question 24

A 10-year-old child with medically refractory spasticity and significant disabling dystonia in all four extremities, face, and neck is being considered for intrathecal baclofen therapy. What is the most appropriate treatment?

- A. Oral baclofen
- B. Physical therapy
- C. Selective dorsal rhizotomy
- D. Intrathecal baclofen pump placement
- E. Deep brain stimulation

Correct answer is D

For a child with severe, medically refractory spasticity and dystonia, intrathecal baclofen pump placement is the most appropriate treatment. This method delivers baclofen directly to the intrathecal space, providing effective relief from spasticity and dystonia with fewer systemic side effects compared to oral baclofen. Physical therapy and selective dorsal rhizotomy are alternative treatments but may not be as effective for severe dystonia involving multiple body regions. Deep brain stimulation is typically used for other movement disorders.[16]

▸▸ Question 25

Premature closure of the metopic suture results in what head shape?

- A. Scaphocephaly
- B. Trigonocephaly
- C. Brachycephaly
- D. Plagiocephaly
- E. Oxycephaly

Correct answer is B

Premature closure of the metopic suture leads to trigonocephaly, characterized by a triangular forehead and closely spaced eyes (hypotelorism). Scaphocephaly results from the premature closure of the sagittal suture, leading to a long, narrow head shape. Brachycephaly is due to the premature closure of both coronal sutures, resulting in a short, wide head. Plagiocephaly involves asymmetrical distortion of the skull, often due to positional factors. Oxycephaly (or turricephaly) refers to a high, tower-like skull, typically resulting from the premature closure of multiple sutures (▶ Fig. 4.6 and ▶ Fig. 4.7).

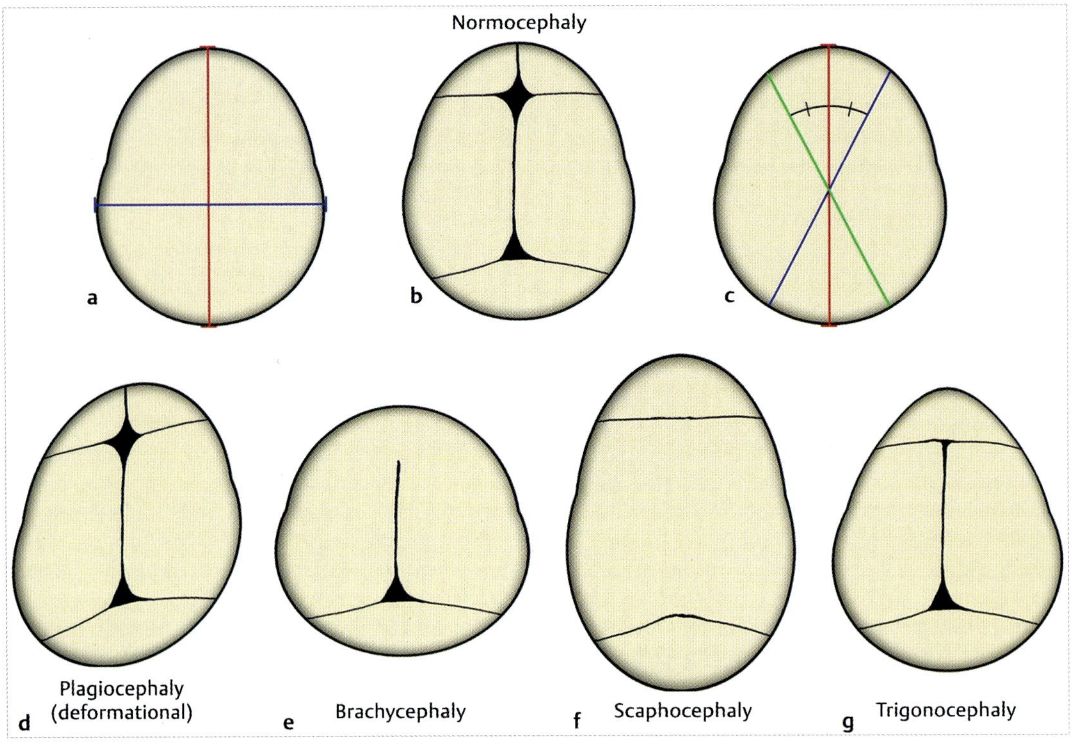

Fig. 4.6 (Source: Reproduced from Positional plagiocephaly. In: Nader R, Sabbagh A, Elbabaa S, Al-Jehani H, Gasco J, Gragnaniello C, eds. Neurosurgery Case Review: Questions and Answers. 2nd ed. New York: Thieme; 2020.)

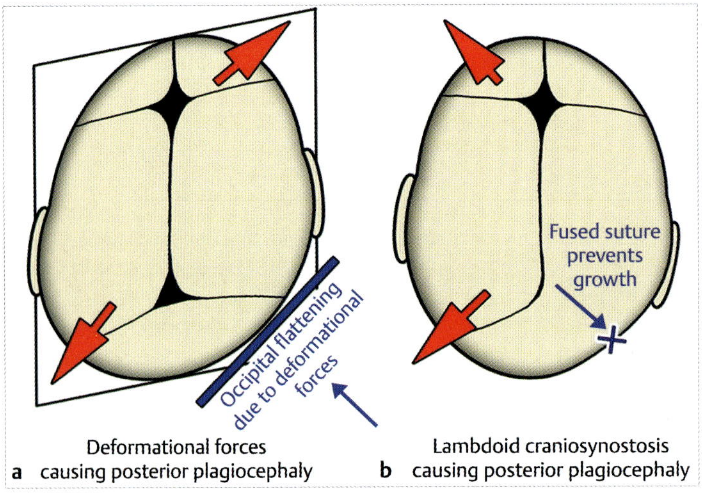

Fig. 4.7 (Source: Reproduced from Positional plagiocephaly. In: Nader R, Sabbagh A, Elbabaa S, Al-Jehani H, Gasco J, Gragnaniello C, eds. Neurosurgery Case Review: Questions and Answers. 2nd ed. New York: Thieme; 2020.)

▸▸ **Question 26**

A 3-year-old child with moyamoya disease is scheduled for an encephaloduroarteriosynangiosis (EDAS) indirect bypass. What is the most common cause of new perioperative neurological deficits?

- A. Hyperperfusion syndrome
- B. Acute ischemic stroke
- C. Hemorrhagic stroke
- D. Anesthetic complications
- E. Infection

Correct answer is A

In patients undergoing indirect revascularization surgery, such as EDAS for moyamoya disease, hyperperfusion syndrome is the most common cause of new perioperative neurological deficits. This condition occurs due to the sudden increase in blood flow to chronically ischemic areas, leading to cerebral edema and hemorrhage. While ischemic and hemorrhagic strokes are also concerns, hyperperfusion syndrome is more specifically related to the surgical revascularization process. Anesthetic complications and infections, although potential perioperative issues, are less common causes of neurological deficits in this context.

▸▸ **Question 27**

Which symptomatic hormone deficiency is most common after pediatric moderate-to-severe traumatic brain injury (TBI)?

- A. Growth hormone deficiency
- B. Thyroid hormone deficiency
- C. Cortisol deficiency
- D. Gonadotropin deficiency
- E. Antidiuretic hormone deficiency

Correct answer is A

Growth hormone deficiency is the most common symptomatic hormone deficiency following moderate-to-severe TBI in children. The pituitary gland is vulnerable to injury, which can lead to hypopituitarism. Thyroid hormone, cortisol, and gonadotropin deficiencies can also occur but are less common than growth hormone deficiency. Antidiuretic hormone deficiency (leading to diabetes insipidus) can be a concern acutely but is not typically a chronic issue post-TBI.

▸▸ **Question 28**

A 12-year-old with Down syndrome has abnormal flexion-extension cervical spine X-rays. The child has no significant neurologic complaints or neck pain. On exam, the child has a full range of motion and no tenderness to palpation. The flexion-extension X-rays show a 7- to 8-mm atlantodental interval in flexion, which reduces to 4 mm in extension. What is the most appropriate next step?

- A. Immediate surgical intervention
- B. MRI to assess for cord compression
- C. Physical therapy and observation
- D. Restriction from contact sports
- E. Repeat X-rays in 6 months

Correct answer is B

In a child with Down syndrome and an increased atlantodental interval, the most appropriate next step is an MRI to assess for spinal cord compression. This is crucial even in the absence of significant neurological symptoms, as the MRI can reveal subclinical findings that might necessitate intervention. Immediate surgical intervention is not warranted without evidence of cord compression. Physical therapy and observation, restriction from contact sports, and repeat X-rays are less urgent steps compared to confirming the absence or presence of cord compression through MRI.

▸▸ **Question 29**

A 10-year-old boy presents with progressive headaches, nausea, and vomiting. MRI reveals a cystic cerebellar mass with an enhancing mural nodule. Histology shows Rosenthal fibers. Which gene mutation is considered to drive this tumor?

- A. IDH1 R132H
- B. H3 K27M
- C. BRAF V600E
- D. TP53
- E. NF1

Correct answer is C

Pilocytic astrocytoma, commonly presenting as a cystic cerebellar mass with an enhancing mural nodule, is typically driven by the BRAF V600E mutation. Histologically, these tumors often contain Rosenthal fibers. While IDH1 R132H and H3 K27M mutations are associated with other types of gliomas, and TP53 mutations are more common

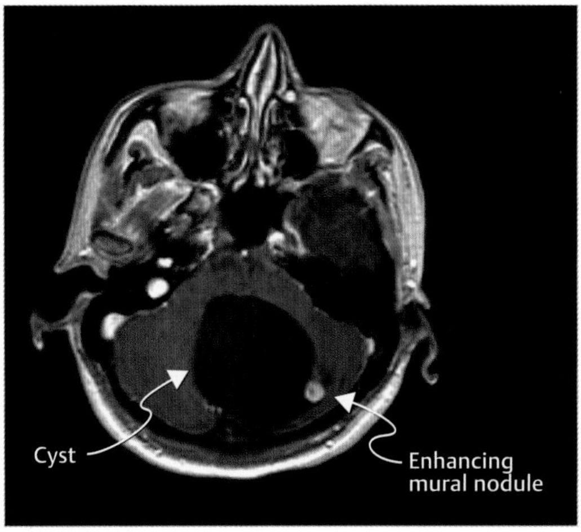

Fig. 4.8 (Source: Reproduced from Imaging. In: Greenberg M, ed. Greenberg's Handbook of Neurosurgery. 10th ed. New York: Thieme; 2023.)

in high-grade gliomas, the BRAF V600E mutation is characteristic of pilocytic astrocytoma. NF1 mutations are associated with neurofibromatosis type 1, which can also predispose to different types of brain tumors, including optic gliomas and pilocytic astrocytomas (▸ Fig. 4.8).

▸▸ Question 30

A 6-month-old infant presents with an asymmetric skull shape. Physical examination reveals unilateral flattening of the occiput and anterior displacement of the ipsilateral ear. What is the most likely diagnosis?

- A. Sagittal synostosis
- B. Metopic synostosis
- C. Positional plagiocephaly
- D. Lambdoid synostosis
- E. Coronal synostosis

Correct answer is C

Positional plagiocephaly is characterized by unilateral flattening of the occiput and anterior displacement of the ipsilateral ear, typically resulting from external pressures on the skull. This condition is often managed conservatively with repositioning and physical therapy. In contrast, craniosynostosis (including sagittal, metopic, lambdoid, and coronal synostosis) involves the premature fusion of cranial sutures, which usually requires surgical intervention. The physical examination findings, along with the clinical history, help differentiate positional plagiocephaly from craniosynostosis.

▸▸ Question 31

A 10-year-old boy with a known genetic diagnosis of von Hippel-Lindau (VHL) disease presents with symptoms of myelopathy. MRI of the spine reveals an intramedullary lesion consistent with a hemangioblastoma. Which of the following is the most appropriate treatment?

- A. Observation and serial imaging
- B. Stereotactic radiosurgery
- C. Chemotherapy
- D. Surgical resection
- E. Immunotherapy

Correct answer is D

In patients with VHL disease who develop symptomatic spinal hemangioblastomas, surgical resection is the most appropriate treatment. These tumors are highly vascular and can cause significant neurological deficits if not treated. Observation is reserved for asymptomatic, small lesions. Stereotactic radiosurgery and chemotherapy are not standard treatments for spinal hemangioblastomas. Immunotherapy is not indicated for this type of tumor. Surgical resection aims to remove the tumor and alleviate compression on the spinal cord (▸ Table 4.2).

▸▸ Question 32

A newborn is noted to have a sacral dimple with a tuft of hair at birth. Ultrasound of the spine is recommended to screen for which of the following conditions?

- A. Diastematomyelia
- B. Spina bifida occulta
- C. Lipomyelomeningocele
- D. Tethered cord syndrome
- E. Meningocele

Correct answer is B

A sacral dimple with a tuft of hair is a cutaneous marker that may be associated with spina bifida occulta, a type of neural tube defect where the vertebral arches fail to close completely. An ultrasound is a noninvasive screening tool used to evaluate the underlying spinal anatomy in

Table 4.2 Associations with VHL disease

Common lesions	Frequency in VHL
Hemangioblastomas	
Cerebellum (solid or cystic)	80%
Retina	41–59%
Brainstem	10–25%
Spinal cord	10–50%
Pancreatic tumors or cysts	22–80%
Renal clear cell Ca and cysts	14–60%
Polycythemia	9–20% of intracranial HGBs
Rare lesions (pertinent to the nervous system)	**Frequency in VHL**
Supratentorial hemangioblastoma	3–6%
Cystadenomas of the broad ligament	10% of 1♀
Papillary cystadenomas of epididymis	25–60% ♂
Endolymphatic sac tumors	10–15%
Adrenal medullary *pheochromocytoma* (tends to be bilateral)	7–24%

Abbreviation: VHL, von Hippel-Lindau.
Source: Reproduced Greenberg's Handbook of Neurosurgery. Greenberg M, ed. 10th Edition. New York: Thieme; 2023.

infants. Diastematomyelia, lipomyelomeningocele, tethered cord syndrome, and meningocele are other potential conditions associated with cutaneous markers, but spina bifida occulta is the most common and typically the initial condition screened for in such presentations.

▸▸ Question 33

A 16-year-old patient with cerebral palsy and severe spasticity is being considered for intrathecal baclofen pump placement. What is the primary goal of this treatment?

- A. Cure of cerebral palsy
- B. Improvement in cognitive function
- C. Reduction of spasticity
- D. Permanent correction of muscle tone
- E. Enhancement of motor skills

Correct answer is C

The primary goal of intrathecal baclofen pump placement in patients with cerebral palsy is to reduce spasticity. This treatment helps manage severe spasticity that is not responsive to oral medications. It can improve comfort, ease of care, and functional abilities, although it does not cure cerebral palsy or permanently correct muscle tone. While improvement in motor skills and cognitive function might be secondary benefits, the main objective is to reduce the spasticity that significantly impacts the patient's quality of life.

▸▸ Question 34

A 7-year-old boy presents with progressive weakness and sensory loss in his lower limbs. MRI of the spine reveals a tethered cord. Which embryological stage is implicated in the development of this condition?

- A. Gastrulation
- B. Neurulation
- C. Somitogenesis
- D. Organogenesis
- E. Neural crest migration

Correct answer is B

Neurulation is the embryological stage during which the neural tube forms, eventually giving rise to the central nervous system. Tethered cord syndrome is associated with defects in neurulation, leading to abnormal fixation of the spinal cord. This condition can result in progressive neurological deterioration due to the tension on the spinal cord. Gastrulation involves the formation of the three germ layers, somitogenesis refers to the formation of somites, and organogenesis is the process where organs develop from the three germ layers. Neural crest migration is essential for the development of peripheral nerves and other structures but is not directly related to tethered cord syndrome.[17]

▸▸ Question 35

A 5-year-old girl with a history of myelomeningocele repair presents with new-onset urinary incontinence and back pain. MRI shows a tethered spinal cord and syringomyelia. What is the most appropriate next step in management?

- A. Observation
- B. Shunt revision
- C. Surgical detethering
- D. Physical therapy
- E. Increase in antispasmodic medication

Correct answer is C

Surgical detethering is the most appropriate next step in managing a patient with a tethered spinal cord and syringomyelia. This intervention aims to release the tethered cord, thereby reducing tension on the spinal cord and alleviating associated symptoms such as back pain and urinary incontinence. Observation and physical therapy would not address the underlying issue. Shunt revision is not indicated unless there is evidence of shunt malfunction. Increasing antispasmodic medication may provide symptom relief but does not treat the tethering itself.

▸▸ Question 36

A 6-year-old boy with Sturge-Weber syndrome presents with a port-wine stain on the face and refractory epilepsy. Which brain findings are most characteristic of this condition?

- A. Leptomeningeal angiomas
- B. Subependymal giant cell astrocytomas
- C. Demyelination of white matter
- D. Focal cortical dysplasia
- E. Arachnoid cysts

Correct answer is A

Leptomeningeal angiomas are the most characteristic brain findings in Sturge-Weber syndrome, a neurocutaneous disorder. These vascular malformations typically affect the leptomeninges and can lead to seizures, stroke-like episodes, and neurological deficits. Subependymal giant cell astrocytomas are associated with tuberous sclerosis, while demyelination of white matter can be seen in various leukodystrophies. Focal cortical dysplasia is a common cause of epilepsy but is not specific to Sturge-Weber syndrome. Arachnoid cysts are fluid-filled sacs that can occur independently of genetic syndromes.

▸▸ Question 37

A 6-month-old male with a history of cutis aplasia presents with rapid head growth and bulging anterior fontanelle. Imaging reveals a significant buildup of cerebrospinal fluid within the ventricles. What is the most likely diagnosis?

- A. Aqueductal stenosis
- B. Arachnoid cyst
- C. Dandy-Walker malformation
- D. Encephalocele
- E. Subdural hematoma

Correct answer is A

Aqueductal stenosis is a common cause of congenital hydrocephalus, characterized by obstruction of cerebrospinal fluid flow at the level of the cerebral aqueduct. This leads to ventriculomegaly, increased intracranial pressure, and rapid head growth in infants. Arachnoid cysts, Dandy-Walker malformation, encephalocele, and subdural hematomas have different presentations and etiologies. Correct diagnosis is crucial for appropriate management, often involving surgical intervention (▸ Fig. 4.9).

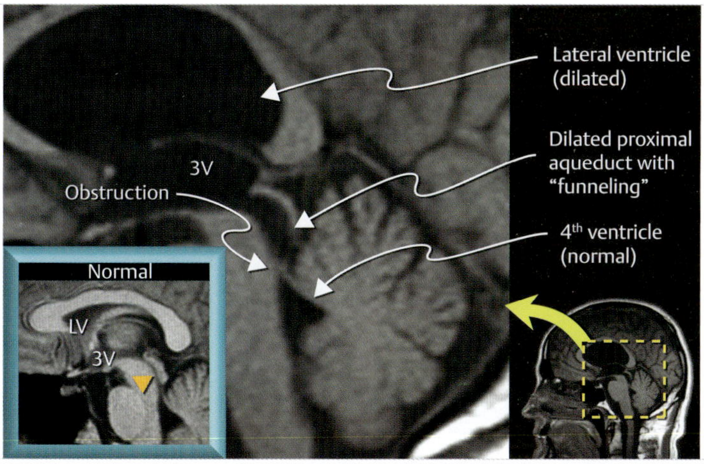

Fig. 4.9 (Source: Reproduced from Evaluation. In: Greenberg M, ed. Greenberg's Handbook of Neurosurgery. 10th ed. New York: Thieme; 2023.)

▸▸ Question 38

A 7-year-old girl with a history of recurrent urinary tract infections presents with back pain and leg weakness. MRI shows an intramedullary spinal cord tumor with enhancement. Which of the following is the most likely diagnosis?

- A. Astrocytoma
- B. Ependymoma
- C. Ganglioglioma
- D. Medulloblastoma
- E. Hemangioblastoma

Correct answer is A

Astrocytoma is the **most common intramedullary spinal cord tumor in children**, typically arising in the cervical or thoracic cord. It presents with symptoms of cord compression, such as back pain, weakness, and sometimes bladder dysfunction. Ependymomas are more common in adults but can occur in children, particularly in the lower spine (conus medullaris or filum terminale). Gangliogliomas are rare and typically cortical. Medulloblastomas arise in the cerebellum. Hemangioblastomas are rare in children and associated with von Hippel-Lindau syndrome.

▸▸ Question 39

A 10-year-old boy presents with a severe headache, nausea, and ataxia. MRI reveals a midline cerebellar mass with heterogeneous enhancement. What is the most likely diagnosis (▸ Fig. 4.10)?

- A. Ependymoma
- B. Pilocytic astrocytoma
- C. Medulloblastoma
- D. Hemangioblastoma
- E. Diffuse intrinsic pontine glioma

Correct answer is C

Medulloblastoma is the most common malignant brain tumor in children and typically presents as a midline cerebellar mass causing obstructive hydrocephalus, headache, nausea, and ataxia. Ependymomas can also be found in the posterior fossa but are less common. Pilocytic astrocytomas are benign cerebellar tumors with cystic components and a mural nodule. Hemangioblastomas are rare in children, often associated with von Hippel-Lindau disease. Diffuse intrinsic pontine gliomas affect the pons and are not midline cerebellar masses.[18]

▸▸ Question 40

Which of the following is a known possible side effect of corpus callosotomy for epilepsy?

- A. Hemiparesis
- B. Memory loss
- C. Split-brain syndrome
- D. Aphasia
- E. Visual field deficits

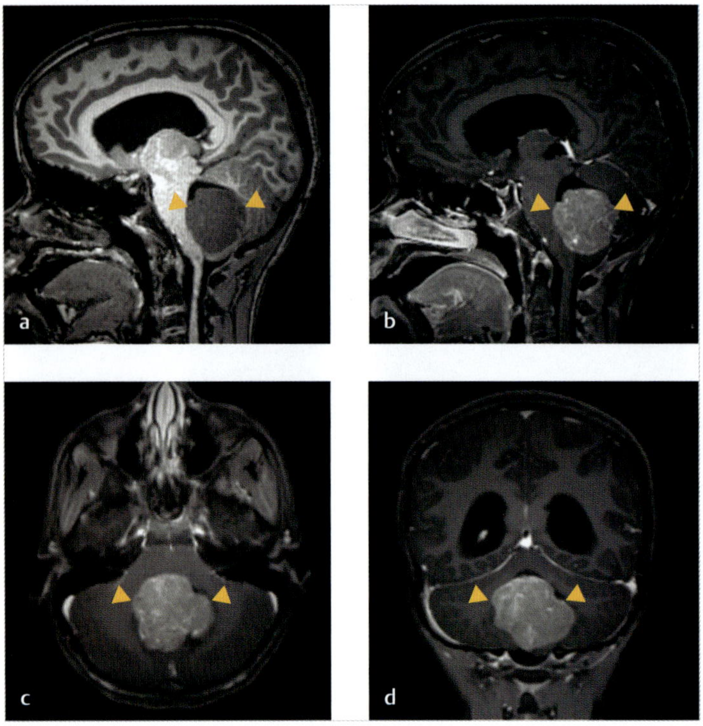

Fig. 4.10 (Source: Reproduced from Evaluation. In: Greenberg M, ed. Greenberg's Handbook of Neurosurgery. 10th ed. New York: Thieme; 2023.)

Correct answer is C

Corpus callosotomy is a palliative surgical procedure for patients with medically refractory epilepsy, particularly those experiencing drop attacks. The procedure involves severing the corpus callosum to prevent seizure propagation between hemispheres. A recognized complication is split-brain syndrome, characterized by a disruption in interhemispheric communication. Symptoms typically include difficulty coordinating tasks that require integration of information from both hemispheres, such as naming objects seen exclusively in the left visual field (anomia), difficulty performing coordinated bimanual tasks, inability to verbally describe stimuli presented to the nondominant hemisphere, and subtle cognitive disconnects during complex tasks. Hemiparesis, memory loss, aphasia, and visual field deficits are less commonly associated with corpus callosotomy and more typically related to other brain surgeries or pathologies.

▸▸ Question 41

A 9-year-old boy with neurofibromatosis type 1 presents with progressive visual loss. MRI reveals an optic pathway glioma. What is the standard treatment for symptomatic optic pathway gliomas in NF1?

- A. Observation
- B. Surgical resection
- C. Chemotherapy
- D. Radiotherapy
- E. Corticosteroids

Correct answer is C

Chemotherapy is the standard treatment for symptomatic optic pathway gliomas in children with neurofibromatosis type 1 (NF1). The most common regimen used is a combination of carboplatin and vincristine. Observation is often appropriate for asymptomatic cases, whereas surgical resection is generally avoided due to high risks, including vision loss. Radiotherapy is discouraged in NF1 due to an increased risk of secondary malignancies. Corticosteroids can provide short-term relief from edema-related symptoms but are not considered definitive treatment.

▸▸ Question 42

A 6-month-old infant presents with macrocephaly, developmental delay, and a tense anterior fontanelle. MRI reveals a large cystic mass in the posterior fossa, fourth ventricular enlargement, and elevated cerebrospinal fluid pressure. What is the most likely diagnosis?

- A. Pilocytic astrocytoma
- B. Dandy-Walker malformation
- C. Ependymoma
- D. Medulloblastoma
- E. Arachnoid cyst

Correct answer is B

Dandy-Walker malformation is characterized by cystic dilation of the fourth ventricle, hypoplasia of the cerebellar vermis, and enlargement of the posterior fossa. These features lead to increased intracranial pressure, macrocephaly, and developmental delays. Pilocytic astrocytomas, ependymomas, and medulloblastomas are neoplastic causes of posterior fossa masses but have different imaging characteristics and clinical presentations. Arachnoid cysts can cause similar symptoms but are typically located in different areas (▸ Fig. 4.11).

▸▸ Question 43

A 4-year-old girl presents with a seizure disorder and intellectual disability. She has multiple hypopigmented macules on her skin. MRI shows cortical tubers and subependymal nodules. What is the most likely diagnosis?

- A. Neurofibromatosis type 1
- B. Sturge-Weber syndrome
- C. Tuberous sclerosis complex
- D. Von Hippel-Lindau disease
- E. Ataxia-telangiectasia

Correct answer is C

Tuberous sclerosis complex (TSC) is characterized by the presence of cortical tubers, subependymal nodules, and hypopigmented macules (ash leaf spots). These features are associated with seizures, intellectual disability, and other systemic manifestations. Neurofibromatosis type 1, Sturge-Weber syndrome, and von Hippel-Lindau disease have different clinical and imaging features.

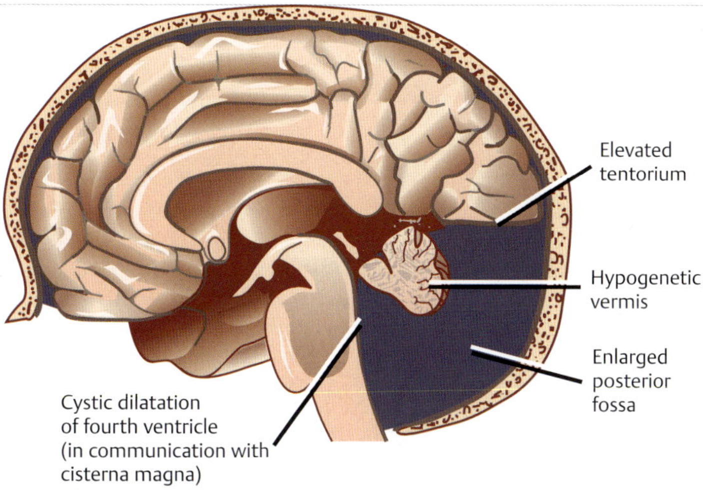

Clinical features

- Characterized by: (1) an enlarged posterior fossa, (2) an elevated tentorial attachment, (3) hypogenesis or agenesis of the cerebellar vermis, and (4) a cystic dilatation of the fourth ventricle
- Associated with hydrocephalus in 90% of cases
- Associated with callosal agenesis in one-third of cases
- May be associated with developmental delay, enlarged head circumference, or signs and symptoms of hydrocephalus

Fig. 4.11 (Source: Reproduced from Dandy-Walker malformation. In: Alberstone C, Benzel E, Jones S, Wang Z, Steinmetz M, eds. Anatomic Basis of Neurologic Diagnosis. 2nd ed. New York: Thieme; 2023.)

Ataxia-telangiectasia is a genetic disorder characterized by progressive cerebellar ataxia, telangiectasias, and immunodeficiency but does not present with cortical tubers and subependymal nodules.

▸▸ Question 44

A 3-year-old boy is evaluated for developmental delay and hypotonia. Genetic testing reveals a deletion on chromosome 15q11-q13. Which of the following conditions is most likely?

- A. Angelman syndrome
- B. Prader-Willi syndrome
- C. Williams syndrome
- D. DiGeorge syndrome
- E. Smith-Magenis syndrome

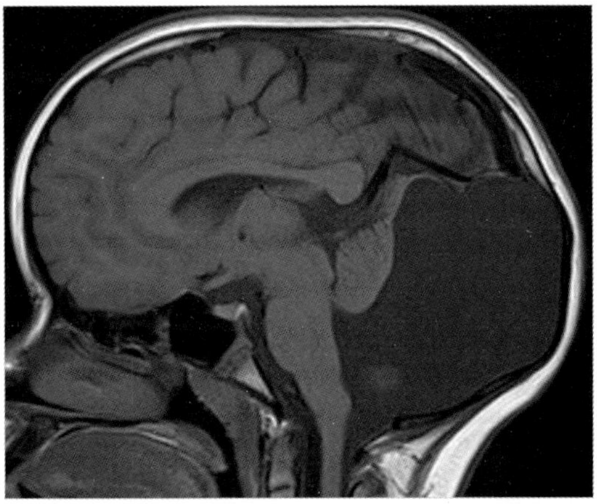

Fig. 4.12 (Source: Reproduced from Dandy-Walker malformation. In: Alberstone C, Benzel E, Jones S, Wang Z, Steinmetz M, eds. Anatomic Basis of Neurologic Diagnosis. 2nd ed. New York: Thieme; 2023.)

Correct answer is B

Prader-Willi syndrome is caused by a deletion on chromosome 15q11-q13 and presents with hypotonia, developmental delays, hyperphagia leading to obesity, and characteristic facial features. Angelman syndrome, also associated with a deletion on chromosome 15q11-q13, presents with severe intellectual disability, ataxia, and a happy demeanor. Williams syndrome, DiGeorge syndrome, and Smith-Magenis syndrome are associated with different genetic abnormalities and clinical features (▶ Fig. 4.12).

▸▸ Question 45

A 10-year-old boy presents with chronic headaches, nausea, and papilledema. MRI reveals a well-circumscribed, enhancing lesion in the pineal region with obstructive hydrocephalus. What is the most likely diagnosis (▶ Fig. 4.13)?

- A. Germinoma
- B. Medulloblastoma
- C. Pineoblastoma
- D. Pilocytic astrocytoma
- E. Ependymoma

Correct answer is A

Germinomas are the most common tumors in the pineal region in children and can cause obstructive hydrocephalus, leading to headaches, nausea, and papilledema. They are typically well-circumscribed and enhance on MRI. Pineoblastomas are also found in the pineal region but are less common. Medulloblastomas are primarily located in the posterior fossa. Pilocytic astrocytomas are usually found in the cerebellum or optic pathways, and ependymomas can arise in the ventricles but are not typically pineal region tumors.

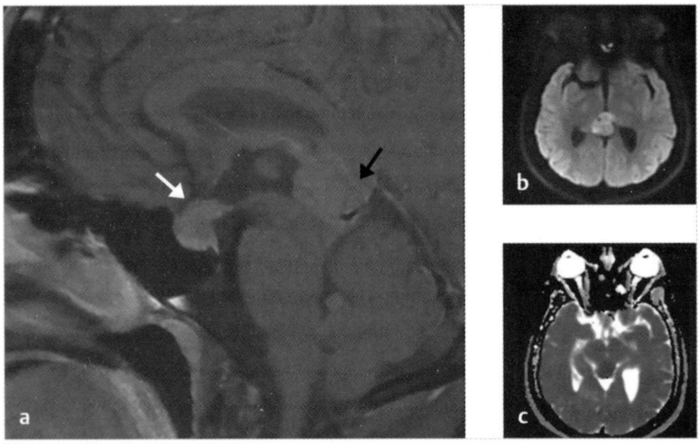

Fig. 4.13 (Source: Reproduced from Germ cell tumors. In: Spetzler R, Kalani M, Lawton M, eds. Surgery of the Brainstem. 1st ed. New York: Thieme; 2019.)

▸▸ Question 46

A 3-year-old girl presents with a rapidly enlarging head circumference, bulging fontanelle, and sunsetting eyes. MRI reveals a large, cystic mass in the cerebellum with an enhancing mural nodule. What is the most likely diagnosis (▸ Fig. 4.14)?

- A. Medulloblastoma
- B. Ependymoma
- C. Pilocytic astrocytoma
- D. Atypical teratoid/rhabdoid tumor (AT/RT)
- E. Choroid plexus carcinoma

Correct answer is C

Pilocytic astrocytoma is a benign tumor commonly found in the cerebellum of young children. It typically presents as a cystic mass with an enhancing mural nodule. Symptoms include increasing head circumference, bulging fontanelle, and sunsetting eyes due to hydrocephalus. Medulloblastomas are malignant and do not typically have a cystic component with a mural nodule. Ependymomas arise from the ependymal lining and have different imaging characteristics. AT/RTs are aggressive tumors that can appear similar but are more heterogeneous. Choroid plexus carcinomas occur within the ventricles and are associated with intraventricular growth.

▸▸ Question 47

A 7-year-old boy with a history of Down syndrome presents with progressive ataxia and weakness. MRI shows atlantoaxial instability. What is the most appropriate next step in management?

- A. Immediate surgical intervention
- B. Cervical collar immobilization
- C. Observation and regular follow-up
- D. Physical therapy
- E. Halo traction

Correct answer is A

In patients with Down syndrome presenting with atlantoaxial instability and progressive neurological symptoms such as ataxia and weakness, immediate surgical stabilization with C1–C2 fusion is indicated. This procedure prevents further neurological deterioration and protects against spinal cord injury. Cervical collar immobilization and halo traction are temporary measures but do not definitively treat the underlying instability. Observation and physical therapy alone are inappropriate given progressive neurological deficits.[19]

▸▸ Question 48

A 5-year-old girl presents with precocious puberty and visual disturbances. MRI reveals a

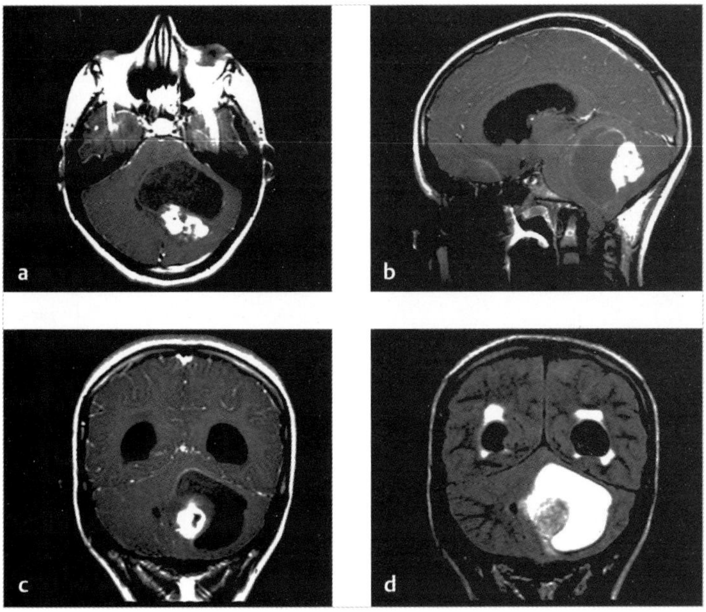

Fig. 4.14 (Source: Reproduced from Perioperative evaluation. In: Spetzler R, Kalani M, Lawton M, eds. Surgery of the Brainstem. 1st ed. New York: Thieme; 2019.)

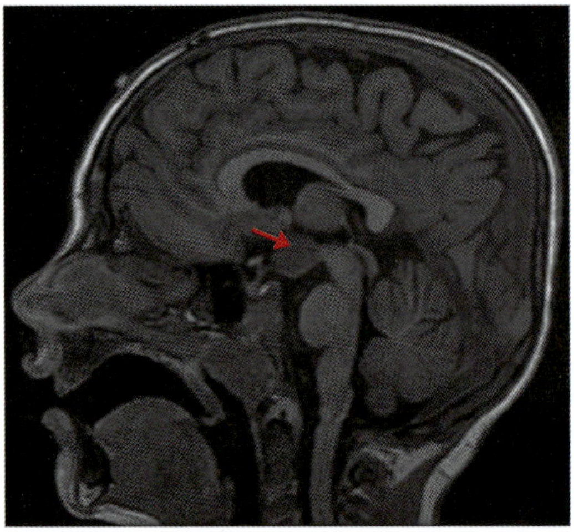

Fig. 4.15 (Source: Reproduced from Congenital malformations. In: Choudhri A, ed. Pediatric Neuroradiology: Clinical Practice Essentials. 1st ed. New York: Thieme; 2016.)

hypothalamic mass. What is the most likely diagnosis (▶ Fig. 4.15)?
- A. Craniopharyngioma
- B. Germinoma
- C. Pilocytic astrocytoma
- D. Hypothalamic hamartoma
- E. Optic pathway glioma

Correct answer is D

Hypothalamic hamartomas are benign congenital lesions that can cause precocious puberty and visual disturbances due to their location. Craniopharyngiomas also present with visual disturbances but typically cause growth failure rather than precocious puberty. Germinomas are malignant and usually present in the pineal or suprasellar regions. Pilocytic astrocytomas are less likely to present with precocious puberty and are more common in the cerebellum. Optic pathway gliomas are associated with visual disturbances but do not typically cause precocious puberty.[20]

▸▸ Question 49

A 12-year-old girl presents with scoliosis and signs of myelopathy. MRI shows an intramedullary spinal cord tumor with syringomyelia. What is the most likely diagnosis?
- A. Ependymoma
- B. Astrocytoma
- C. Hemangioblastoma
- D. Ganglioglioma
- E. Meningioma

Correct answer is B

Astrocytomas are the most common intramedullary spinal cord tumors in children and can present with scoliosis and myelopathy. These tumors often cause syringomyelia, a cystic dilation of the spinal cord. Ependymomas are also common spinal cord tumors but are more frequently found in adults. Hemangioblastomas are rare in children and more often associated with von Hippel-Lindau disease. Gangliogliomas and meningiomas are less common in the spinal cord.

▸▸ Question 50

A previously healthy 3-year-old boy presents with rapidly progressive enlargement of his head circumference, irritability, a tense and bulging fontanelle, and impaired upward gaze (Parinaud syndrome). MRI demonstrates a large, heterogeneous pineal-region mass causing marked obstructive hydrocephalus. Which tumor is the most likely diagnosis?
- A. Pineoblastoma
- B. Germinoma
- C. Pilocytic astrocytoma
- D. Craniopharyngioma
- E. Medulloblastoma

Correct answer is A

Pineoblastomas are highly aggressive primitive neuroectodermal tumors located in the pineal region. They characteristically cause rapidly progressive obstructive hydrocephalus by compressing the cerebral aqueduct, resulting in accelerated head growth, bulging fontanelle, and classic Parinaud syndrome (impaired upward gaze). Germinomas, also arising in the pineal region, typically present in older children and adolescents, exhibiting slower progression with more insidious symptoms such as chronic headaches, subtle visual symptoms, and delayed onset of hydrocephalus. They are generally less aggressive.

Pilocytic astrocytomas usually arise in the cerebellum or optic pathways and are slow-growing tumors.

Craniopharyngiomas occur in the suprasellar region, affecting visual fields and pituitary function, not typically presenting with pineal-region symptoms.

Medulloblastomas originate in the posterior fossa (cerebellum) and usually cause ataxia and symptoms related to cerebellar compression, rather than Parinaud syndrome.

▸▸ Question 51

A 2-year-old girl with a history of seizure disorder presents with new-onset focal seizures. MRI shows a cortical lesion suggestive of focal cortical dysplasia. What is the definitive treatment for this condition?

- A. Antiepileptic drug therapy
- B. Ketogenic diet
- C. Cortical resection of the lesion
- D. Vagus nerve stimulation
- E. Deep brain stimulation

Correct answer is C

Focal cortical dysplasia is a common cause of medically refractory epilepsy in children. The definitive treatment is surgical resection of the epileptogenic focus, which can lead to seizure freedom in many patients. Antiepileptic drug therapy and the ketogenic diet may help manage seizures but do not address the underlying structural abnormality. Vagus nerve stimulation and deep brain stimulation are additional options for refractory epilepsy but are less effective than resection in focal cortical dysplasia.

▸▸ Question 52

A 5-year-old boy presents with left-sided hemiparesis and seizures. MRI reveals a large, infiltrative brain tumor crossing the midline. Biopsy shows cells with 1p/19q co-deletion. What is the most likely diagnosis?

- A. Glioblastoma
- B. Anaplastic astrocytoma
- C. Oligodendroglioma
- D. Ependymoma
- E. Medulloblastoma

Correct answer is C

Oligodendrogliomas are characterized by the presence of oligodendroglial cells and the co-deletion of chromosomes 1p and 19q. These tumors are typically slow-growing but can present with seizures and focal neurological deficits. Glioblastomas and anaplastic astrocytomas are more aggressive and do not typically have 1p/19q co-deletion. Ependymomas arise from the ependymal lining and have different histological features. Medulloblastomas are pediatric tumors found in the posterior fossa.

▸▸ Question 53

A 9-year-old girl presents with headaches, visual disturbances, and hormonal imbalances. MRI reveals a suprasellar mass compressing the optic chiasm. What is the most likely diagnosis (▸ Fig. 4.16)?

- A. Craniopharyngioma
- B. Germinoma
- C. Pilocytic astrocytoma
- D. Pineoblastoma
- E. Ependymoma

Correct answer is A

Craniopharyngiomas are common suprasellar tumors in children who can present with headaches, visual disturbances, and endocrine dysfunction due to their proximity to the optic chiasm and pituitary gland. Germinomas can also occur in the suprasellar region but are less common. Pilocytic astrocytomas are more typically found in the cerebellum. Pineoblastomas are located in the pineal region, and ependymomas

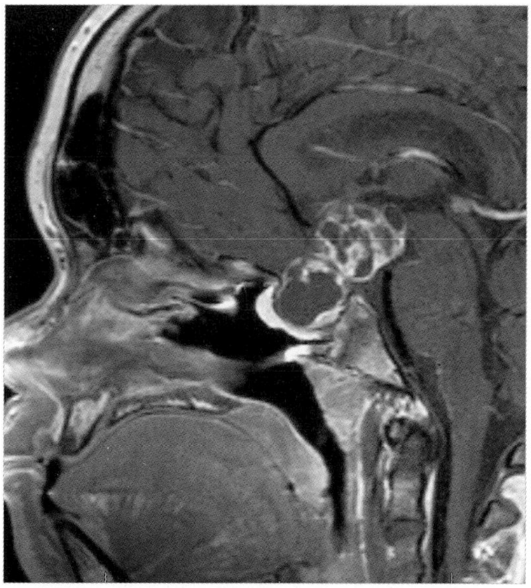

Fig. 4.16 (Source: Reproduced from Transplanum/Transtuberculum (suprasellar) approach. In: Hanna E, DeMonte F, eds. Comprehensive Management of Skull Base Tumors. 2nd ed. New York: Thieme; 2021.)

usually arise from the ependymal lining of the ventricles or spinal cord.

▸▸ Question 54

A 4-year-old boy presents with irritability, lethargy, and difficulty with upward gaze. MRI shows a mass in the pineal region causing obstructive hydrocephalus. What is the most appropriate next step in management?

- A. Stereotactic biopsy
- B. Endoscopic third ventriculostomy (ETV)
- C. Ventriculoperitoneal shunt placement
- D. Radiation therapy
- E. Chemotherapy

Correct answer is B

In the acute management of obstructive hydrocephalus caused by a pineal region mass, endoscopic third ventriculostomy is often preferred to immediately relieve hydrocephalus. This procedure creates an alternative pathway for cerebrospinal fluid flow. Stereotactic biopsy may be performed later for diagnosis, and ventriculoperitoneal shunt placement is another option but less preferred initially. Radiation therapy and chemotherapy are not first-line treatments for hydrocephalus management.

▸▸ Question 55

A 5-year-old boy presents with new-onset seizures and developmental delay. MRI reveals a cortical malformation suggestive of focal cortical dysplasia (FCD). Which subtype is specifically characterized by the presence of balloon cells?

- A. Type I
- B. Type IIa
- C. Type IIb
- D. Type III
- E. Type IV

Correct answer is C

FCD type IIb is characterized by the presence of balloon cells, which are abnormal, large cells with an eccentric nucleus and eosinophilic cytoplasm. This subtype is often associated with refractory epilepsy and requires surgical intervention. FCD type I features architectural abnormalities without balloon cells, type IIa shows dysmorphic neurons without balloon cells, type III is associated with another principal lesion, and type IV includes tumors.

▸▸ Question 56

A 10-year-old girl presents with a slowly enlarging, painless mass at the right skull convexity. Imaging reveals a lytic lesion with sclerotic margins in the temporal bone. Biopsy shows eosinophilic granuloma. What is the most likely diagnosis (▸ Fig. 4.17)?

- A. Osteosarcoma
- B. Ewing sarcoma
- C. Langerhans cell histiocytosis
- D. Chordoma
- E. Fibrous dysplasia

Correct answer is C

Langerhans cell histiocytosis (LCH) can present as a lytic bone lesion, particularly in the skull. Eosinophilic granuloma is a localized form of LCH, often seen in children and characterized by a solitary, lytic lesion with a well-defined border.

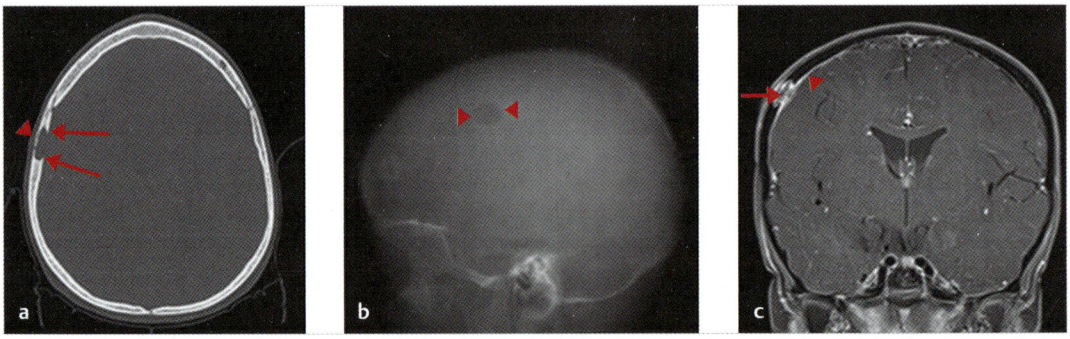

Fig. 4.17 (Source: Reproduced from Solitary radiolucent skull lesion without sclerotic margins in children. In: Tsementzis S, ed. Differential Diagnosis in Neurology and Neurosurgery: A Clinician's Pocket Guide. 2nd ed. Stuttgart: Thieme; 2019.)

Osteosarcoma and Ewing sarcoma are more aggressive bone tumors with different histological features. Chordomas are typically found in the clivus or sacrococcygeal area, and fibrous dysplasia presents as a ground-glass appearance on imaging.

▸▸ Question 57

A 12-year-old girl presents with chronic headaches and visual disturbances. MRI reveals an enlarged pituitary gland with a cystic component. Laboratory tests show elevated prolactin levels. What is the most likely diagnosis?

- A. Craniopharyngioma
- B. Pituitary adenoma
- C. Rathke cleft cyst
- D. Germinoma
- E. Hypothalamic hamartoma

Correct answer is B

Pituitary adenomas, particularly prolactinomas, can present with headaches, visual disturbances, and elevated prolactin levels due to compression of the pituitary stalk or direct hormone secretion. Craniopharyngiomas are more likely to cause hypopituitarism and diabetes insipidus. Rathke cleft cysts are usually nonsecretory and asymptomatic unless large. Germinomas and hypothalamic hamartomas have different clinical and imaging features.

▸▸ Question 58

A 5-year-old girl with a history of recurrent otitis media and recent mastoiditis presents with fever, irritability, and swelling behind her ear. MRI of the brain reveals a well-defined, ring-enhancing lesion with significant surrounding edema in the temporal lobe adjacent to the mastoid bone. What is the most likely diagnosis?

- A. Epidural abscess
- B. Brain abscess
- C. Subdural empyema
- D. Otitic hydrocephalus
- E. Mastoiditis

Correct answer is B

A brain abscess commonly occurs as a complication of chronic ear infections or mastoiditis due to contiguous spread of infection. It typically presents on imaging as a well-defined, ring-enhancing lesion with central necrosis and surrounding vasogenic edema. When the abscess involves the temporal lobe, it often results from direct extension of infection from the mastoid or middle ear. In contrast, an epidural abscess is located between the skull and dura and generally lacks the distinct ring enhancement and parenchymal involvement seen in brain abscesses. A subdural empyema involves infection in the subdural space and usually appears as a crescent-shaped collection along the brain surface, without a focal intraparenchymal mass or ring enhancement. Otitic hydrocephalus refers to increased intracranial pressure secondary to chronic middle ear infection but is not associated with a focal mass lesion. Mastoiditis alone is limited to inflammation or infection of the mastoid air cells and surrounding soft tissues and does not produce a ring-enhancing lesion within the temporal lobe. Given the patient's clinical history and characteristic imaging findings, the diagnosis of a brain abscess is most consistent.

▸▸ Question 59

A 6-year-old boy presents with a large, non-tender abdominal mass and hypertension. Imaging shows a mass arising from the adrenal gland. What is the most likely diagnosis?

- A. Wilms tumor
- B. Neuroblastoma
- C. Hepatoblastoma
- D. Rhabdomyosarcoma
- E. Adrenocortical carcinoma

Correct answer is B

Neuroblastoma is the most common extracranial solid tumor in children, often arising from the adrenal gland. It can present with an abdominal mass and hypertension due to catecholamine secretion. Wilms tumor also presents with an abdominal mass but typically originates from the kidney. Hepatoblastoma arises from the liver, rhabdomyosarcoma from muscle, and adrenocortical carcinoma from the adrenal cortex but is less common.

▸▸ Question 60

A 7-year-old girl presents with a sudden onset of severe headache, vomiting, and decreased level of consciousness. CT scan shows a large cerebellar hemorrhage. What is the most likely underlying condition?

- A. Arteriovenous malformation
- B. Moyamoya disease
- C. Cavernous malformation
- D. Hemophilia
- E. Brain tumor

Correct answer is A

Arteriovenous malformations (AVMs) are a common cause of intracranial hemorrhage in children and can present with a sudden onset of severe headache, vomiting, and altered consciousness. Cavernous malformations can also cause hemorrhage but typically present with smaller bleeds. Moyamoya disease is associated with ischemic strokes, and hemophilia causes bleeding but is less likely to present with isolated intracerebral hemorrhage. Brain tumors can cause hemorrhage but usually present with additional focal neurological signs or symptoms.

▸▸ Question 61

A 6-month-old infant presents with macrocephaly and developmental delay. MRI shows diffuse cerebral white matter changes. What is the most likely diagnosis?

- A. Adrenoleukodystrophy
- B. Krabbe disease
- C. Canavan disease
- D. Metachromatic leukodystrophy
- E. Pelizaeus-Merzbacher disease

Correct answer is C

Canavan disease is a leukodystrophy characterized by diffuse cerebral white matter changes, macrocephaly, and developmental delay in infancy. It results from a deficiency in the enzyme aspartoacylase. Adrenoleukodystrophy, Krabbe disease, metachromatic leukodystrophy, and Pelizaeus-Merzbacher disease are other leukodystrophies but have different clinical and imaging features.

▸▸ Question 62

A 2-year-old boy presents with difficulty walking, frequent falls, and calf hypertrophy. Genetic testing reveals a mutation in the *DMD* gene. What is the most likely diagnosis?

- A. Becker muscular dystrophy
- B. Duchenne muscular dystrophy
- C. Limb-girdle muscular dystrophy
- D. Congenital myopathy
- E. Spinal muscular atrophy

Correct answer is B

Duchenne muscular dystrophy (DMD) is characterized by progressive muscle weakness, calf hypertrophy, and difficulty walking, typically presenting in early childhood. It is caused by mutations in the *DMD* gene encoding dystrophin. Becker muscular dystrophy has a similar but milder and later onset. Limb-girdle muscular dystrophy affects the hip and shoulder muscles. Congenital myopathies present with hypotonia and muscle weakness from birth, and spinal muscular atrophy is a motor neuron disease.

▸▸ Question 63

A 2-year-old boy presents with progressive macrocephaly, developmental delays, and signs of increased intracranial pressure. MRI reveals a large posterior fossa arachnoid cyst causing significant mass effect on adjacent structures. What is the most appropriate initial treatment?

- A. Observation
- B. Shunt placement
- C. Endoscopic fenestration
- D. Craniotomy and cyst resection
- E. Radiation therapy

Correct answer is C

The most appropriate initial treatment for a symptomatic posterior fossa arachnoid cyst is endoscopic fenestration, which creates an opening in the cyst wall to allow cerebrospinal fluid drainage and relieve mass effect. This minimally invasive approach typically provides immediate symptom relief and improvement in intracranial pressure.

Observation would be appropriate only if the cysts were small, stable, and asymptomatic. Shunt placement may be considered if endoscopic fenestration fails or if symptoms recur despite fenestration. Craniotomy with cyst resection is more invasive and reserved for complex or refractory cases not amenable to endoscopic treatment. Radiation therapy is not indicated for benign lesions such as arachnoid cysts.

▸▸ Question 64

A 7-year-old girl with a history of tuberous sclerosis presents with new-onset seizures. MRI shows multiple cortical tubers and subependymal nodules. Which gene mutation is most commonly associated with this condition?

- A. NF1
- B. TSC1
- C. PTEN
- D. VHL
- E. TP53

Correct answer is B

Tuberous sclerosis complex (TSC) is commonly associated with mutations in the *TSC1* or *TSC2* genes. It presents with cortical tubers, subependymal nodules, and seizures. NF1 mutations are linked to neurofibromatosis type 1. PTEN mutations cause Cowden syndrome. VHL mutations are seen in von Hippel-Lindau disease. TP53 mutations are associated with Li-Fraumeni syndrome.

▸▸ Question 65

A 12-year-old boy presents with progressive lower extremity weakness, sensory changes, and urinary difficulties. MRI reveals a heterogeneously enhancing intradural mass centered at the conus medullaris and filum terminale. What is the most likely diagnosis?

- A. Myxopapillary ependymoma
- B. Astrocytoma
- C. Ganglioglioma
- D. Hemangioblastoma
- E. Medulloblastoma

Correct answer is A

Myxopapillary ependymoma is the most common tumor of the conus medullaris, cauda equina, and filum terminale, particularly in children and young adults. It typically presents with progressive lower extremity weakness, sensory loss, and bladder or bowel dysfunction. MRI usually shows a heterogeneously enhancing mass in the lower spinal cord or filum, sometimes with associated cysts or hemorrhage.

Although astrocytomas are more common in the thoracic or cervical spinal cord, they are less frequent in the conus. Gangliogliomas and hemangioblastomas are rare in this location. Medulloblastomas are exclusively cerebellar tumors and do not arise in the spinal cord.

▸▸ Question 66

A 5-year-old girl presents with progressive vision loss and precocious puberty. MRI shows an enhancing suprasellar mass compressing the optic chiasm. What is the most likely diagnosis?

- A. Craniopharyngioma
- B. Germinoma
- C. Pilocytic astrocytoma
- D. Pineoblastoma
- E. Meningioma

Correct answer is A

Craniopharyngiomas are benign epithelial tumors that typically arise in the suprasellar region and can compress the optic chiasm, leading to vision loss. They are also associated with endocrine disturbances, such as precocious puberty. Germinomas and pineoblastomas are germ cell tumors that can occur in the suprasellar region but are less common. Pilocytic astrocytomas are typically found in the cerebellum. Meningiomas are rare in children and usually occur outside the suprasellar region.

References

[1] Kulkarni AV, Drake JM, Mallucci CL, Sgouros S, Roth J, Constantini S; Canadian Pediatric Neurosurgery Study Group. Endoscopic third ventriculostomy in the treatment of childhood hydrocephalus. J Pediatr 2009;155(2):254–259.e1

[2] Bhattacharjee M, Hicks J, Langford L, et al. Central nervous system atypical teratoid/rhabdoid tumors of infancy and childhood. Ultrastruct Pathol 1997;21(4):369–378

[3] Holliday MA, Segar WE. The maintenance need for water in parenteral fluid therapy. Pediatrics 1957;19(5): 823–832

[4] Cohen MM Jr, Kreiborg S. New indirect method for estimating the birth prevalence of the Apert syndrome. Int J Oral Maxillofac Surg 1992;21(2):107–109

[5] Katouni K, Nikolaou A, Mariolis T, et al. Syndromic craniosynostosis: a comprehensive review. Cureus 2023;15(12): e50448

[6] Northcott PA, Korshunov A, Witt H, et al. Medulloblastoma comprises four distinct molecular variants. J Clin Oncol 2011;29(11):1408–1414

[7] Taylor MD, Northcott PA, Korshunov A, et al. Molecular subgroups of medulloblastoma: the current consensus. Acta Neuropathol 2012;123(4):465–472

[8] Maria BL, Hoang KB, Tusa RJ, et al. "Joubert syndrome" revisited: key ocular motor signs with magnetic resonance imaging correlation. J Child Neurol 1997;12(7):423–430

[9] Ackerman LL, Menezes AH. Spinal congenital dermal sinuses: a 30-year experience. Pediatrics 2003;112(3, Pt 1):641–647

[10] Franz DN, Belousova E, Sparagana S, et al. Efficacy and safety of everolimus for subependymal giant cell astrocytomas associated with tuberous sclerosis complex (EXIST-1): a multicentre, randomised, placebo-controlled phase 3 trial. Lancet 2013;381(9861):125–132[Erratum in: Lancet. 2013 Jan 12;381(9861):116. PMID: 23158522]

[11] Adzick NS, Thom EA, Spong CY, et al; MOMS Investigators. A randomized trial of prenatal versus postnatal repair of myelomeningocele. N Engl J Med 2011;364(11):993–1004

[12] Luyken C, Blümcke I, Fimmers R, et al. The spectrum of long-term epilepsy-associated tumors: long-term seizure and tumor outcome and neurosurgical aspects. Epilepsia 2003;44(6):822–830

[13] Di Rocco F, Arnaud E, Renier D. Evolution in the frequency of nonsyndromic craniosynostosis. J Neurosurg Pediatr 2009;4(1):21–25

[14] Roberts D, Brown J, Medley N, Dalziel SR. Antenatal corticosteroids for accelerating fetal lung maturation for women at risk of preterm birth. Cochrane Database Syst Rev 2017;3 (3):CD004454

[15] Constine LS, Woolf PD, Cann D, et al. Hypothalamic-pituitary dysfunction after radiation for brain tumors. N Engl J Med 1993;328(2):87–94 [Erratum in: N Engl J Med 1993; 328(16):1208. PMID: 8416438]

[16] Hasnat MJ, Rice JE. Intrathecal baclofen for treating spasticity in children with cerebral palsy. Cochrane Database Syst Rev 2015;2015(11):CD004552

[17] Lew SM, Kothbauer KF. Tethered cord syndrome: an updated review. Pediatr Neurosurg 2007;43(3):236–248

[18] Packer RJ, Cogen P, Vezina G, Rorke LB. Medulloblastoma: clinical and biologic aspects. Neuro Oncol 1999;1(3):232–250

[19] Atlantoaxial instability in Down syndrome. Lancet 1989;1 (8628):24

[20] Carballo Cuello CM, De Jesus O. Hypothalamic hamartoma. In: StatPearls [Internet]. Treasure Island, FL: StatPearls Publishing; 2025. PMID: 32809498

5 Functional/Epilepsy Neurosurgery

Syed I. Khalid, Nate Pertsch, Sepehr Sani, Francesco Pucci, Konstantin Slavin

▸▸ Question 1

A 75-year-old woman is receiving oxcarbazepine to treat trigeminal neuralgia. This patient is at greatest risk for developing which of the following?

- A. Hyponatremia
- B. Hyperkalemia
- C. Hypernatremia
- D. Hypokalemia
- E. Hyperammonemia

Correct answer is A

Oxcarbazepine is associated with the risk of developing hyponatremia, particularly in elderly patients and women. This is due to its antidiuretic hormone-like effect, which can cause water retention and dilutional hyponatremia. Hyperkalemia, hypernatremia, hypokalemia, and hyperammonemia are not typically associated with oxcarbazepine use. Hyperammonemia is associated with valproic acid use.

▸▸ Question 2

A 27-year-old woman with chronic low back pain is evaluated because of a gradual recurrence of pain and a new onset of leg numbness. Her back pain has been treated successfully for the past 3 years with an intrathecal morphine infusion via an implanted pump that delivers 15 mg/day. Which of the following is the most likely explanation for the current symptoms?

- A. Pump malfunction
- B. Catheter dislodgement
- C. Tolerance to morphine
- D. Intrathecal granuloma formation
- E. Spinal stenosis progression

Correct answer is D

Intrathecal granuloma formation is a relatively common (~2–3%) complication of chronic intrathecal opioid therapy and should be considered when a patient with a long-standing device develops recurrence of pain or signs of myelopathy. Small granulomas can be managed with catheter replacement, although large granulomas with neurologic deficit may require decompression and resection. Pump malfunction and catheter dislodgement can cause loss of pain control but are less likely to present with a new onset of leg numbness. Tolerance to morphine would present with a recurrence of pain but not with numbness. Spinal stenosis progression is possible but less likely to coincide with the specific history of intrathecal morphine use.

▸▸ Question 3

A 52-year-old man presents with a history of episodic severe, unilateral headache that is associated with nasal congestion and rhinorrhea. The headaches last for about 30 minutes and occur multiple times per day. Which of the following is the next appropriate therapeutic intervention?

- A. Nasal decongestant
- B. Oxygen therapy
- C. Intranasal lidocaine
- D. Greater occipital nerve block
- E. Sphenopalatine ganglion stimulation

Correct answer is B

Cluster headaches are characterized by severe, unilateral orbital, supraorbital, or temporal pain, often described as sharp or piercing, accompanied by ipsilateral autonomic symptoms such as lacrimation, nasal congestion or rhinorrhea, conjunctival injection, ptosis, and miosis. Episodes typically last 15 to 180 minutes and occur in clusters, with attacks happening up to eight times daily. The condition predominantly affects men more than women, usually beginning in young to middle adulthood. Misdiagnosis as a sinus headache or migraine is common due to overlapping autonomic symptoms.

The first-line acute treatments for cluster headaches include high-flow oxygen therapy (100% oxygen at 12–15 L/min via non-rebreather mask for 15–20 minutes) and subcutaneous sumatriptan. Additional acute therapies such as intranasal lidocaine, sphenopalatine ganglion (SPG) blocks or stimulation, or greater occipital nerve blocks may be considered as adjunctive treatments or in refractory cases.

Preventive therapy focuses on reducing the frequency and intensity of cluster episodes, with verapamil (starting dose approximately 240 mg/day and titrated upward based on response and tolerability) established as the first-line preventive medication. Glucocorticoids (e.g., prednisone) can serve as bridge therapy, providing rapid relief while awaiting the preventive medication's therapeutic effect. For refractory chronic cluster headaches, advanced interventions such as sphenopalatine ganglion stimulation, SPG blockade, or surgical treatments (e.g., nerve ablation) may be explored.

▸▸ Question 4

A 65-year-old man reports brief episodes of stabbing, sharp unilateral facial pain radiating to the right lower lip. The pain is triggered by activities such as chewing and brushing his teeth. Light tactile stimulation in front of the right ear elicits the pain upon evaluation in the clinic. He has no left-sided pain, no cervical pain, and no headaches. Which of the following medications is considered the first-line treatment?

- A. Amitriptyline
- B. Gabapentin
- C. Carbamazepine
- D. Baclofen
- E. Pregabalin

Correct answer is C

Carbamazepine is the first-line pharmacological treatment for trigeminal neuralgia, effectively reducing the frequency and severity of painful episodes. It acts by stabilizing voltage-gated sodium channels in their inactivated state, thereby decreasing neuronal excitability and pain signal transmission. Alternative agents such as gabapentin, pregabalin, and baclofen are often employed as second-line treatments or adjunct therapies when carbamazepine is insufficient or poorly tolerated. In contrast, amitriptyline, a tricyclic antidepressant, is typically used for other forms of neuropathic pain (e.g., diabetic neuropathy, post-herpetic neuralgia) rather than trigeminal neuralgia.

▸▸ Question 5

A 65-year-old man presents with brief, sharp, and stabbing episodes of unilateral facial pain radiating to the lower lip. The pain is triggered by activities such as chewing and brushing his teeth. Light tactile stimulation in front of the ear elicits pain during clinical evaluation. Based on the International Classification of Headache Disorders (ICHD-3), which of the following diagnostic criteria must be met to confirm classical trigeminal neuralgia?

- A. Pain is bilateral and lasts continuously for hours
- B. Pain is dull and non-radiating
- C. Pain is unilateral, brief (lasting from a fraction of a second to 2 minutes), and triggered by innocuous stimuli
- D. Pain is associated with autonomic symptoms such as nasal congestion and tearing
- E. Pain is always refractory to pharmacologic therapy

Correct answer is C

Classical trigeminal neuralgia is characterized by brief, recurrent episodes of severe unilateral facial pain, often described as stabbing, sharp, or electric shock-like. It is typically triggered by innocuous stimuli such as touch, chewing, or speaking. The pain lasts from a fraction of a second to 2 minutes and is confined to the distribution of one or more branches of the trigeminal nerve. Bilateral pain (**A**) and dull pain (**B**) do not fit trigeminal neuralgia. Autonomic symptoms (**D**) are more typical of cluster headaches. Refractoriness to treatment (**E**) may occur but is not required for diagnosis.

ICHD-3 diagnostic criteria for classical trigeminal neuralgia:

1. Paroxysms of unilateral facial pain in the distribution of the trigeminal nerve
2. Pain duration: A fraction of a second to 2 minutes per episode
3. Pain characteristics: Severe, sharp, stabbing, or shock-like
4. Precipitated by stimuli such as light touch or chewing
5. No significant neurologic deficit on examination (for idiopathic cases)

▸▸ Question 6

A 48-year-old man presents with a 1-year history of severe facial pain. He describes intense, sharp, stabbing pain localized to the left deep ear, posterior tongue, and tonsillar region. Pain episodes last seconds but occur multiple times per day and are frequently triggered by swallowing. He reports significant weight loss due to avoiding eating. Carbamazepine initially provided partial relief, but his symptoms have progressively worsened despite medication. What is the most appropriate definitive treatment?

- A. Vagus rhizotomy
- B. Microvascular decompression of the nervus intermedius
- C. Radiofrequency ablation
- D. Gamma Knife radiosurgery
- E. Microvascular decompression of cranial nerve IX

Correct answer is E

This patient's clinical presentation is characteristic of glossopharyngeal neuralgia, a disorder causing recurrent episodes of severe, sharp, stabbing pain within regions innervated by the glossopharyngeal nerve (cranial nerve IX). Typical pain locations include the deep ear, posterior tongue, throat, and tonsillar region. Episodes are brief, lasting seconds to minutes, and commonly triggered by swallowing, chewing, speaking, or coughing, often resulting in significant weight loss due to avoidance behaviors.

Initial management usually involves pharmacological therapy, such as carbamazepine or baclofen. When medical therapy is insufficient or ineffective, the most appropriate definitive surgical treatment is microvascular decompression (MVD) of cranial nerve IX. During this procedure, vascular compression of the glossopharyngeal nerve is identified and relieved, providing long-term pain resolution. If no clear vascular compression is found intraoperatively, a selective rhizotomy of cranial nerve IX may be considered.

Alternative treatments such as Gamma Knife radiosurgery or radiofrequency ablation might be considered in select patients, but MVD remains the gold standard definitive therapy due to superior long-term pain control and lower recurrence rates.

Thus, the correct answer is (E) Microvascular decompression of cranial nerve IX.[1]

▸▸ Question 7

A 55-year-old woman with trigeminal neuralgia undergoes percutaneous radiofrequency rhizotomy through the foramen ovale. Postoperatively, she experiences significant pain relief. What is the most likely adverse event from this procedure?

- A. Anesthesia dolorosa
- B. Diminished corneal reflex and keratitis
- C. Cutaneous facial numbness
- D. Masseter weakness
- E. Meningitis

Correct answer is C

Percutaneous radiofrequency rhizotomy is a procedure used to treat trigeminal neuralgia by targeting the trigeminal nerve (cranial nerve V). This procedure can result in pain relief, but mild facial numbness is typical due to the lesioning of sensory fibers. More concerning are corneal numbness (V_1), which can lead to blindness due to unnoticed injury to the eye, and anesthesia dolorosa—a rare severe deafferentation pain associated with lesioning the trigeminal nerve. Additionally, masseter weakness is possible due to injury to the motor branch of V_3. Complications are avoided by test doses to ensure on target effects before permanent lesioning and controlling depth of radiofrequency electrode in foramen ovale to target the appropriate trigeminal branch (▸ Fig. 5.1).[2]

▸▸ Question 8

A 60-year-old woman presents with a history of chronic low back pain that radiates to her left leg. MRI reveals lumbar spinal stenosis at L4–L5. She undergoes a lumbar epidural steroid injection with significant pain relief. Which of the following best describes the mechanism of action of epidural steroid injections?

- A. Blocking nerve conduction
- B. Reducing inflammation
- C. Muscle relaxation
- D. Dissolving scar tissue
- E. Increasing blood flow

Correct answer is B

Epidural steroid injections are used to treat radicular pain by delivering anti-inflammatory medication directly to the epidural space, thereby reducing inflammation around the nerve roots. This can help alleviate pain and improve function in conditions such as lumbar spinal stenosis.[3]

▸▸ Question 9

A 35-year-old woman with multiple sclerosis experiences severe spasticity in all extremities unresponsive to oral medications. Which of the

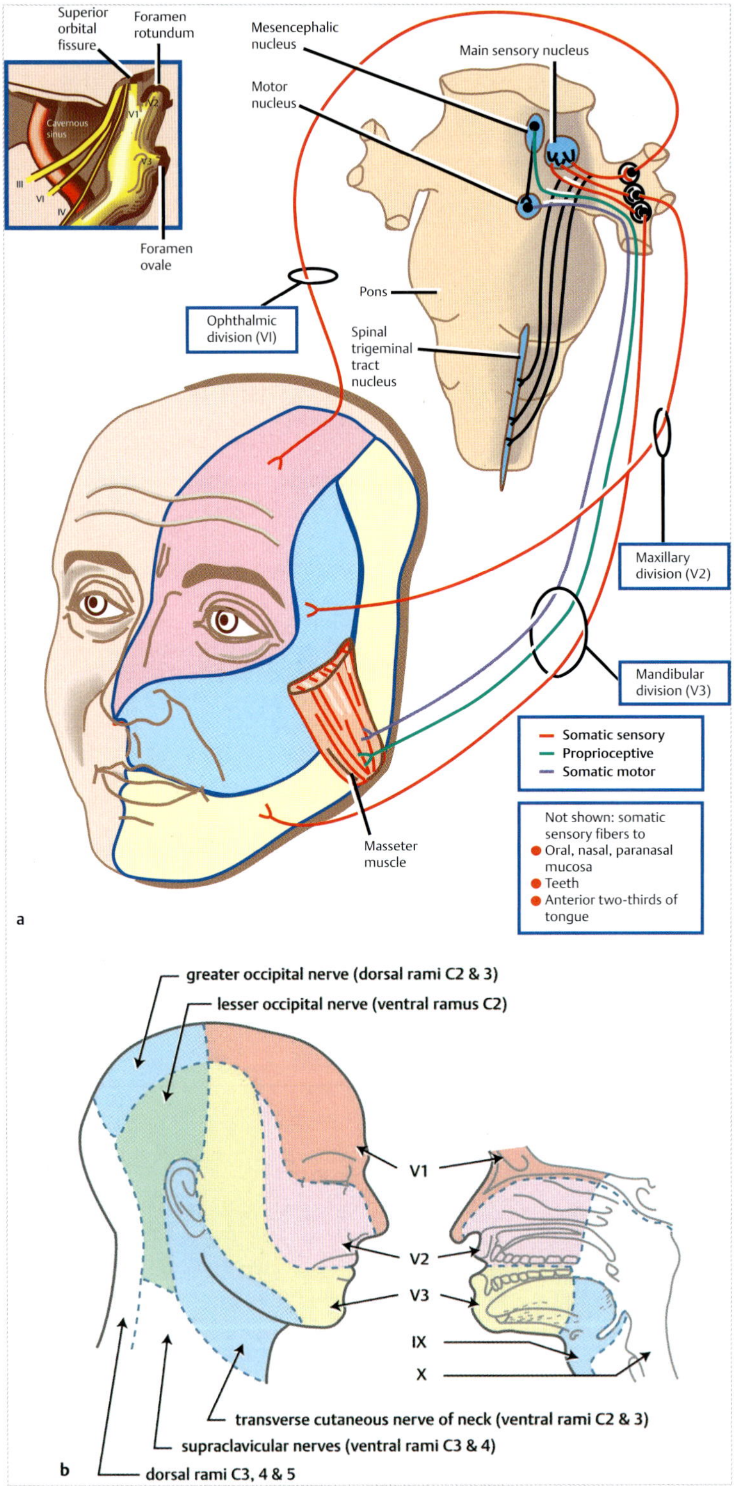

Fig. 5.1 (Source: Part a is reproduced from Applied anatomy. In: Greenberg M, ed. Greenberg's Handbook of Neurosurgery. 10th Edition. New York: Thieme; 2023. Part b is reproduced from The Trigeminal Nerve. In: Alberstone C, Benzel E, Jones S, Wang Z, Steinmetz M, Anatomic Basis of Neurologic Diagnosis. 2nd Edition. New York: Thieme; 2023)

following treatments is most appropriate for managing her spasticity?
- A. Selective lumbosacral dorsal rhizotomy
- B. Physical therapy
- C. Intrathecal baclofen pump
- D. Intrathecal diazepam
- E. Botulinum toxin injections

Correct answer is C

For patients with severe spasticity unresponsive to oral medications, an intrathecal baclofen pump can provide significant relief. This device delivers baclofen directly into the cerebrospinal fluid, allowing for lower doses and reduced systemic side effects compared to oral administration.

▸▸ Question 10

A 68-year-old man with a history of cancer presents with severe, intractable mechanical back pain due to vertebral metastases. Which of the following procedures is most likely to provide immediate pain relief?
- A. Radiotherapy
- B. Vertebroplasty
- C. Chemotherapy
- D. Physical therapy
- E. Oral opioids

Correct answer is B

Vertebroplasty involves the percutaneous injection of polymethylmethacrylate (PMMA) bone cement into a vertebral body weakened by metastatic disease. This intervention provides rapid analgesia by stabilizing micro-fractures and halting the movement of bone fragments, thus alleviating pain caused by the metastatic infiltration of the vertebra. In patients with painful vertebral metastases, vertebroplasty is preferred over conservative management due to its potential to provide immediate and significant pain relief, improving quality of life.[4]

▸▸ Question 11

A 55-year-old man presents with severe, persistent right-sided facial pain following a dental procedure 1 year ago. He describes a continuous burning, aching sensation in the right lower jaw and cheek, accompanied by intermittent sharp, stabbing pain episodes lasting several seconds. The pain occurs multiple times per day and can be triggered by chewing or gentle touch. He reports significant distress and weight loss due to fear of triggering pain episodes. Carbamazepine initially provided partial relief, but symptoms have progressively worsened. What is the most likely diagnosis?
- A. Trigeminal neuralgia type I
- B. Trigeminal neuralgia type II
- C. Trigeminal neuropathic pain
- D. Glossopharyngeal neuralgia
- E. Geniculate neuralgia

Correct answer is C

This patient's presentation is consistent with trigeminal neuropathic pain, characterized by continuous pain (often burning, aching, or throbbing) combined with intermittent sharp, stabbing episodes in the trigeminal nerve distribution (cranial nerve V). It typically follows direct injury or trauma to the trigeminal nerve, such as dental procedures, facial surgery, trauma, or nerve damage from infections.

Differential diagnoses:
- Trigeminal neuralgia type I (classic trigeminal neuralgia) involves brief, severe electric shock-like episodes lasting seconds to minutes without persistent pain between episodes. Triggers often include minor stimuli such as talking, eating, or touching the face.
- Trigeminal neuralgia type II (atypical trigeminal neuralgia) includes a persistent background aching pain combined with sharp exacerbations but typically does not have a clear precipitating event like nerve injury or trauma.
- Glossopharyngeal neuralgia involves sharp, stabbing pain in the ear, posterior tongue, tonsillar region, or throat, typically triggered by swallowing or speaking, without continuous pain.
- Geniculate neuralgia (nervus intermedius neuralgia) presents as sharp, stabbing pain localized primarily in or around the ear canal, often accompanied by lacrimation or altered taste.

The clear history of continuous neuropathic pain following a dental procedure combined with episodic exacerbations distinguishes trigeminal neuropathic pain (option **C**) as the correct diagnosis.

▸▸ Question 12

A 60-year-old woman presents with severe, intermittent episodes of stabbing pain in her inner ear, throat, tonsillar area, and base of her tongue. The pain is triggered by swallowing. Which of the following is the most likely diagnosis?

- A. Trigeminal neuralgia
- B. Glossopharyngeal neuralgia (GPN)
- C. Eagle syndrome
- D. Geniculate neuralgia
- E. Temporal arteritis

Correct answer is B

GPN manifests as episodic, severe, sharp pain localized to the areas innervated by the glossopharyngeal nerve, including the throat, tonsillar fossa, base of the tongue, and sometimes the ear. The pain is often triggered by swallowing, speaking, or coughing. Etiologies include idiopathic origins, vascular compression, or lesions such as tumors. Management typically begins with anticonvulsants like carbamazepine. Refractory cases may benefit from microvascular decompression or nerve sectioning (▶ Fig. 5.2).[5]

▸▸ Question 13

A 45-year-old man presents with brief episodes of severe, electric shock-like pain on the left side of his face, exacerbated by a light touch of the cheek. MRI shows areas of high signal T2/FLAIR signal intensity and contrast enhancement in the pons near the trigeminal root entry zone. What is the most likely diagnosis?

- A. Trigeminal neuralgia type 2
- B. Atypical facial pain
- C. Trigeminal neuropathic pain
- D. Symptomatic trigeminal neuralgia
- E. Post-herpetic neuralgia

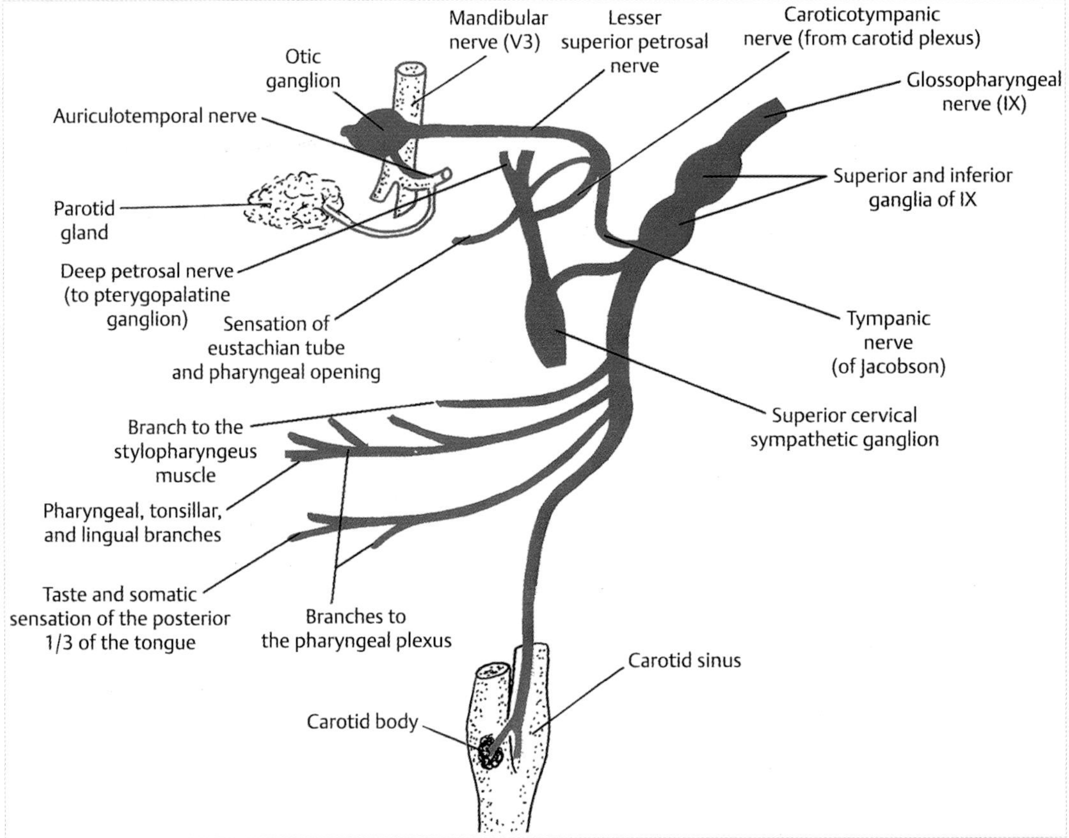

Fig. 5.2 (Source: Reproduced from XV Cranial nerves. In: Citow J, Macdonald R, Refai D, Citow J, Macdonald R, eds. Comprehensive Neurosurgery Board Review. 2nd ed. New York: Thieme; 2009.)

Correct answer is D

Trigeminal neuralgia secondary to multiple sclerosis (MS), also known as symptomatic trigeminal neuralgia, occurs due to demyelination within the trigeminal nerve root or the pontine root entry zone. This demyelination disrupts normal signal conduction, leading to ectopic axonal activity and ephaptic transmission, which causes paroxysmal, lancinating facial pain. The pain is often triggered by light touch or trivial stimuli and is refractory to typical analgesics. MRI is essential in diagnosing MS-related TN, revealing characteristic demyelinating plaques.

The Burchiel Classification of Trigeminal Neuralgia

The Burchiel classification divides TN into distinct subtypes. Classical TN (Type 1) presents with sharp, electric shock-like pain with pain-free intervals, often caused by vascular compression. TN Type 2 (TN2) features a combination of constant, aching pain and paroxysms. Symptomatic TN, as seen in this case, is secondary to underlying pathologies such as MS or tumors, with MRI findings confirming the cause. Trigeminal neuropathic pain results from trauma or nerve injury and is characterized by constant, burning discomfort.

In this patient, the MRI findings of demyelinating lesions near the trigeminal root entry zone strongly suggest symptomatic trigeminal neuralgia secondary to MS, making (option **D**) Symptomatic trigeminal neuralgia the correct answer.

▸▸ Question 14

A 35-year-old man with severe trigeminal neuralgia is undergoing gamma knife radiosurgery. Which of the following best describes the mechanism by which gamma knife radiosurgery alleviates pain?

- A. Immediately lysing nerve fibers
- B. Increasing blood flow to the trigeminal nerve
- C. Reducing inflammation around the trigeminal nerve
- D. Inducing axonal degeneration of the trigeminal nerve root
- E. Blocking neurotransmitter release at synapses

Correct answer is D

Gamma knife radiosurgery for trigeminal neuralgia delivers a high dose of focused radiation to the trigeminal nerve root at the root entry zone. This precise targeting creates a lesion that disrupts the transmission of pain signals without significant collateral damage. The lesioning effect leads to axonal degeneration and demyelination, reducing aberrant pain transmission. Gamma knife radiosurgery is a minimally invasive option that provides durable pain relief for many patients, with the benefit of fewer complications compared to open surgical approaches. However, the full benefit is delayed due to the time required for axonal degeneration to manifest after radiosurgery.[6]

▸▸ Question 15

A 60-year-old man with Parkinson disease (PD) presents with severe bradykinesia, rigidity, and tremor despite optimal medical therapy. He was initially responsive to levodopa therapy. Now, he experiences significant on-off motor fluctuations with increasing medial therapy. Which of the following is the most appropriate next step in management?

- A. Increase the dose of levodopa
- B. Add a dopamine agonist
- C. Deep brain stimulation (DBS)
- D. Physical therapy
- E. Botulinum toxin injections

Correct answer is C

DBS is an effective treatment for patients with PD who experience significant bradykinesia, rigidity, and tremor despite optimal medical therapy. DBS involves the surgical implantation of electrodes into specific brain regions, such as the subthalamic nucleus or globus pallidus internus, which are then connected to a pulse generator that delivers electrical impulses. This intervention helps modulate the abnormal neural activity associated with PD, thereby reducing symptoms and improving quality of life. DBS is typically considered when pharmacological treatments fail to provide adequate symptom control or cause intolerable side effects (▸ Fig. 5.3).[7]

▸▸ Question 16

A 45-year-old woman with medically refractory epilepsy is evaluated for surgical intervention. Video-EEG monitoring localizes the seizure focus to the left mesial temporal lobe. MRI demonstrates abnormalities within the left hippocampus, including loss of volume, loss of internal

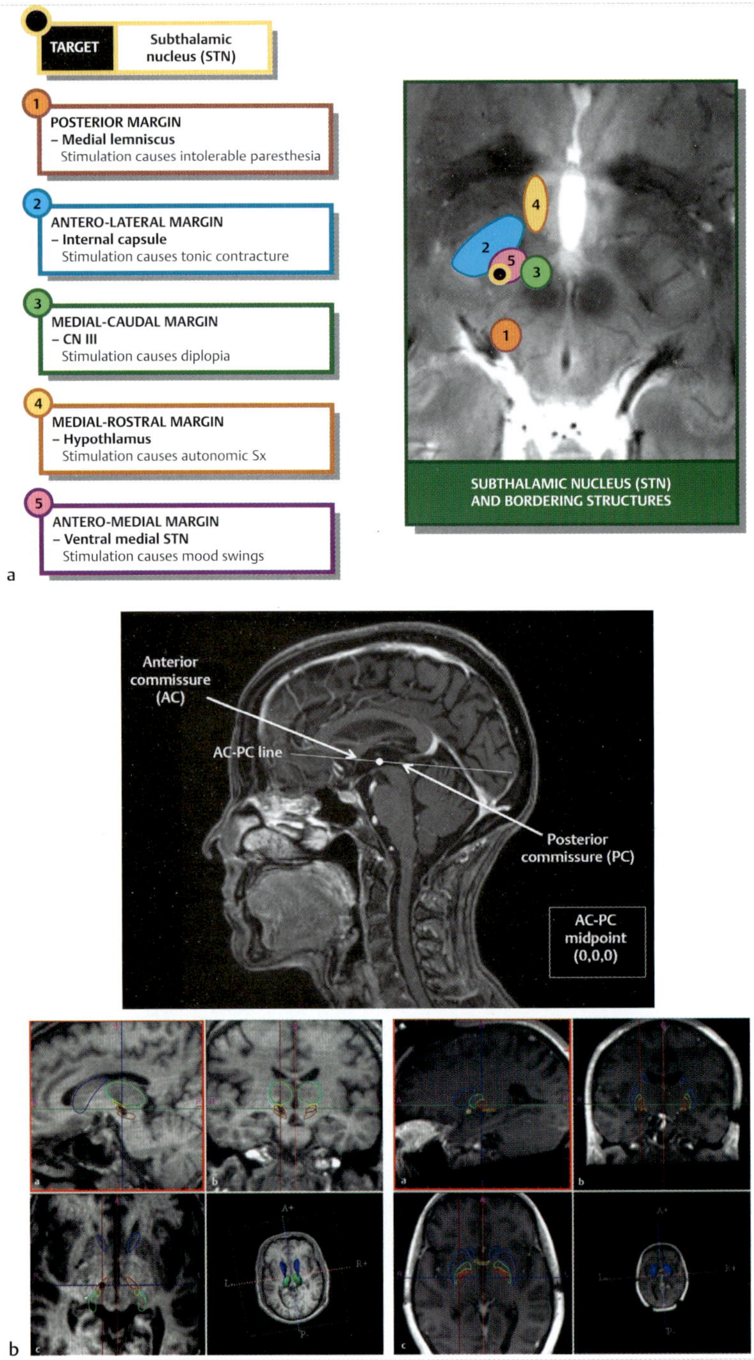

Fig. 5.3 (Source: Part a is reproduced from Subthalamic Nucleus (STN). In: Alberstone C, Benzel E, Jones S, Wang Z, Steinmetz M, ed. Anatomic Basis of Neurologic Diagnosis. 2nd Edition. New York: Thieme; 2023. Part b is reproduced from Nuclei Targeting. In: Kanekar S, ed. Imaging of Neurodegenerative Disorders. 1st Edition. New York: Thieme; 2015. Part c is reproduced from Source: Therapeutic Mechanisms of Movement Disorder Surgery. In: Bakay R, ed. Movement Disorder Surgery: The Essentials. 1st Edition. New York: Thieme; 2008.)

(*Continued*)

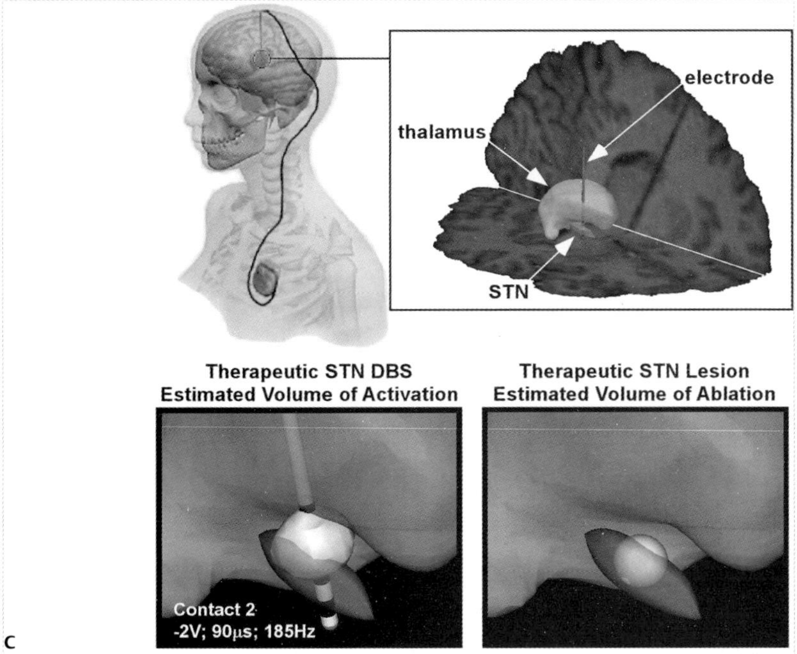

Fig. 5.3 (*Continued*)

architecture, and increased T2/FLAIR signal. Wada results suggested left language dominance and bilateral memory representation. In order to potentially minimize any cognitive effects, the patient would like to pursue a selective resection of the left mesial temporal lobe and spare the basolateral cortex. Which of the following is *not* a reported surgical approach for selective amygdalohippocampectomy (SAH)?

- A. Transcortical
- B. Transsylvian
- C. Subtemporal
- D. Supracerebellar transtentorial
- E. Transfrontal isthmus

Correct answer is E

Temporal lobectomy is a well-established surgical intervention for patients with medically refractory epilepsy localized to the mesial temporal lobe. It involves resection of the anterior temporal lobe, including the hippocampus and amygdala, which are common sites of seizure origination. This procedure has a high success rate in achieving seizure freedom or significant seizure reduction, particularly when the seizure focus is well-defined through video-EEG monitoring and imaging studies such as MRI.

SAH is an alternative approach that focuses on removing the seizure focus while sparing surrounding cortical areas to potentially minimize cognitive side effects. Various surgical approaches to SAH include the following:

Transcortical: Involves accessing the mesial temporal structures via a direct cortical incision.

Transsylvian: Utilizes the sylvian fissure as a natural corridor to reach the amygdala and hippocampus.

Subtemporal: Accesses the mesial temporal lobe by approaching beneath the temporal lobe, avoiding cortical incision.

Supracerebellar transtentorial: A less common approach, typically used for lesions in the posterior hippocampus or parahippocampal gyrus, avoiding cortical damage.

The transfrontal isthmus approach, however, is not a reported method for SAH. This approach is typically utilized to access the insular cortex, which lies in a different anatomical region and is unrelated to mesial temporal lobe epilepsy surgery (▶ Fig. 5.4).[8]

▸▸ Question 17

A 30-year-old woman with severe obsessive-compulsive disorder (OCD) has not responded to multiple trials of medications and cognitive-behavioral therapy. Which of the following functional neurosurgical procedures can be considered for her condition?

- A. Deep brain stimulation of the subthalamic nucleus
- B. Anterior cingulotomy
- C. Vagal nerve stimulation
- D. Gamma Knife posterior capsulotomy
- E. Temporal lobectomy

Correct answer is B

Anterior cingulotomy is a functional neurosurgical procedure used to treat severe, treatment-refractory OCD. The procedure involves creating lesions in the anterior cingulate cortex, which is implicated in the pathophysiology of OCD. This intervention aims to disrupt the abnormal circuits involved in the excessive anxiety and compulsive behaviors characteristic of OCD. Anterior cingulotomy has been shown to reduce symptoms in patients who do not respond to conventional treatments such as pharmacotherapy and cognitive-behavioral therapy.[9]

▸▸ Question 18

A 27-year-old female with neurofibromatosis type 2 has bilateral vestibular schwannomas. The left is intracanalicular with hearing preservation. The right is 4.5 cm with brainstem compression, with some auditory dysfunction. However, she has serviceable hearing in the right ear and can use a phone on that side. You are monitoring brainstem auditory evoked responses (BAERs) during a retrosigmoid approach for tumor resection. Which gray matter site in the auditory pathway is the first to receive bilateral (binaural) input?

- A. Cochlear nucleus
- B. Superior olivary complex
- C. Inferior colliculus
- D. Medial geniculate nucleus (MGN)
- E. Heschl gyrus

Correct answer is B

Binaural auditory input is first integrated in the superior olivary complex (SOC), a gray matter structure located in the brainstem. The SOC plays a crucial role in localizing sound through interaural time and intensity differences, essential for spatial hearing. It is part of the ascending auditory pathway, where signals from the cochlear nuclei on both sides of the brainstem converge.

Auditory Pathway

(**A**) Cochlear nucleus: This is the first relay station in the central auditory pathway, where auditory nerve fibers synapse. It processes monaural input (signals from one ear only).

(**B**) Superior olivary complex: This is the first structure to integrate binaural input, essential for sound localization. It sends projections to higher auditory centers via the lateral lemniscus.

(**C**) Inferior colliculus: Located in the midbrain, it processes auditory signals from the SOC and integrates sound localization information before transmitting signals to the thalamus.

(**D**) Medial geniculate nucleus: A relay station in the thalamus, it processes auditory information before it is sent to the auditory cortex.

(**E**) Heschl gyrus: The primary auditory cortex in the temporal lobe, responsible for the perception and interpretation of sound (▸ Fig. 5.5).

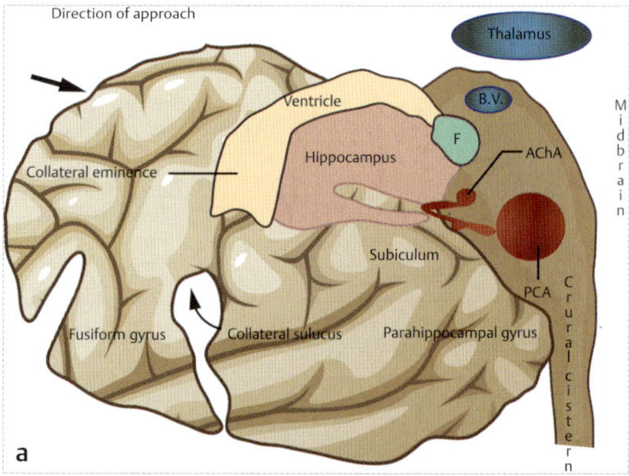

Fig. 5.4 (Source: Part a is reproduced from 6.6 Lateral Lobectomy. In: Baltuch G, Cukiert A, ed. Operative Techniques in Epilepsy Surgery. 2nd Edition. New York: Thieme; 2019. Part b is reproduced from 6.7 Microsurgical Resection of the Mesial Temporal Lobe. In: Baltuch G, Cukiert A, ed. Operative Techniques in Epilepsy Surgery. 2nd Edition. New York: Thieme; 2019.)

(Continued)

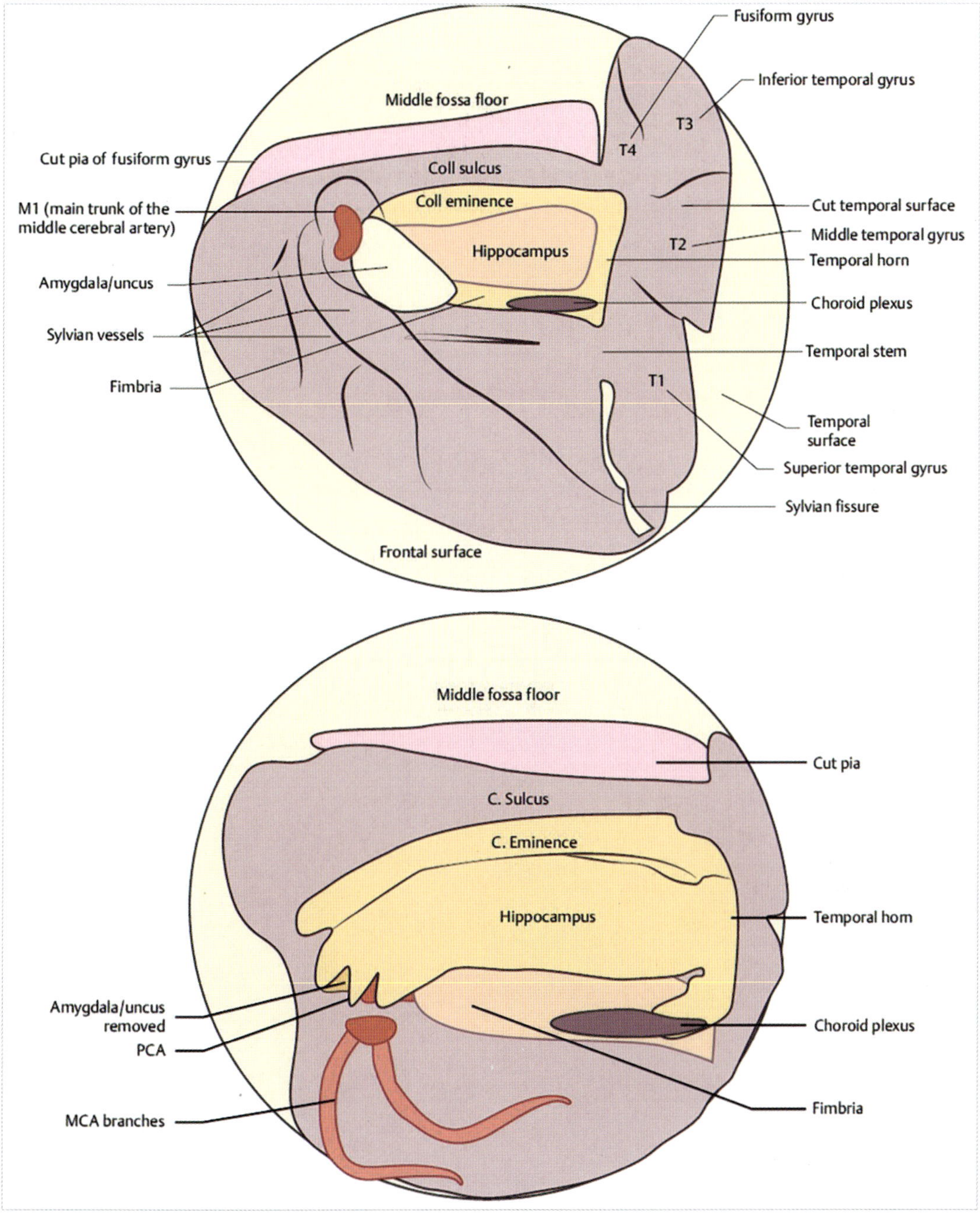

Fig. 5.4 (*Continued*)

(Continued)

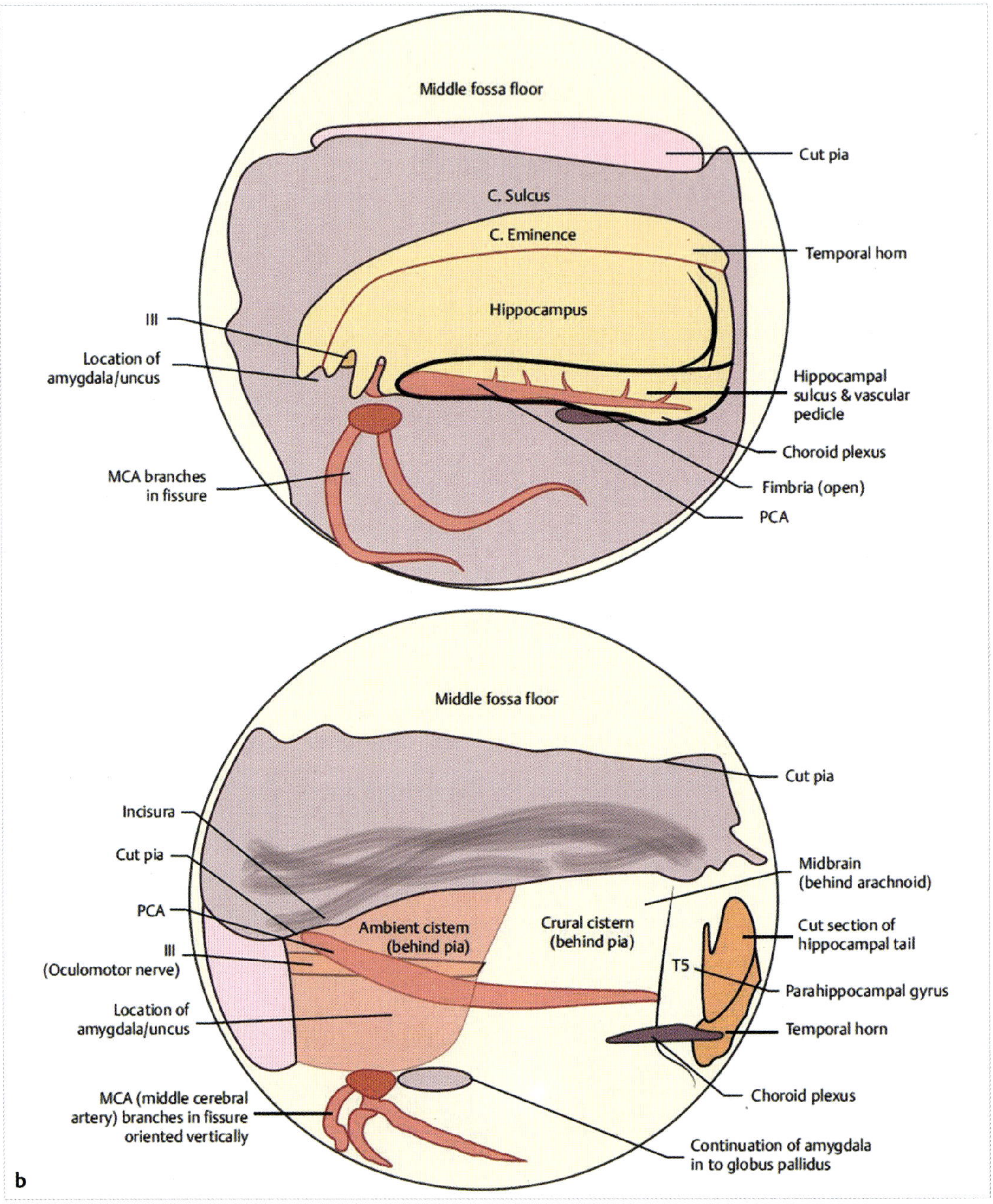

Fig. 5.4 (*Continued*)

(*Continued*)

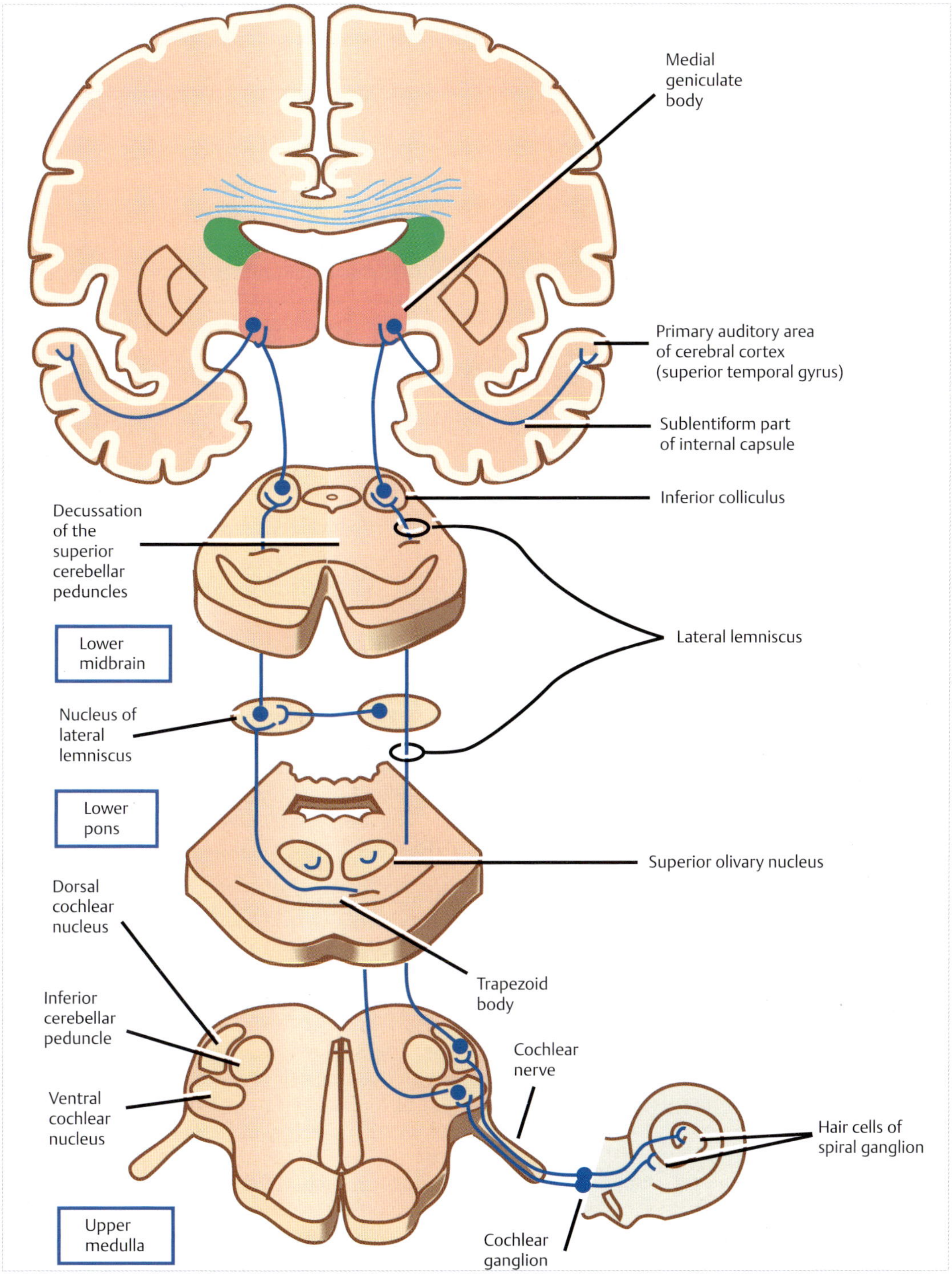

Fig. 5.5 (Source: Reproduced from Brainstem. In: Alberstone C, Benzel E, Jones S, Wang Z, Steinmetz M, ed. Anatomic Basis of Neurologic Diagnosis. 2nd ed. New York: Thieme; 2023.)

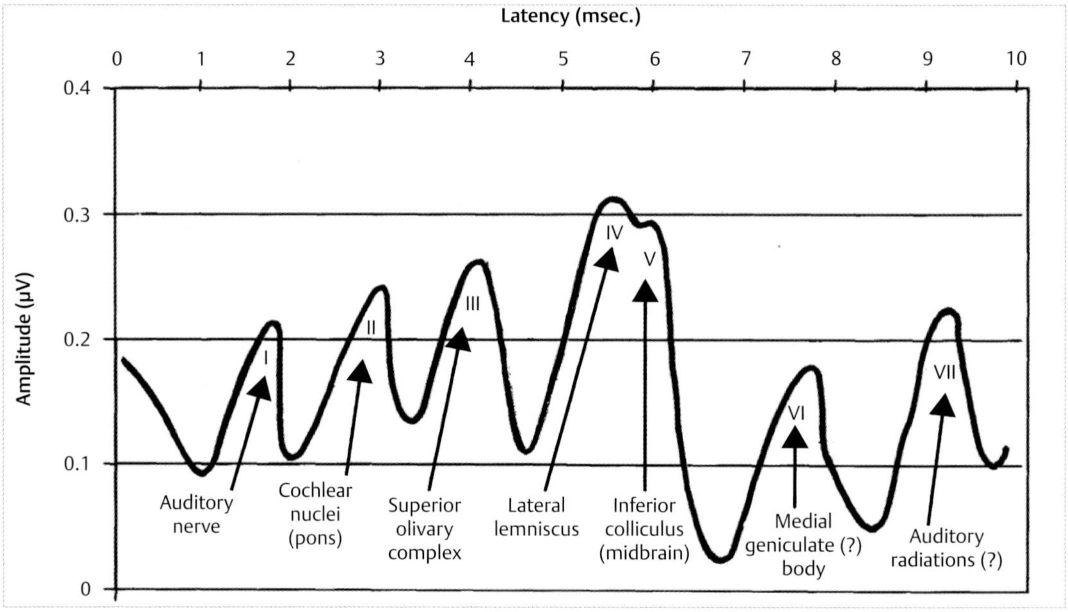

Fig. 5.6 (Source: Reproduced from Peripheral nerve. In: Citow J, Macdonald R, Puffer R, Khalid S, Carter B, Cohen A, Spinner R, Refai D, eds. Comprehensive Neurosurgery Board Review. 3rd ed. New York: Thieme; 2019.)

Brainstem Auditory Evoked Responses

During vestibular schwannoma surgery, BAERs are monitored to preserve auditory function. BAERs are generated by sequential activation of the auditory pathway (► Fig. 5.6):

1. Wave I: Action potential of the auditory nerve.
2. Wave II: Cochlear nucleus activity.
3. Wave III: Superior olivary complex.
4. Wave IV/V: Lateral lemniscus and inferior colliculus.

In this patient, BAER monitoring focuses on the preservation of the auditory pathway during the retrosigmoid approach for tumor resection. The superior olivary complex, as the first site of binaural integration, is critical for maintaining sound localization and auditory function.

▸▸ Question 19

50-year-old woman with essential tremor (ET) that is refractory to medications is considered for surgical treatment. Which of the following is the most appropriate surgical intervention for her condition?

- A. Pallidotomy
- B. Vagal nerve stimulator
- C. Deep brain stimulation (DBS) of the ventral intermediate nucleus of the thalamus
- D. Motor cortex stimulation
- E. Deep brain stimulation of the subthalamic nucleus

Correct answer is C

DBS of the ventral intermediate nucleus (VIM) of the thalamus is the preferred surgical treatment for patients with essential tremor (ET) that is refractory to medical therapy. The VIM is a critical relay station for the dentatorubrothalamic tract, a prominent tremor circuit, and DBS in this region can effectively reduce tremor severity. MR-guided focused ultrasound (MRgFUS) thalamotomy is an emerging treatment with the same target. DBS offers the advantage of being adjustable and reversible, while MRgFUS is incisionless with no need for battery changes. Both interventions have been shown to significantly improve tremor control and quality of life in patients with ET. DBS of the subthalamic nucleus is utilized in Parkinson disease to address bradykinesia and rigidity in addition to tremor (► Fig. 5.7).

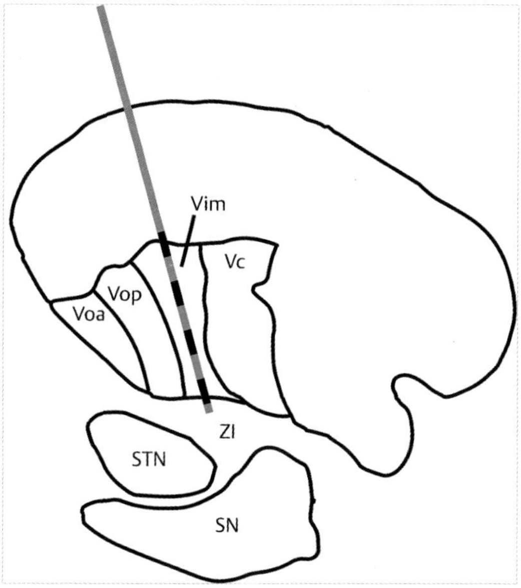

Fig. 5.7 (Source: Reproduced from Microelectrode recordings. In: Gross R, Boulis N, eds. Neurosurgical Operative Atlas: Functional Neurosurgery. 3rd ed. New York: Thieme; 2018.)

► Fig. 5.8 shows the pathophysiology of tremor. The basal ganglia and cerebellum have separate pathways to the thalamus. The globus pallidus internus sends inhibitory gamma-aminobutyric acid (GABA)-ergic fibers to the ventrolateral thalamus anterior nucleus (restraining motor cortical activity), whereas the cerebellar nuclei send excitatory glutamatergic innervation to ventrolateral thalamus posterior nucleus (facilitating motor cortical activity). Subthalamic nucleus functions as a connection hub to conduct signals to the motor cortex in tremor pathophysiology. The left side of the diagram illustrates the links between basal ganglia and motor cortex (blue), which are involved in Parkinson disease. The right side of the diagram demonstrates the links between the cerebellum and motor cortex (orange) that are responsible for ET. Subthalamic nucleus anatomically connects the cerebellum to basal ganglia (black arrow) and is thought to be responsible for the shared tremor mechanisms between Parkinson disease and ET. DBS at deep brain nucleus (subthalamic nucleus, globus pallidus), ketamine, levodopa, and propofol reduces the hyperactivity of cerebellothalamocortical circuit, resulting in an antitremor effect (arrows indicating sites of action). GPi, internal part of the globus pallidus; GPe, external part of the globus pallidus; ILN, thalamic intralaminar nucleus; IO, inferior olive; RN, red nucleus; STN, subthalamic nucleus; VLa, anterior part of the ventrolateral thalamus; VLp, posterior part of the ventrolateral thalamus; ILN, thalamic intralaminar nuclei; SNc, substantia nigra pars compacta; DBS, deep brain stimulation; DBN, deep brain nucleus; PD, Parkinson disease.[10]

►► **Question 20**

A 65-year-old man with Parkinson disease underwent deep brain stimulation (DBS) of the subthalamic nucleus (STN). Intraoperative microelectrode recording demonstrated a 5-mm tract of robust multiunit spiking activity above the planned target. Passive limb movement did drive increased neuronal spiking activity during microelectrode recording. With macrostimulation, he experiences some improvement in left upper extremity tremor, but he also experiences dysarthria and muscle contractions on the left side of his face at the same stimulation parameter. Before completing the operation, what adjustment should be made to the position of the DBS lead to optimize the therapeutic window of stimulation?

- A. The lead should be moved 2 mm lateral
- B. The lead should be moved 2 mm medial
- C. The lead should be moved 2 mm posterior
- D. The lead should be moved 2 mm dorsal
- E. The lead should be moved 2 mm ventral

Correct answer is B

Electrode placement in DBS for Parkinson disease requires precise targeting of the STN. When the electrode is placed too lateral or anteriorly in the STN, it can affect the internal capsule, leading to dysarthria and involuntary muscle contractions (dystonia) due to stimulation of corticobulbar fibers. The internal capsule contains motor fibers that can cause these symptoms if inadvertently stimulated (► Table 5.1).[11]

►► **Question 21**

A 70-year-old woman with Parkinson disease treated with deep brain stimulation (DBS) of the subthalamic nucleus (STN) presents with new-onset diplopia and worsening balance. Imaging confirms the electrode is suboptimally placed.

Table 5.1 Structures adjacent to the subthalamic nucleus and symptoms resulting from stimulation spread during deep brain stimulation

Anatomical context	Structures	Symptoms and associated tracts	Symptoms
Above STN	Zona incerta, thalamus	–	–
Below STN	Substantia nigra pars reticulata	–	–
Anterior to STN	Internal capsule, fields of Forel	Internal capsule	Dysarthria, muscle contractions (dystonia), hemiparesis
Posterior to STN	Red nucleus, substantia nigra pars compacta	Red nucleus	Involuntary movements such as tremor, worsening dyskinesia
Lateral to STN	Internal capsule	Internal capsule	Motor symptoms such as hemiparesis, dysarthria
Medial to STN	Hypothalamus	Hypothalamus	Autonomic dysfunction (e.g., changes in blood pressure, heart rate)

Note: Recognition of these anatomical relationships guides electrode placement and programming optimization to maximize therapeutic benefit while minimizing stimulation-induced side effects.

Which structure is most likely being stimulated to cause these symptoms?
- A. Red nucleus
- B. Internal capsule
- C. Zona incerta
- D. Optic tract
- E. Hypothalamus

Correct answer is A

In DBS for Parkinson disease, improper placement of the electrode in relation to STN can result in off-target stimulation of adjacent structures, leading to unintended side effects.

The red nucleus, located medially and posteriorly to the STN, is a common structure affected when the electrode is misaligned medially. Stimulation of the red nucleus can result in diplopia (double vision) due to its proximity to oculomotor pathways and worsening balance or ataxia due to its involvement in motor coordination within the rubrospinal tract (▶ Table 5.2).[12]

▸▸ Question 22

When treating dystonia with deep brain stimulation (DBS), typically the globus pallidus internus (GPi) is targeted. What is the primary reason for targeting the GPi in dystonia?
- A. To improve motor function by modulating thalamic output
- B. To reduce tremor by inhibiting the red nucleus
- C. To control dystonia by altering the output of the basal ganglia
- D. To alleviate pain by stimulating sensory pathways
- E. To enhance cognitive function by modulating the prefrontal cortex

Correct answer is C

The GPi is the thalamic receiving zone for outflow from the basal ganglia and plays an important role in the pathophysiology of dystonia. By modulating the abnormal output signals of the GPi, DBS can help control dystonic movements. This has a separate effect from targeting thalamic outputs (for motor function and tremor), sensory pathways (for pain), or the prefrontal cortex (for cognitive function).[13,14]

▸▸ Question 23

A 70-year-old woman with essential tremor is scheduled for magnetic resonance focused ultrasound (MRgFUS) thalamotomy targeting the ventral intermediate nucleus (VIM) of the thalamus. Which of the following are potential complications of MRgFUS targeting this area?
- A. Dysarthria and impaired balance
- B. Involuntary movements

Table 5.2 Anatomical relationships of the subthalamic nucleus and pathophysiology of DBS's side effects

Structure	Relative position to STN	Symptoms of off-target stimulation	Reason
Red nucleus	Medial and slightly posterior	Diplopia, worsening balance, or ataxia	Involvement in motor coordination (rubrospinal tract) and proximity to oculomotor pathways
Oculomotor nucleus	Medial	Diplopia	Direct stimulation of cranial nerve nuclei affecting extraocular muscles
Internal capsule	Lateral	Motor contractions, dysarthria	Activation of corticospinal or corticobulbar fibers
Zona incerta	Anterior	Autonomic disturbances, somatosensory effects	Modulates autonomic and sensory integration pathways
Optic tract	Inferior	Visual disturbances (e.g., phosphenes)	Involvement in visual processing pathways

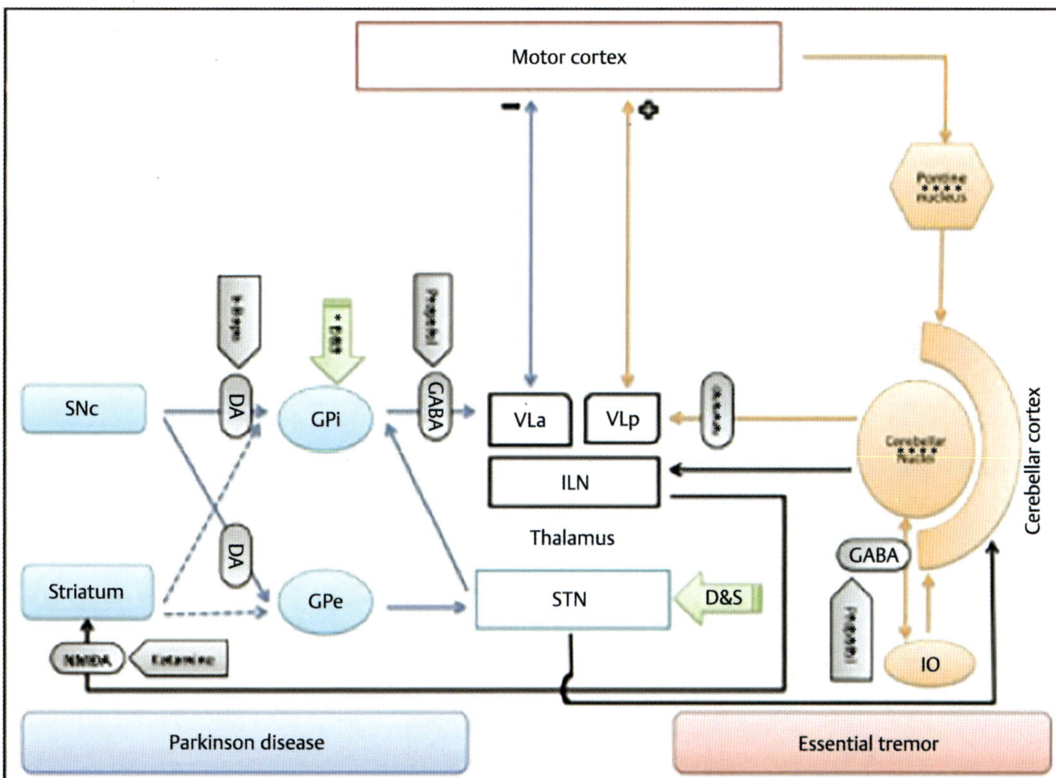

Fig. 5.8 (Source: Reproduced from Chui J, Alamri R, Bihari F et al. Propofol reduces microelectrode-recording artefacts caused by Parkinsonian tremor during deep brain stimulation. J Neuroanaesthesiol Crit Care 2018;05(01):21–25.)

- C. Hemiparesis
- D. Autonomic dysfunction
- E. Visual disturbances

Correct answer is A

MRgFUS targeting the VIM of the thalamus for essential tremor can sometimes cause dysarthria and impaired balance, which may be temporary or permanent. Other complications such as hemiparesis, involuntary movements, and autonomic dysfunction are less common but can occur if lesioning affects different adjacent structures.[15]

▸▸ Question 24

A 68-year-old man with Parkinson's disease who had deep brain stimulation (DBS) of the subthalamic nucleus (STN) now experiences autonomic dysfunction, including significant changes in blood pressure and heart rate. Where is the likely misplacement of the DBS lead?

- A. Anterior to the STN
- B. Posterior to the STN
- C. Medial to the STN
- D. Lateral to the STN
- E. Inferior to the STN

Correct answer is C

The hypothalamus is medial to the STN and is involved in autonomic functions. Stimulation or misplacement of the DBS lead anteromedially into the hypothalamus can result in autonomic dysfunction, such as changes in blood pressure and heart rate. Lateral or anterolateral placement would affect the internal capsule, posteromedial placement would involve the red nucleus, lateral placement would also affect the internal capsule, and inferior placement would involve the substantia nigra pars reticulata. ▸ Fig. 5.9 shows that the subthalamic nucleus is a small, almond-shaped structure just lateral to the red nucleus. Off-target stimulation effects can provide a clue about which direction the electrode should be moved in.

▸▸ Question 25

A patient with Parkinson's disease underwent bilateral deep brain stimulation (DBS) of the subthalamic nucleus (STN) with successful intraoperative identification of the dorsolateral sensorimotor portion of the nucleus. Upon initiating stimulation, the patient experiences a reduction in both rigidity and tremor. However, she also experiences severe dyskinesias. Which is the first step that should be undertaken to alleviate the dyskinesia?

- A. Increase the amplitude
- B. Decrease the amplitude
- C. Change the frequency to below 100 Hz
- D. Decrease the pulse width
- E. Switch to constant voltage mode

Correct answer is B

Dyskinesias after DBS of the STN are often a result of overstimulation. Amplitude is the strength or power of the signal being delivered. Decreasing the amplitude of the stimulation can decrease tissue penetrance and reduce excessive stimulation, or stimulation of adjacent structures, and thereby alleviate the dyskinesias. Reducing the frequency

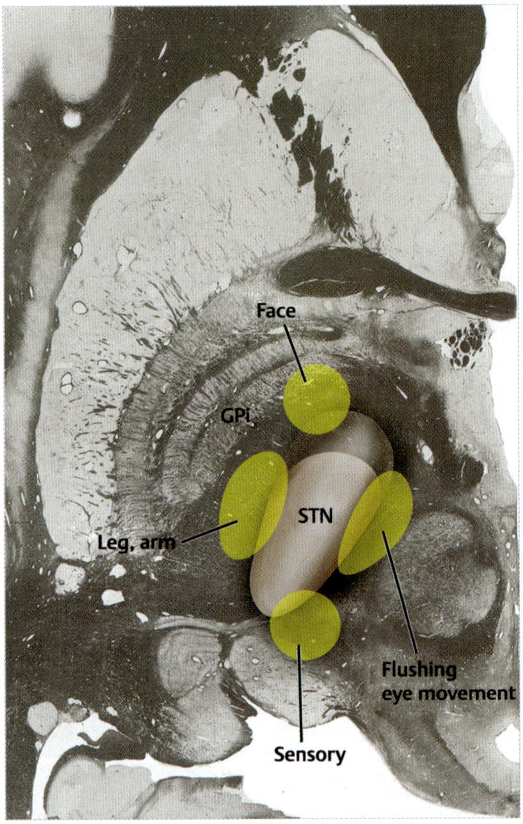

Fig. 5.9 (Source: Reproduced from Direct (image-guided) targeting. In: Anderson W, ed. Deep Brain Stimulation: Techniques and Practices. 1st ed. New York: Thieme; 2019.)

and pulse width may also help, but the first step typically involves reducing the amplitude.[16]

▸▸ Question 26

A 68-year-old man with Parkinson's disease has experienced worsening symptoms despite optimal medical therapy. He is now considered a candidate for deep brain stimulation (DBS) of the subthalamic nucleus (STN). During intraoperative microelectrode recording, a robust tract of spiking activity and kinesthetic cells are identified. When macrostimulation is performed, the patient experiences persistent severe contralateral paresthesias in the face and upper extremity, which do not attenuate with time. Stimulation of what structure is responsible for the adverse effects?

- A. Internal capsule
- B. Vc thalamus
- C. Vim thalamus
- D. Medial lemniscus
- E. Zona incerta

Correct answer is D

When planning DBS of the STN, precise placement of the electrode is essential to maximize therapeutic effects and minimize side effects. Adverse effects often arise from off-target stimulation of nearby structures.

In this case, persistent severe contralateral paresthesias in the face and upper extremity are indicative of stimulation near the medial lemniscus, a structure responsible for transmitting somatosensory information (e.g., touch and proprioception). The lead is too posterior in this scenario and must be moved anteriorly to avoid stimulating the medial lemniscus (▸ Table 5.3).[17]

▸▸ Question 27

A 30-year-old woman with medically refractory epilepsy undergoes a right anterior temporal lobectomy. Postoperatively, she experiences new visual field deficits. Which of the following visual field deficits is most likely associated with this surgery?

- A. Bitemporal hemianopsia
- B. Left homonymous hemianopsia
- C. Left homonymous inferior quadrantanopia
- D. Left homonymous superior quadrantanopia
- E. Superior quadrantanopia affecting the left eye

Table 5.3 Anatomical relationships of the subthalamic nucleus and stimulation-induced side effects during deep brain stimulation

Anatomical context	Structures	Symptoms and associated tracts	Symptoms
Above STN	Zona incerta, Thalamus	–	–
Below STN	Substantia nigra pars reticulata	–	–
Anterior to STN	Internal capsule, fields of Forel	Internal capsule	Dysarthria, muscle contractions (dystonia), hemiparesis
Posterior to STN	Red nucleus, substantia nigra pars compacta	Red nucleus	Involuntary movements such as tremor, worsening dyskinesia
Lateral to STN	Internal capsule	Internal capsule	Motor symptoms such as hemiparesis, dysarthria
Medial to STN	Hypothalamus	Hypothalamus	Autonomic dysfunction (e.g., changes in blood pressure, heart rate)

Note: This table summarizes the neural structures surrounding the STN in each anatomical direction and the clinical symptoms that may result from inadvertent current spread during DBS. Understanding these spatial relationships is essential for interpreting stimulation-induced side effects and guiding programming adjustments. Structures anterior and lateral to the STN (internal capsule, fields of Forel) produce motor symptoms including dysarthria, dystonic contractions, and hemiparesis when stimulated. Posterior spread to the red nucleus and substantia nigra pars compacta may paradoxically worsen involuntary movements, while medial spread to the hypothalamus can cause autonomic instability.

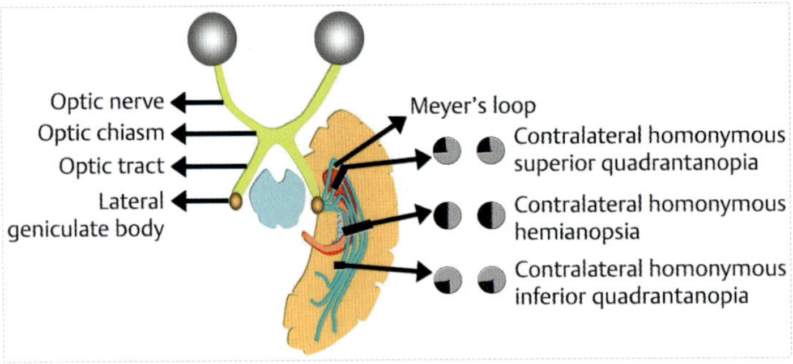

Fig. 5.10 (Source: Reproduced from Temporal lobe epilepsy. In: Nader R, Sabbagh A, Elbabaa S, Al-Jehani H, Gasco J, Gragnaniello C, eds. Neurosurgery Case Review: Questions and Answers. 2nd ed. New York: Thieme; 2020.)

Correct answer is D

An anterior temporal lobectomy can affect the optic radiation, particularly Meyer loop, which courses through the temporal lobe. Damage to this area typically results in a contralateral superior quadrantanopia, often referred to as a "pie in the sky" visual field defect. This occurs because Meyer loop carries visual information from the superior quadrant of the contralateral visual field (▸ Fig. 5.10).[8]

▸▸ Question 28

A 22-year-old man with intractable epilepsy is being evaluated for potential surgical intervention. MRI is negative for a lesion. Video EEG suggests bilateral temporal lobe epilepsy. The patient underwent deep brain stimulation (DBS) of the anterior nucleus of the thalamus (ANT). Which of the following is true regarding this therapy?

- A. Patients must be carefully monitored for worsening depression and suicidal ideation
- B. An extraventricular approach is associated with the greatest accuracy of lead placement, with 90% of cases having at least one DBS contact within the ANT
- C. The majority of patients who undergo DBS of the ANT for epilepsy have > 80% seizure reduction
- D. The portion of the ANT posterior to the mammillothalamic tract should be targeted when placing the DBS leads to result in the greatest seizure reduction
- E. ANT DBS is FDA-approved as a first-line treatment for drug-resistant epilepsy

Correct answer is A

DBS of the anterior nucleus of the thalamus is an FDA-approved therapy for patients with intractable epilepsy, particularly for cases involving multifocal or bilateral seizures. The ANT is a key node in the limbic system, and its stimulation is thought to modulate seizure activity through its connections to the hippocampus and cortex.

Key points about ANT DBS:

1. *Efficacy*: Although long-term studies have shown that patients undergoing ANT DBS often experience significant seizure reduction, the majority achieve 50 to 70% seizure reduction, not > 80%, over time. Seizure outcomes tend to improve gradually, with maximal effects often observed years after implantation.
2. *Targeting*: The anterior portion of the ANT, anterior to the mammillothalamic tract, is targeted for the best seizure outcomes. This region has stronger connectivity to limbic circuits involved in epilepsy modulation. Accurate lead placement is crucial, but no approach guarantees 90% of DBS contacts within the ANT. Errors can occur with both extraventricular and transventricular approaches, requiring intraoperative imaging or postoperative confirmation.
3. *Neuropsychiatric risks*: A critical consideration with ANT DBS is the risk of worsening depression, anxiety, and suicidal ideation, which necessitates preoperative psychiatric evaluation and close postoperative monitoring. The stimulation of the limbic-related circuitry in the thalamus may contribute to these effects.
4. *Therapy management*: Stimulation parameters are adjusted postoperatively to balance seizure control with side effects. These parameters often include low-frequency stimulation to avoid adverse neuropsychiatric outcomes.

▸▸ Question 29

A 24-year-old female underwent surgery for drug-resistant epilepsy. Seizures began in childhood and were initially responsive to antiseizure medication. There was a fulminant recurrence in early adulthood, highly resistant to medication. Video EEG showed right lateralized ictal and interictal epileptiform activity, more prominent in sleep. MRI demonstrated a lesion with blurring of the gray–white junction and a transmantle sign. PET showed a concordant area of focal-decreased FDG uptake. The patient underwent a resection with image guidance and intraoperative electrocorticography. The pathology showed a focal cortical dysplasia (FCD) type IIb. What is the statistically most likely location of the lesion in this patient?

- A. Superior frontal sulcus
- B. Central sulcus
- C. Superior temporal sulcus
- D. Intraparietal sulcus
- E. Parieto-occipital fissure

Correct answer is A

FCD type IIb is a well-established cause of drug-resistant epilepsy, commonly identified through a combination of clinical, imaging, and pathological findings. This type of FCD is characterized by specific neuroimaging features, including the following:

- MRI findings: Blurring of the gray–white matter junction; reflects disorganized cortical and subcortical structure
- Transmantle sign: A tapering hyperintense signal extending from the cortex to the ventricle on T2/FLAIR, highly specific for FCD type IIb.
- PET findings: Focal decreased FDG uptake; corresponds to hypometabolism in the epileptogenic zone and often aligns with the MRI lesion
- Pathology: FCD type IIb is histologically characterized by dysmorphic neurons and balloon cells, correlating with high seizure resistance to medical therapy.

The frontal lobe, particularly near the superior frontal sulcus, is statistically the most common location for FCD type IIb. Other less frequent areas include the central sulcus, temporal lobe, or parietal regions. Accurate localization of the epileptogenic zone through a multimodal approach (MRI, PET, video EEG, and intraoperative electrocorticography) is essential for achieving successful surgical outcomes.

▸▸ Question 30

A 45-year-old man with intractable seizures undergoes evaluation for epilepsy surgery. Video-EEG monitoring localizes the seizure focus to the left mesial temporal lobe. Which of the following is the most likely finding on histopathological examination of the resected tissue?

- A. Low-grade astrocytoma
- B. Segmental loss of pyramidal neurons in CA1 and CA4 region of the hippocampus
- C. Segmental loss of pyramidal neurons CA3 region of the hippocampus
- D. Heterotopic and dysplastic neurons in the hippocampal formation
- E. Sinusoidal vessels surrounded by hemosiderin

Correct answer is B

Hippocampal sclerosis is the most common histopathological finding in patients with mesial temporal lobe epilepsy, serving as a hallmark of the condition. It is characterized by segmental neuronal loss, primarily in the CA1 and CA4 regions of the hippocampus, with relative sparing of CA3. This neuronal degeneration is accompanied by reactive gliosis, evidenced by GFAP+(glial fibrillary acidic protein-positive) astrogliosis, reflecting the chronic nature of the pathology.

The development of hippocampal sclerosis is often linked to an initial precipitating event, such as febrile seizures, status epilepticus, or hypoxia, which initiates neuronal injury and contributes to the formation of an epileptogenic focus. Patients with hippocampal sclerosis frequently have drug-resistant mesial temporal lobe epilepsy, making surgical intervention an important treatment option.

MRI findings commonly associated with hippocampal sclerosis include hippocampal atrophy and increased T2/FLAIR signal intensity, which provide preoperative clues to the diagnosis. Surgical procedures, such as anterior temporal lobectomy or selective amygdalohippocampectomy, often lead to significant seizure reduction, with many patients achieving seizure freedom.

While other findings, such as low-grade gliomas or cortical dysplasia, may occasionally be observed in epilepsy cases, the hallmark histopathological feature in this context is segmental loss of pyramidal neurons in CA1 and CA4 regions, along with GFAP+astrogliosis, confirming hippocampal sclerosis. ▶ Fig. 5.11 shows a coronal FLAIR image in a patient with known left mesial temporal sclerosis, showing a small left hippocampus (red arrow), abnormally increased signal, and a loss of internal architecture.[18]

▸▸ Question 31

A 28-year-old woman with intractable epilepsy undergoes vagus nerve stimulation (VNS). Which of the following is *not* related to mechanisms of action?

- A. Increase catecholamine release from the locus coeruleus
- B. Activation of efferent fibers of within the cervical portion of the vagus nerve
- C. Modulation of thalamic activity
- D. Activation of the nucleus tractus solitarius (NTS)
- E. Upregulation of serotonin release from the midline raphe nuclei

Correct answer is B

VNS primarily exerts its antiepileptic effects through the activation of afferent fibers within the cervical portion of the vagus nerve, rather than efferent fibers. When afferent fibers are stimulated, signals are transmitted to the NTS in the brainstem, which serves as a central hub projecting to various brain regions, including the locus coeruleus, thalamus, and midline raphe nuclei. This interconnected network modulates brain activity by increasing catecholamine release from the locus coeruleus, upregulating serotonin release from the midline raphe nuclei, and modulating thalamic activity. These changes collectively decrease cortical excitability and suppress seizure activity, providing therapeutic effects in epilepsy. The role of efferent fibers, which are associated with parasympathetic outputs to peripheral organs, is minimal and not significant in the anticonvulsant effects of VNS. Understanding these mechanisms highlights the importance of the afferent pathways in the success of VNS therapy for managing epilepsy.[19]

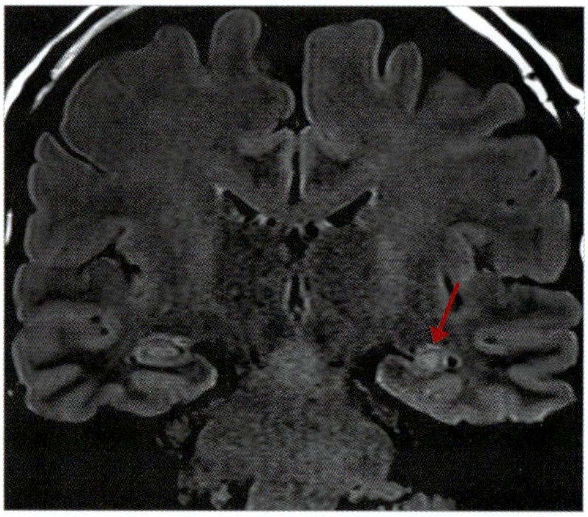

Fig. 5.11 (Source: Reproduced from Medial temporal lobe epilepsy. In: Alberstone C, Benzel E, Jones S, Wang Z, Steinmetz M, eds. Anatomic Basis of Neurologic Diagnosis. 2nd ed. New York: Thieme; 2023.)

▸▸ Question 32

A 70-year-old woman is experiencing new-onset left hemiballismus. MRI reveals a lesion in the right subthalamic nucleus. Which pathway is most likely disrupted, leading to her symptoms?

- A. Direct pathway of the basal ganglia
- B. Indirect pathway of the basal ganglia
- C. Corticospinal tract
- D. Spinothalamic tract
- E. Reticulospinal tract

Correct answer is B

Hemiballismus is typically caused by a lesion in the subthalamic nucleus, which disrupts the indirect pathway of the basal ganglia. This pathway normally inhibits unwanted movements, and its disruption leads to hyperkinetic movements such as hemiballismus (▸ Fig. 5.12).[20]

▸▸ Question 33

Which neurotransmitter is primarily released by neurons of the substantia nigra pars compacta and is critical in the pathophysiology of Parkinson disease?

- A. Dopamine
- B. Acetylcholine
- C. Serotonin
- D. GABA
- E. Glutamate

Correct answer is A

Dopamine is the primary neurotransmitter released by neurons of the substantia nigra pars compacta. In Parkinson's disease, the loss of these dopaminergic neurons leads to the characteristic motor symptoms due to decreased dopamine levels in the striatum.

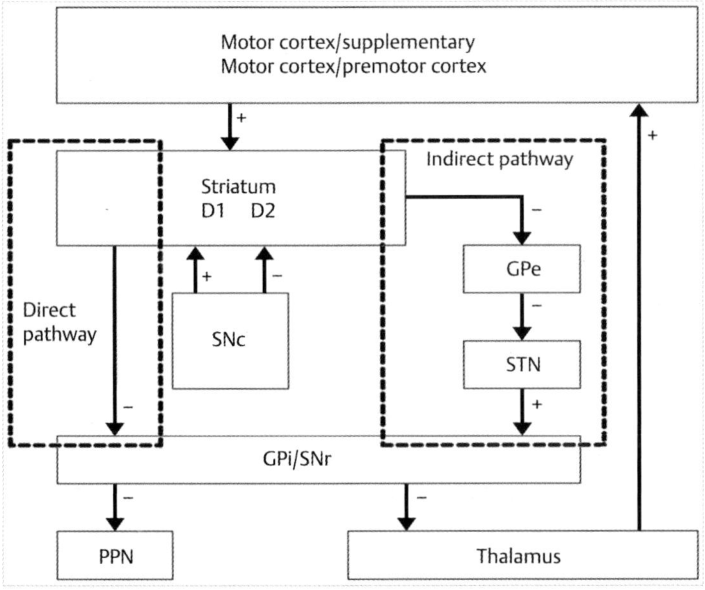

Fig. 5.12 (Source: Reproduced from Indications and pathophysiology. In: Gasco J, Nader R, eds. The Essential Neurosurgery Companion. 1st ed. New York: Thieme; 2012.)

▸▸ Question 34

A patient presents with refractory essential tremor. Which of the following brain regions is commonly targeted in deep brain stimulation (DBS) and MR-guided focused ultrasound for this condition?

- A. Subthalamic nucleus
- B. Globus pallidus interna
- C. Ventral intermediate nucleus of the thalamus
- D. Pedunculopontine nucleus
- E. Caudate nucleus

Correct answer is C

The ventral intermediate nucleus (VIM) of the thalamus is the most common target for DBS in patients with essential tremor. This area is involved in the cerebellar–thalamic–cortical loop, which is critical for the modulation of tremor.[21] ▸ Fig. 5.13 shows a schematic diagram of thalamic somatotopy. Tremor reduction is best targeting Vim, specifically the aspect including the "arm" and "hand" regions. Primary foot kinesthetics are suggestive of lateral position, while primarily, the face and jaw kinesthetic neurons are suggestive of medial electrode positioning. Electrodes placed too posteriorly will generate sustained paresthesias with stimulation due to the proximity to Vca. Thalamic structures are labeled using the Hassler classification of human thalamic anatomy: Ce, centromedian nucleus; Lpo, lateral posterior; Pf, parafasicular nucleus; Vca, ventral caudalis anterior; Vcp, ventral caudalis posterior; Vim, ventral intermediate nucleus; Voa, ventral oralis anterior. Extra-thalamic anatomy: Cd, caudate; Fx, fornix; Pul, pulvinar; Put, putamen.

▸▸ Question 35

A 33-year-old female with obsessive-compulsive disorder is evaluated by your center's multidisciplinary review board for potential surgical candidacy. She has severe symptoms despite medication and cognitive behavioral therapy with exposure and response prevention. The treatment team and patient elect for bilateral deep brain stimulation targeting the ventral capsule/ventral striatum. Which dopaminergic brain center provides input to the ventral striatum, part of a circuit implicated in reward and addiction?

- A. Substantia nigra pars compacta
- B. Ventral tegmental area
- C. Median raphe nucleus
- D. Arcuate nucleus of the hypothalamus
- E. Nucleus accumbens

Correct answer is B

Deep brain stimulation targeting the ventral capsule and ventral striatum is an emerging treatment for severe, refractory obsessive-compulsive

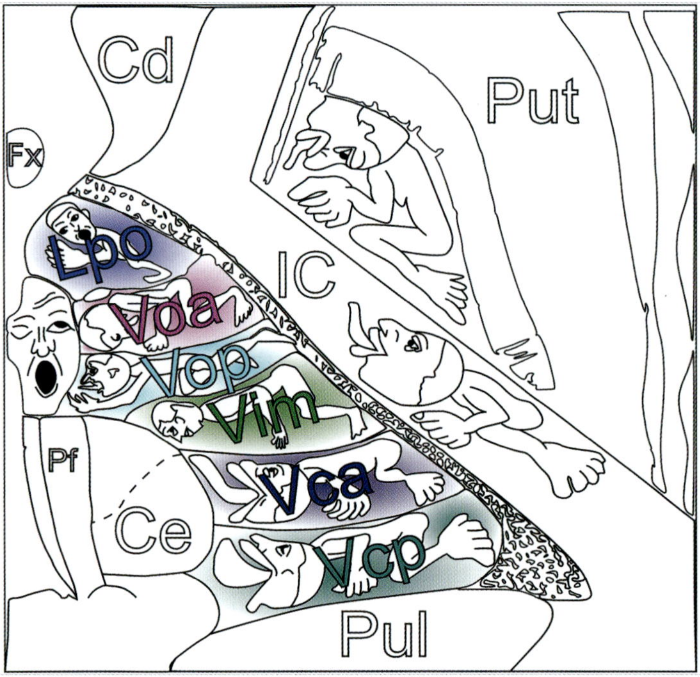

Fig. 5.13 (Source: Reproduced from Neuronal Responses During MER (Fig. 9.3). In: Anderson W, ed. Deep Brain Stimulation: Techniques and Practices. 1st Edition. New York: Thieme; 2019.)

disorder. This brain region is a key component of the cortico-striatal-thalamo-cortical circuit, which is hyperactive in obsessive-compulsive disorder and plays a central role in regulating reward, motivation, and compulsive behaviors. The ventral tegmental area, a structure in the midbrain, provides dopaminergic input to the ventral striatum. This connection is critical for reward processing, addiction, and reinforcement learning. Dysregulation in these circuits contributes to the compulsive and repetitive behaviors seen in obsessive-compulsive disorder.

The therapeutic effects of deep brain stimulation in this region are thought to stem from its ability to disrupt abnormal activity within these neural circuits, restoring a more balanced function. In contrast, other dopaminergic centers, such as the substantia nigra pars compacta, primarily regulate motor control through projections to the dorsal striatum. Similarly, the median raphe nucleus and the arcuate nucleus of the hypothalamus are associated with serotonin regulation and hypothalamic–pituitary axis functions, respectively, rather than directly influencing the ventral striatum.

The ventral tegmental area's role in modulating dopamine release highlights its importance in the reward and habit-forming circuits implicated in obsessive-compulsive disorder. For this reason, the ventral tegmental area is the correct answer, emphasizing its contribution to the therapeutic effects of deep brain stimulation targeting the ventral capsule and ventral striatum.

▸▸ Question 36

During deep brain stimulation (DBS) surgery, microelectrode recordings are used to differentiate between neurons in the subthalamic nucleus (STN) and those in the substantia nigra pars reticulata (SNr). Which of the following best describes the electrophysiologic firing pattern differences between these areas?

- A. STN neurons exhibit irregular, high-frequency bursts; SNr neurons show regular, tonic firing
- B. STN neurons exhibit regular, tonic firing; SNr neurons show irregular, high-frequency bursts
- C. Both STN and SNr neurons exhibit irregular, high-frequency bursts
- D. Both STN and SNr neurons show regular, tonic firing
- E. STN neurons exhibit low-frequency bursts; SNr neurons show regular, tonic firing

Correct answer is A

Microelectrode recordings typically show that STN neurons exhibit irregular, high-frequency bursts, whereas SNr neurons demonstrate regular, tonic firing. These distinct firing patterns help neurosurgeons accurately identify target areas during DBS surgery.[22] ▶ Fig. 5.14 shows a typical microelectrode recording physiological signatures of structures encountered. (**a**) Thalamus. (**b**) Zona incerta. (**c**) Subthalamic nucleus. (**d**) Substantia nigra pars reticularis.

▸▸ Question 37

A 68-year-old man with Parkinson disease is undergoing DBS surgery targeting the subthalamic nucleus (STN). During intraoperative microelectrode recording, a 4-mm length tract of multiunit spiking activity is identified just above the planned target depth. During intraoperative behavioral testing, passive limb movement did not drive any of the neuronal spiking activity. Intraoperative macroelectrode stimulation did result in moderate tremor suppression. Postoperatively, the patient reports increased depression and anxiety. When the stimulation is turned off, these symptoms improve; however, his tremor returns to his preoperative levels. Which of the following areas is most likely responsible for his stimulation-related adverse effects?

- A. Dorsolateral STN
- B. Ventromedial STN
- C. Nucleus accumbens
- D. Ventral pallidum
- E. Mediodorsal thalamus

Correct answer is B

The ventral subthalamic nucleus (STN) is involved in limbic circuits, and stimulation in this area can lead to increased depression and anxiety. Identification of the STN activity by microelectrode recording but without identification of kinesthetic cells may indicate electrode position within either the associative or limbic STN, rather than the sensorimotor STN (dorsolateral). The limbic STN has projections to the ventral pallidum. Careful targeting and adjustment of the stimulation parameters are required to minimize these side effects.[23]

▸▸ Question 38

A 60-year-old woman with Parkinson disease undergoes DBS of the globus pallidus interna (GPi). Which of the following is *false* regarding the primary output projections of the GPi?

- A. The GPi is the primary output nucleus of both the direct and indirect basal ganglia pathways
- B. The ventral anterior (VA) nucleus of the thalamus is the primary target of GPi efferent fibers
- C. The ansa lenticularis preferentially provides input to the anterior ventralis oralis (Voa) nucleus of the thalamus
- D. The thalamic fasciculus provides input to both the anterior and posterior ventralis oralis (Voa and Vop) nuclei of the thalamus
- E. GPi projections travel directly to the spinal cord to modulate motor function

Correct answer is C

Both the direct and indirect basal ganglia pathways ultimately converge on the GPi, which in turn provides GABAergic output to the VA nucleus of the thalamus. In the Hassler nomenclature, this nucleus is referred to as the ventralis oralis (Vo) and is divided into anterior and posterior segments (Voa, Vop). The ansa lenticularis conveys GPi output to the Vop, and the lenticular fasciculus conveys GPi output to the Voa. The ansa lenticularis and lenticular fasciculus (Forel's field H2) converge to form the thalamic fasciculus (Forel's field H1) prior to their input into the VA thalamus.

▸▸ Question 39

Which of the following is *not* true regarding the trisynaptic hippocampal circuit?

- A. Entorhinal cortex provides input to the dentate gyrus via the perforant path
- B. Dentate gyrus granule cells project to the CA3 region via mossy fibers

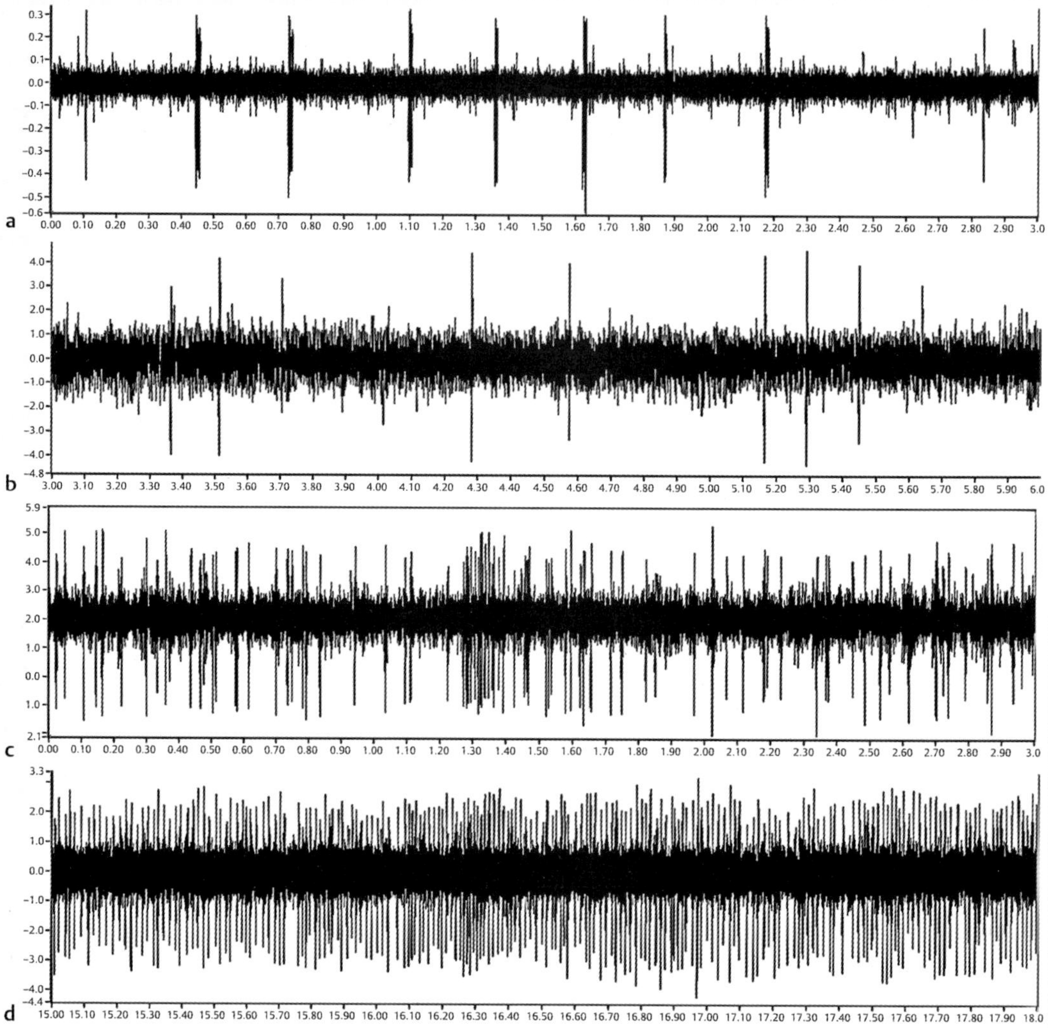

Fig. 5.14 (Source: Reproduced from Physiological target localization. In: Gross R, Boulis N, eds. Neurosurgical Operative Atlas: Functional Neurosurgery. 3rd ed. New York: Thieme; 2018.)

- C. CA3 pyramidal cells provide input to CA1 pyramidal cells
- D. CA1 pyramidal neurons project to the subiculum via Shaffer collaterals
- E. The subiculum projects fibers through the alveus and fimbria into the fornix.

Correct answer is D

The trisynaptic hippocampal circuit is a fundamental pathway involved in memory processing and spatial navigation. It begins with input from the entorhinal cortex, which projects to the dentate gyrus via the perforant path. Granule cells in the dentate gyrus then send excitatory projections, called mossy fibers, to the pyramidal cells in the CA3 region. The CA3 pyramidal cells further project to the CA1 pyramidal cells via the Schaffer collateral pathway, completing the core of the trisynaptic loop.

However, CA1 pyramidal neurons do not project to the subiculum via Schaffer collaterals, as stated in option **D**. Instead, Schaffer collaterals are the axonal projections that connect CA3 to CA1. CA1 pyramidal neurons send their output to the subiculum and entorhinal cortex, forming an essential component of the hippocampal output system. The subiculum, in turn, projects fibers through the alveus and fimbria into the fornix, which connects the hippocampus to other brain regions involved in memory and cognition.

This circuit plays a critical role in integrating and relaying information, allowing the hippocampus to function as a hub for memory formation and retrieval. Understanding the precise pathways and synaptic connections within the hippocampus is essential for grasping its role in both normal cognitive processes and pathological states such as epilepsy or Alzheimer disease.

▸▸ Question 40

A 67-year-old male with Parkinson disease underwent bilateral deep brain stimulation (DBS) targeting the subthalamic nucleus (STN). Which of the following is *not* a putative therapeutic mechanism?

- A. Antidromic stimulation of axons of the hyperdirect pathway, whose cell bodies are in the motor cortex
- B. Local suppression of STN neuronal activity
- C. Reduction of pathological synchronized oscillatory activity within the basal ganglia and motor cortex in the gamma range
- D. Concomitant stimulation of neighboring pallidofugal fibers
- E. Downstream reduction in GABAergic output from the GPi to the ventral anterior thalamus

Correct answer is C

DBS of the STN is a well-established treatment for Parkinson disease, primarily alleviating motor symptoms by modulating abnormal neuronal activity within the basal ganglia circuitry. The therapeutic mechanisms of DBS involve multiple pathways, and understanding these is critical for optimizing its effects.

1. *Antidromic stimulation*: DBS can stimulate axons of the hyperdirect pathway, whose cell bodies reside in the motor cortex. This stimulation likely disrupts abnormal patterns of activity and reestablishes more physiologic signaling.
2. *Local suppression of STN neuronal activity*: High-frequency stimulation may suppress overactive STN neurons, mitigating their excitatory drive onto downstream structures like the globus pallidus interna (GPi).
3. *Concomitant stimulation of neighboring pallidofugal fibers*: DBS may incidentally stimulate nearby fibers of the pallidum, influencing motor pathways and contributing to its therapeutic effects.
4. *Downstream effects on GABAergic output*: DBS reduces the excessive inhibitory output from the GPi to the ventral anterior thalamus, thereby improving thalamocortical activity and restoring motor control.

The correct option, (**C**) Reduction of pathological synchronized oscillatory activity within the basal ganglia and motor cortex in the gamma range, highlights a misunderstanding of the oscillatory activity associated with Parkinson disease. Pathological synchronization in Parkinson disease is predominantly observed in the beta frequency range (13–30 Hz) rather than the gamma range (> 30 Hz). Beta oscillations are correlated with motor impairment, and their reduction is a key therapeutic effect of DBS. Gamma activity, on the other hand, is typically associated with normal motor function and may even increase as motor symptoms improve with effective DBS therapy.

▸▸ Question 41

A 70-year-old woman with Parkinson disease is being evaluated for DBS. Which of the following symptoms is least likely to improve with DBS of the subthalamic nucleus?

- A. Tremor
- B. Bradykinesia
- C. Rigidity
- D. Postural instability
- E. Dyskinesias

Correct answer is D

Postural instability is often less responsive to DBS of the subthalamic nucleus compared with other symptoms such as resting tremor, bradykinesia, and rigidity, and may require additional therapeutic approaches.[24]

▸▸ Question 42

A 27-year-old female with drug-resistant epilepsy undergoes a presurgical evaluation. She is found to have a cavernous malformation in the right temporal pole, with concordant video EEG evaluation. You perform a craniotomy and "lesionectomy" with resection of the cavernous malformation and hemosiderin-laden tissue immediately around the malformation. Before surgery, the patient experienced weekly seizures consisting of a foul smell, a sensation of epigastric rising, impaired awareness, and ipsilateral automatisms. Historically, before medical optimization, she would experience progression to generalized tonic-clonic seizures. After surgery, the patient experienced an initial 3 months of seizure freedom. However, now she experiences episodes every 2 to 3 months. They consist of a foul smell of burnt rubber that lasts for tends of seconds, without any further progression. She maintains awareness during these episodes. She takes her antiseizure medication as prescribed. What is the Engel classification of her surgical outcome?

- A. Engel Class I
- B. Engel Class II
- C. Engel Class III
- D. Engel Class IV
- E. Not classifiable

Correct answer is A

The Engel classification is a standardized system for assessing outcomes after epilepsy surgery, focusing on seizure frequency and severity. The classification ranges from Engel Class I, representing excellent seizure control, to Engel Class IV, indicating minimal or no benefit from surgery.

In this case, the patient's outcome aligns with **Engel Class I**, which includes patients who achieve freedom from disabling seizures. This classification encompasses the following subcategories:

- **Class IA:** Completely seizure-free, including auras, for at least 2 years postoperatively.
- **Class IB:** Free from disabling seizures but may experience occasional auras.
- **Class IC:** No disabling seizures but auras occur only in the first 2 years after surgery.
- **Class ID:** No disabling seizures but nocturnal seizures may occur.

This patient's episodes of a foul smell lasting seconds without further progression are classified as auras, which are not considered "disabling seizures." Her overall reduction in seizure frequency and absence of progression to generalized tonic-clonic seizures following surgery fulfill the criteria for Engel Class I, specifically Class IB due to the presence of occasional auras.

The surgical outcome demonstrates significant improvement, reflecting the efficacy of lesionectomy in cases where seizure foci are associated with structural lesions such as cavernous malformations.

▸▸ Question 43

One potential anatomical site of neuromodulatory intervention for drug-resistant epilepsy is the anterior nucleus of the thalamus (ANT). Which of the following is *true* regarding the connectivity of this nucleus?

- A. The mammillothalamic tract contains efferent projections from the ANT to the hypothalamus
- B. The ANT preferentially has connectivity with the orbitofrontal cortex and cingulate cortex
- C. The ANT preferentially has connectivity with the sensorimotor cortex
- D. The ANT has robust direct projections to the anterior temporal neocortex
- E. The ANT receives its primary direct input via the fornix.

Correct answer is B

The ANT is a key structure in the limbic system, with critical roles in memory, emotional processing, and seizure modulation. The ANT is a common target for neuromodulatory interventions, such as deep brain stimulation, in drug-resistant epilepsy.

1. Connectivity with the limbic system:
    - The ANT is heavily interconnected with the orbitofrontal cortex and cingulate cortex, regions associated with emotional regulation and decision-making. These connections are integral to its role in modulating seizures and limbic network activity.
    - It also has reciprocal connections with the hippocampal formation, mediated via the mammillothalamic tract, which conveys input from the mammillary bodies of the hypothalamus to the ANT.
2. Input and output pathways:
    - The mammillothalamic tract provides primary input to the ANT from the mammillary bodies.
    - The ANT projects efferent fibers to the cingulate gyrus, forming part of the Pape

circuit, a neural loop involved in emotion and memory processing.

3. Misconceptions clarified:
   - The mammillothalamic tract does not carry efferent projections from the ANT to the hypothalamus but rather afferent input to the ANT.
   - The ANT is not primarily connected to the sensorimotor cortex or anterior temporal neocortex; its connectivity is predominantly within the limbic system.
   - While the fornix carries critical information between the hippocampus and other brain regions, it does not serve as the primary direct input to the ANT.

These connections highlight the ANT's central role in the limbic network, supporting its use as a neuromodulation target in epilepsy management. This deep understanding of its connectivity is vital for optimizing interventions and predicting outcomes in neuromodulatory therapies.

▸▸ Question 44

Which of the following statements regarding focal cortical dysplasia (FCD) as a cause of drug-resistant epilepsy is *false*?

- A. Focal cortical dysplasia is the leading pathological finding in pediatric patients who undergo resection for drug-resistant epilepsy
- B. FCD type 2 often has highly focal decreased FDG uptake on interictal PET
- C. FCD type 2B is often preferentially located at the bottom of a sulcus, as opposed to the crown of the gyrus.
- D. Patients who undergo surgery for resection of FCD type 2A have a greater chance of seizure freedom than patients who undergo resection of FCD type 2B.
- E. FCD type 2B contains both dysmorphic neurons and large cells with pale eosinophilic cytoplasm known as balloon cells

Correct answer is D

FCD is the leading pathological diagnosis in pediatric patients undergoing resective surgery for drug-resistant epilepsy. It is also a significant finding in adult epilepsy cases, though less common. FCD Type 2 (especially Type 2B) is associated with characteristic imaging features, such as blurring of the gray–white matter junction and the "transmantle sign" on MRI. On interictal PET, FCD Type 2 often demonstrates highly focal areas of decreased FDG uptake, aiding in localization. FCD Type 2B is distinguished by the presence of dysmorphic neurons and balloon cells. Balloon cells are large cells with pale eosinophilic cytoplasm, a hallmark feature of this subtype. Patients with FCD Type 2B generally have a better chance of achieving seizure freedom following surgical resection compared to patients with FCD Type 2A. This improved outcome is due to the more localized and well-demarcated nature of FCD Type 2B lesions, making complete resection more achievable.

Key features and surgical considerations for FCD types are outlined below:

FCD type	Features
FCD Type 1	• Histology: Mild abnormalities in cortical lamination and neuronal organization without dysmorphic neurons or balloon cells • Imaging: Subtle findings, often with normal MRI. May show mild cortical thickening • Location: Found in any cortical region • Surgical Outcome: Variable, generally less favorable compared to FCD Type 2
FCD Type 2A	• Histology: Presence of dysmorphic neurons but no balloon cells • Imaging: Blurring of the gray–white matter junction, but transmantle sign is less common • Location: Any cortical region, but less commonly at the bottom of a sulcus • Surgical outcome: Seizure outcomes are better than FCD Type 1 but less favorable than FCD Type 2B
FCD Type 2B	• Histology: Dysmorphic neurons and balloon cells, which are large cells with pale eosinophilic cytoplasm • Imaging: Blurring of the gray–white matter junction with a transmantle sign (T2 hyperintensity extending to the ventricle) • Location: Often preferentially ocated at the bottom of a sulcus • Surgical outcome: High likelihood of seizure freedom with complete resection

▸▸ Question 45

A 28-year-old woman with medically refractory epilepsy undergoes a preoperative workup that localizes her seizure focus to the left mesial temporal lobe. The patient would like to pursue the surgery, which offers her the greatest chance of complete seizure freedom (on medication) at 1-year follow-up postoperatively. Which would be the most appropriate recommendation?

- A. Vagus nerve stimulation
- B. Stereotactic laser amygdalohippocampotomy
- C. Anterior temporal lobectomy
- D. Responsive neurostimulation (RNS) targeting the left hippocampus and amygdala
- E. Selective amygdalohippocampectomy (SAH)

Correct answer is C

Anterior temporal lobectomy is the most effective surgical intervention for patients with medically refractory epilepsy localized to the mesial temporal lobe. This procedure has a high success rate in achieving seizure freedom.

▸▸ Question 46

During resection of a vestibular schwannoma, the neurophysiology specialist reports a clinically significant alteration in the brainstem auditory evoked response (BAER). Maintenance of wave I and other waveform is *mostly* correlated with postoperative hearing preservation? Which is the anatomical generator of this waveform?

- A. Wave III, cochlear nucleus
- B. Wave III, superior olivary complex
- C. Wave V, lateral lemniscus
- D. Wave V, inferior colliculus
- E. Wave VII, acoustic radiation

Correct answer is D

Preservation of Wave I and wave V is most strongly correlated with postoperative hearing preservation. Wave I of the BAER is generated by the compound action potential of the vestibulocochlear nerve. Wave V of the BAER is primarily generated by the inferior colliculus. BAERs are used to assess the integrity of the auditory pathways from the ear to the brainstem (▸ Fig. 5.14 and ▸ Table 5.4).[25]

▸▸ Question 47

A 62-year-old male was referred to a neurologist for a hyperkinetic movement disorder. He has constant, wide-amplitude, and violent involuntary movement involving primarily the proximal left upper extremity. What is the most likely underlying etiology of the patient's condition?

- A. Lesion of the subthalamic nucleus
- B. Degeneration of the substantia nigra pars compacta
- C. Pathological oscillatory activity in the cerebello-thalamo-cortical network
- D. Autoimmune inflammation with detectable antiphospholipid antibodies
- E. Loss of GABAergic medium spiny neurons in the neostriatum

Correct answer is A

Hemiballismus is characterized by involuntary, violent, flinging movements of the limbs, typically caused by a lesion in the subthalamic nucleus. This region is crucial for regulating motor activity, and its dysfunction leads to disinhibition of motor pathways. Parkinson disease is caused by degeneration of the substantial nigra pars compacta. Dysfunction of the cerebellar motor network is

Table 5.4 BAER waveform generators and clinical significance

BAER wave	Generator	Clinical significance
Wave I	Auditory nerve (distal)	Assessing peripheral hearing function
Wave II	Auditory nerve (proximal)	Identifying nerve lesions or damage
Wave III	Cochlear nucleus	Evaluating brainstem function
Wave IV	Superior olivary complex	Assessing midbrain auditory pathways
Wave V	Inferior colliculus	Monitoring the integrity of the central auditory pathway

Source: Citow J, Macdonald R, Refai D, eds. Comprehensive Neurosurgery Board Review. 2nd ed. New York: Thieme; 2009.

responsible for postural tremor in essential tremor patients. Antiphospholipid antibody syndrome may present with chorea, a hyperkinetic movement disorder. Huntington disease is typically a genetic condition resulting in trinucleotide repeat expansion and neuronal loss in the striatum and chorea.

▸▸ Question 48

Which of the following is *not* a listed indication for intrathecal drug delivery in chronic pain by the Polyanalgesic Consensus Conference?

- A. Cancer-related pain
- B. Complex regional pain syndrome
- C. Severe fibromyalgia
- D. Failed back surgery syndrome
- E. Intractable post-herpetic neuralgia

Correct answer is B

Intrathecal drug delivery systems provide a targeted approach for managing severe, chronic pain conditions that are refractory to conventional therapies. Indications for this treatment, as outlined by the Polyanalgesic Consensus Conference, include:

- Cancer-related pain
- Failed back surgery syndrome
- Intractable post-herpetic neuralgia
- Chronic pancreatitis pain
- Complex regional pain syndrome type II (with confirmed nerve injury)

These systems deliver medication directly to the spinal cord, offering improved pain control while minimizing systemic side effects. While there are reports of intrathecal therapy being utilized for fibromyalgia in select cases, it is not a standard or widely accepted indication within current guidelines due to the condition's diffuse nature and differing pathophysiology. Thus, "severe fibromyalgia" is not officially listed as an indication by the Polyanalgesic Consensus Conference, making it the correct answer.

Intrathecal therapy should be reserved for carefully selected patients whose pain severely impacts their quality of life and who have not responded to more conservative measures. Proper patient selection and adherence to evidence-based indications are critical for optimizing outcomes.[26]

▸▸ Question 49

A 57-year-old man has severe, intractable left lower extremity pain from an osseous sarcoma. You plan to perform a percutaneous radiofrequency cordotomy guided by intraoperative CT myelography. Which of the following statements about this procedure is *true*?

- A. Because the patient has only lower extremity pain, the procedure should be performed at the T10 segmental level
- B. The ablation probe should be positioned anterior to the dentate ligament to avoid damaging fibers of the lateral corticospinal tract
- C. The ablation procedure targets the left (ipsilateral) sensory fibers of the dorsal column
- D. The ablation procedure targets the left (ipsilateral) sensory fibers of the spinothalamic tract
- E. Central hyperventilation is a known risk of unilateral cordotomy

Correct answer is B

Percutaneous radiofrequency cordotomy is a neurosurgical procedure performed to relieve unilateral, severe, and refractory pain (often cancer-related) by selectively ablating fibers of the spinothalamic tract, which transmit pain and temperature sensations.

The correct answer (**B**) emphasizes the necessity of positioning the ablation probe anterior to the dentate ligament, which safely targets the contralateral spinothalamic tract located in the anterolateral quadrant of the spinal cord. This approach avoids injury to the lateral corticospinal tract, situated dorsolaterally, which mediates voluntary motor function. Incorrect placement posterior to the dentate ligament risks motor deficits due to damage to these motor fibers. (**A**) For lower extremity pain relief, the cordotomy should typically be performed at the upper cervical spinal segments (usually C1–C2), because the spinothalamic tract fibers are well localized there. (**C** and **D**) Cordotomy targets the contralateral spinothalamic tract (pain/temperature), not ipsilateral fibers or dorsal column fibers, which carry fine touch and proprioception. (**E**) Central hypoventilation syndrome (Ondine's curse) is associated primarily with bilateral cordotomy due to the disruption of autonomic respiratory pathways, not unilateral procedures.

Thus, precise anatomical targeting is critical in cordotomy to achieve effective pain relief while avoiding inadvertent damage to the lateral corticospinal tract.

▸▸ Question 50

Which of the following is the mostly likely primary mechanism by which spinal cord stimulation (SCS) alleviates chronic pain?
- A. Inhibition of pain transmission in the dorsal horn
- B. Direct stimulation of the pain pathways
- C. Activation of descending inhibitory pathways
- D. Modulation of cortical pain perception
- E. Stimulation of peripheral nerves

Correct answer is A

SCS alleviates chronic pain primarily by inhibiting pain transmission within the dorsal horn of the spinal cord, a mechanism grounded in Melzack and Wall's Gate Control Theory of Pain. This theory posits that nonpainful stimuli can "close the gate" to painful signals, preventing them from reaching the brain. SCS achieves this by directly stimulating dorsal horn interneurons, such as islet cells, which release inhibitory neurotransmitters such as GABA, effectively dampening nociceptive signal transmission. Additionally, SCS may engage the descending antinociceptive system, a network of pathways that suppress pain by amplifying inhibitory signals, further contributing to its pain-relieving effects. Neuroimaging studies have also revealed cortical and thalamic changes in patients undergoing SCS; however, the precise causal relationship between these changes and therapeutic outcomes remains uncertain. These mechanisms collectively highlight the multifaceted approach of SCS in modulating pain, emphasizing both local spinal and broader central nervous system effects.[27]

▸▸ Question 51

You are performing deep brain stimulation (DBS) surgery targeting the ventral intermediate nucleus for a patient with essential tremor. Intraoperative test stimulation results in significant tremor suppression of the contralateral upper extremity at a threshold of 1.5 mA. At a threshold of 4 mA, the patient has persistent contralateral paresthesia of the upper extremity and face. There is no dysarthria or capsular effects related to stimulation up to 4 mA. You deem this a satisfactory location for the DBS lead. Which of the following is *true* regarding the sensorimotor thalamus?
- A. The external segment of the ventral caudalis nucleus (Vc) contains the somatotopic representation of the contralateral face
- B. The ventral intermediate nucleus (Vim) has more robust connectivity with premotor cortex than primary motor cortex
- C. Placement of the DBS lead at a Y coordinate 15% of the AC-PC distance anterior to the posterior commissure will typically result in good tremor suppression without stimulation-related adverse effects
- D. The ventral oralis nucleus (Vo) projects to the primary sensory cortex
- E. Placement of the DBS lead at an X coordinate 11 mm lateral to the wall of the third ventricle will typically target representation of the contralateral upper extremity and result in good tremor suppression

Correct answer is E

The sensorimotor thalamus, including the ventral intermediate nucleus (Vim), is a critical target for DBS in patients with essential tremor. The Vim lies within a region often referred to as the quadrilateral nucleus complex, which also includes the ventral caudal nucleus (Vc), ventral oralis posterior (Vop), and ventral oralis anterior (Voa). Accurate placement within the Vim can result in effective tremor suppression with minimal side effects.

Answer **E** is correct because placement of the DBS lead approximately 11 mm lateral to the third ventricle wall targets the contralateral upper extremity representation within the Vim, leading to good tremor suppression (▸ Table 5.5).

▸▸ Question 52

You are performing deep brain stimulation (DBS) surgery targeting the globus pallidus pars interna for the treatment of primary dystonia. You have placed the DBS lead and performed intraoperative test stimulation. The patient describes luminescent purple orbs in her visual field. Stimulation of which structure is most likely responsible?
- A. Optic nerve
- B. Optic chiasm

Table 5.5 Quadrilateral sensorimotor thalamus

Nucleus	Key connections	Function/Role	Clinical relevance
Ventral intermediate nucleus (Vim)	Connected to primary motor cortex and cerebellum via the dentato-rubro-thalamic tract	Suppresses tremor effectively at low DBS stimulation thresholds	Targeted for tremor control; incorrect placement risks sensory or capsular side effects
Ventral caudal nucleus (Vc)	Contains somatotopic sensory representations (e.g., contralateral face medial)	Processes sensory information	Incorrect DBS placement here can result in sensory paresthesia
Ventral oralis posterior and anterior nuclei (Vop, Voa)	Project to premotor and supplementary motor areas	Involved in motor planning and coordination rather than tremor suppression	Not ideal for tremor suppression; targeting these areas may lead to ineffective tremor management

- C. Optic tract
- D. Lateral geniculate nucleus
- E. Fibers of the optic radiation

Correct answer is C

During DBS procedures targeting structures such as the globus pallidus pars interna, unintended stimulation of adjacent neural pathways can lead to various sensory phenomena. In this case, the patient experiences phosphenes, which are the perception of light without any actual light entering the eye. Phosphenes often manifest as luminescent orbs, flashes, or streaks in the visual field and are typically induced by stimulation of the visual pathways.

The optic tract is the most likely structure responsible for eliciting phosphenes during DBS. The optic tract carries visual information from the optic chiasm to the lateral geniculate nucleus of the thalamus. Its proximity to the globus pallidus pars interna means that electrical stimulation intended for the pallidal region can inadvertently activate the optic tract fibers, resulting in the perception of phosphenes.

▸▸ Question 53

You are performing deep brain stimulation (DBS) surgery for a patient with Parkinson disease. The target is the subthalamic nucleus (STN). You are performing awake intraoperative microelectrode recording. When making your stereotactic trajectory, you place the target at the bottom of the STN at its junction with the substantia nigra pars reticulata. At a distance of 10 mm above the target depth, you encounter neuronal single-unit spiking activity, which is sparse and highly distinct from background activity. Passive limb movement does not drive this spiking activity. Which is the most likely location of the tip of the microelectrode?

- A. Subthalamic nucleus
- B. Thalamic reticular nucleus
- C. Zona incerta
- D. Ventral intermediate thalamus
- E. White matter

Correct answer is B

Accurate electrode placement during DBS for Parkinson disease is essential for optimal therapeutic outcomes. The thalamic reticular nucleus (TRN) is situated just dorsal to the STN and is characterized by sparse, highly distinct neuronal spiking that remains uninfluenced by passive limb movements, as described in this scenario. In contrast, the STN typically exhibits more robust and motor-responsive neuronal activity. Recognizing the electrophysiological signatures of surrounding structures, such as the TRN, is crucial to avoid misplacement. The zona incerta lies further dorsally and has different spiking patterns, while the ventral intermediate thalamus is usually targeted for essential tremor rather than Parkinson disease. Understanding these distinctions ensures precise targeting of the STN, thereby enhancing the efficacy of DBS therapy and minimizing potential side effects.

▸▸ Question 54

A 32-year-old male is being evaluated for drug-resistant epilepsy. Video EEG confirms right lateralized interictal and ictal activity. Clinically, the patient describes a sensation in his throat and coughing prior to loss of awareness. On video EEG, the first clinical sign you see is clonic jerking movements involving the left lower face. MRI and PET are normal. You formulate a hypothesis primarily involving the right frontal operculum. You recommend stereoelectroencephalography (stereo-EEG) in order to map the epileptogenic zone. Which of the following is *not* a potential reason to choose stereo-EEG over craniotomy with subdural grid implantation when evaluating a patient for long-term intracranial seizure monitoring?

- A. Stereo-EEG can better sample regions of the brain, including the depth of sulci, the operculum and insula, the mesial temporal lobe, and other midline structures than subdural grid placement
- B. The composite rate of surgical complications is less with stereo-EEG than with craniotomy for subdural grid placement in contemporary usage
- C. Bilateral investigations can be performed with stereo-EEG when indicated
- D. Placement of multiple depth electrodes for stereo-EEG has higher spatial sampling resolution and therefore allows for better functional brain mapping including, for example, language function
- E. Stereo-EEG is minimally invasive and has a better short-term recovery

Correct answer is D

Stereo-EEG is favored over subdural grid implantation for several reasons, including its ability to sample deep brain structures like the insula and mesial temporal lobe, lower surgical complication rates, the capability for bilateral monitoring, and its minimally invasive nature, leading to quicker recovery times. However, option **D** is *not* a valid reason because while stereo-EEG provides excellent access to deep and medial structures, subdural grids offer superior spatial resolution for surface areas of the brain, which is essential for detailed functional mapping such as language areas. Functional brain mapping for cortical functions is typically better achieved with subdural grids rather than stereo-EEG, making option **D** the correct answer.[28]

▸▸ Question 55

A 65-year-old woman is at your clinic for a second opinion regarding surgical management of her facial pain. Ten years ago, she developed symptoms of classical trigeminal neuralgia, including shock-like pain in the mandibular distribution of her right trigeminal nerve, which was paroxysmal and had cutaneous triggers. She initially responded to carbamazepine, but later required escalating doses without relief. She underwent multiple percutaneous radiofrequency rhizotomies at an outside healthcare system. Today, she reports that she is completely numb on the right side of her lower face. On exam, she is unable to identify light touch to the right V2 and V3 distributions on exam with her eyes closed. Despite this, she has severe burning pain in the same distribution, which is constant and debilitating. Which of the following surgical options do you recommend for the patient?

- A. Microvascular decompression
- B. Percutaneous gangliolysis by mechanical balloon compression
- C. Gamma Knife targeting the cisternal segment of the trigeminal nerve
- D. Peripheral trigeminal nerve stimulation
- E. Motor cortex stimulation

Correct answer is E

This patient presents with atypical trigeminal neuralgia characterized by constant burning pain despite previous surgical interventions that resulted in facial numbness. Traditional surgical options such as microvascular decompression or percutaneous rhizotomies may be less effective in cases where pain becomes constant and neuropathic. Motor cortex stimulation is indicated for refractory trigeminal pain, especially when peripheral treatments have failed, as it modulates central pain pathways to provide relief. This approach is suitable for patients who have exhausted other surgical options and continue to experience debilitating pain. Understanding the transition from peripheral to central neuromodulation therapies is crucial for managing complex cases of trigeminal neuralgia effectively.

▸▸ Question 56

A 46-year-old woman with severe spasticity related to multiple sclerosis underwent placement of an intrathecal pump for baclofen drug delivery 4 years ago. Her current dose is 300 µg/day. She presented to the emergency room with increasing spasticity, itching, fever, tachycardia, and delirium. Her surgical sites appear well healed without signs of infection. You interrogate the pump, and there are no alarms or concerning findings. Which is the appropriate medical therapy to administer next?

- A. Enteral baclofen
- B. Benzodiazepines
- C. Cyproheptadine
- D. Dantrolene
- E. A, B, and C

Correct answer is E

The patient's symptoms suggest baclofen withdrawal, a potentially life-threatening condition often resulting from pump malfunction or discontinuation. Baclofen withdrawal can present with increased spasticity, autonomic instability (fever, tachycardia), and neurological symptoms (delirium). Immediate management includes reinstating baclofen therapy, which can be achieved through enteral administration if the intrathecal pump is compromised. Additionally, benzodiazepines and cyproheptadine may be used to manage spasticity and autonomic symptoms. Monitoring creatine kinase levels is important to assess for rhabdomyolysis, and if medical therapy is insufficient, surgical exploration of the pump may be necessary.

▸▸ Question 57

A 68-year-old woman presents with left facial pain. She describes sharp pain radiating from the front of the left ear to below the left eye and to the upper lip. The pain is episodic, lasting seconds. The pain is triggered by a light touch to the face or a breeze on the face when the patient goes outside. There is no contralateral pain, no cervical pain, and no other headaches. The patient initially had improvement with oxcarbazepine, but now her pain is progressing in severity and frequency despite medical therapy. The patient expresses a strong desire to be pain-free. She underwent high-resolution MRI of the skull base (including MR cisternography), and there was no clear evidence of an artery impinging on the left trigeminal nerve over its intradural course. What is the most appropriate recommendation?

- A. No surgical treatment is recommended
- B. Microvascular decompression
- C. Percutaneous radiofrequency rhizotomy
- D. Stereotactic radiosurgery
- E. Trigeminal nerve stimulation

Correct answer is B

In cases of Type 1 trigeminal neuralgia, characterized by sharp, episodic facial pain triggered by stimuli like light touch or breeze, medical therapy with anticonvulsants such as oxcarbazepine is first-line. However, when pain becomes refractory to medication, surgical options are considered. Microvascular decompression (option **B**) is the preferred surgical treatment even if MRI does not show a clear neurovascular conflict, as it addresses the underlying nerve compression and offers the best chance for long-term pain relief. Other surgical interventions, such as radiofrequency rhizotomy or stereotactic radiosurgery, may be considered based on patient-specific factors, but microvascular decompression remains the most appropriate recommendation for patients desiring definitive pain relief.

▸▸ Question 58

You are evaluating a patient for deep brain stimulation (DBS) for Parkinson disease. When the patient takes levodopa-carbidopa 25/100 mg, he develops severe dyskinesia. Which of the following statements regarding target selection is *true*?

- A. Bilateral GPi stimulation is the best target choice since it will allow for a reduction in the total daily levodopa dosage required by the patient
- B. Bilateral GPi DBS typically results in a greater short-term cognitive decline compared to subthalamic nucleus (STN) stimulation
- C. STN DBS is superior to GPi DBS in improvement in UPDRS score and quality-of-life metrics
- D. Bilateral STN DBS has a high probability of resulting in severe dyskinesias at low stimulation amplitudes
- E. Bilateral STN DBS is a favored stimulation target since there is a lower incidence of depression compared to GPi stimulation

Correct answer is D

DBS for Parkinson disease commonly targets the STN or GPi. STN DBS is effective in improving motor symptoms and allows for significant reductions in levodopa dosage, but it can increase the risk of dyskinesias, particularly if stimulation settings are not carefully managed. In contrast, GPi DBS is associated with better control of dyskinesias and tends to have a lower risk of inducing severe involuntary movements. Therefore, in patients who develop severe dyskinesias, such as the one described, bilateral STN DBS may exacerbate these symptoms at low stimulation amplitudes, making option **D** the correct statement.

References

[1] Okon II, Menon SS, Osama M, et al. Microvascular decompression: a contemporary update. BMC Surg 2025;25(1):20

[2] Yoon KB, Wiles JR, Miles JB, Nurmikko TJ. Long-term outcome of percutaneous thermocoagulation for trigeminal neuralgia. Anaesthesia 1999;54(8):803–808

[3] Manchikanti L, Cash KA, McManus CD, Damron KS, Pampati V, Falco FJ. A randomized, double-blind controlled trial of lumbar interlaminar epidural injections in central spinal stenosis: 2-year follow-up. Pain Physician 2015;18(1):79–92

[4] Barr JD, Barr MS, Lemley TJ, et al. Percutaneous vertebroplasty for pain relief and spinal stabilization. Spine (Phila Pa 1976) 2000;25(8):923–928

[5] Chen J, Sindou M. Vago-glossopharyngeal neuralgia: a literature review of neurosurgical experience. Acta Neurochir (Wien) 2015;157(2):311–321

[6] Régis J, Tuleasca C, Resseguier N, et al. Long-term safety and efficacy of Gamma Knife surgery in classical trigeminal neuralgia: a 497-patient historical cohort study. J Neurosurg 2016;124(4):1079–1087

[7] Weaver FM, Follett K, Stern M, et al; CSP 468 Study Group. Bilateral deep brain stimulation vs best medical therapy for patients with advanced Parkinson disease: a randomized controlled trial. JAMA 2009;301(1):63–73

[8] Wiebe S, Blume WT, Girvin JP, Eliasziw M; Effectiveness and Efficiency of Surgery for Temporal Lobe Epilepsy Study Group. A randomized, controlled trial of surgery for temporal-lobe epilepsy. N Engl J Med 2001;345(5):311–318

[9] Sheth SA, Neal J, Tangherlini F, et al. Limbic system surgery for treatment-refractory obsessive-compulsive disorder: a prospective long-term follow-up of 64 patients. J Neurosurg 2013;118(3):491–497

[10] Deuschl G, Bain P, Brin M. Consensus statement of the Movement Disorder Society on Tremor. Ad Hoc Scientific Committee. Mov Disord 1998;13(Suppl 3):2–23

[11] Krack P, Batir A, Van Blercom N, et al. Five-year follow-up of bilateral stimulation of the subthalamic nucleus in advanced Parkinson's disease. N Engl J Med 2003;349 (20):1925–1934

[12] Moro E, Esselink RJ, Xie J, Hommel M, Benabid AL, Pollak P. The impact on Parkinson's disease of electrical parameter settings in STN stimulation. Neurology 2002;59(5):706–713

[13] Larsh T, Wu SW, Vadivelu S, Grant GA, O'Malley JA. Deep brain stimulation for pediatric dystonia. Semin Pediatr Neurol 2021;38:100896

[14] Lozano AM, Kumar R, Gross RE, et al. Globus pallidus internus pallidotomy for generalized dystonia. Mov Disord 1997;12(6):865–870

[15] Mohammed N, Patra D, Nanda A. A meta-analysis of outcomes and complications of magnetic resonance-guided focused ultrasound in the treatment of essential tremor. Neurosurg Focus 2018;44(2):E4 [Erratum in: Neurosurg Focus. 2018;45(1):E16]

[16] Volkmann J, Moro E, Pahwa R. Basic algorithms for the programming of deep brain stimulation in Parkinson's disease. Mov Disord 2006;21(Suppl 14):S284–289

[17] Schuurman PR, Bosch DA, Bossuyt PM, et al. A comparison of continuous thalamic stimulation and thalamotomy for suppression of severe tremor. N Engl J Med 2000;342 (7):461–468

[18] Blümcke I, Pauli E, Clusmann H, et al. A new clinico-pathological classification system for mesial temporal sclerosis. Acta Neuropathol 2007;113(3):235–244

[19] Ben-Menachem E, Mañon-Espaillat R, Ristanovic R, et al. Vagus nerve stimulation for treatment of partial seizures: 1. A controlled study of effect on seizures. First International Vagus Nerve Stimulation Study Group. Epilepsia 1994;35 (3):616–626

[20] Albin RL, Young AB, Penney JB. The functional anatomy of basal ganglia disorders. Trends Neurosci 1989;12(10):366–375

[21] Benabid AL, Pollak P, Gao D, et al. Chronic electrical stimulation of the ventralis intermedius nucleus of the thalamus as a treatment of movement disorders. J Neurosurg 1996;84(2):203–214

[22] Hutchison WD, Allan RJ, Opitz H, et al. Neurophysiological identification of the subthalamic nucleus in surgery for Parkinson's disease. Ann Neurol 1998;44(4):622–628

[23] Temel Y, Kessels A, Tan S, Topdag A, Boon P, Visser-Vandewalle V. Behavioural changes after bilateral subthalamic stimulation in advanced Parkinson disease: a systematic review. Parkinsonism Relat Disord 2006;12 (5):265–272

[24] Limousin P, Krack P, Pollak P, et al. Electrical stimulation of the subthalamic nucleus in advanced Parkinson's disease. N Engl J Med 1998;339(16):1105–1111

[25] Oh T, Nagasawa DT, Fong BM, et al. Intraoperative neuromonitoring techniques in the surgical management of acoustic neuromas. Neurosurg Focus 2012;33(3):E6

[26] Deer TR, Pope JE, Hayek SM, et al. The Polyanalgesic Consensus Conference (PACC): recommendations for intrathecal drug delivery: guidance for improving safety and mitigating risks. Neuromodulation 2017;20 (2):155–176

[27] Melzack R, Wall PD. Pain mechanisms: a new theory. Science 1965;150(3699):971–979

[28] Katz JS, Abel TJ. Stereoelectroencephalography versus subdural electrodes for localization of the epileptogenic zone: What is the evidence? Neurotherapeutics 2019;16 (1):59–66

6 Trauma and Critical Care

Syed I. Khalid, Aladine Elsamadicy, Faten El Ammar, Mariyam Humayun, Jared M. Davis, Ciro Ramos-Estebanez

▸▸ Question 1

A 68-year-old female with a history of chronic kidney disease presents with nausea, headache, and confusion. Her serum sodium is 118 mEq/L, serum osmolality is 260 mOsm/kg, and urine osmolality is 550 mOsm/kg. She is euvolemic on examination. Which condition is most likely responsible for her hyponatremia?

- A. Diabetes insipidus
- B. Cerebral salt wasting
- C. Syndrome of inappropriate antidiuretic hormone secretion (SIADH)
- D. Hyperglycemia
- E. Pseudohyponatremia

Correct answer is C

SIADH is characterized by the inappropriate secretion of antidiuretic hormone, resulting in water retention and dilutional hyponatremia. The high urine osmolality in the presence of low serum osmolality and hyponatremia supports the diagnosis of SIADH. SIADH is commonly associated with various conditions, including CNS disorders, malignancies, and pulmonary diseases.

Pseudohyponatremia (**E**) occurs in conditions like hyperlipidemia or hyperproteinemia, where measured serum sodium is low but serum osmolality is normal. Diabetes insipidus (**A**) leads to hypernatremia due to an inability to concentrate urine. Cerebral salt wasting (**B**) results in hypovolemic hyponatremia and is mainly distinguished from SIADH by the volume status. Hyperglycemia (**D**) can cause hyponatremia but would typically present with an elevated serum osmolality due to the osmotic effect of glucose. ▸ Fig. 6.1 shows etiologies of hyponatremia.

▸▸ Question 2

A 45-year-old woman with a history of epilepsy on chronic carbamazepine therapy presents with confusion and generalized weakness. Her serum sodium is 118 mEq/L, serum osmolality is 260 mOsm/kg, and urine osmolality is 550 mOsm/kg. What is the most likely cause of her hyponatremia?

- A. Psychogenic polydipsia
- B. Syndrome of inappropriate antidiuretic hormone secretion (SIADH)
- C. Diuretic use
- D. Hypothyroidism
- E. Cerebral salt wasting

Correct answer is B

Carbamazepine is known to induce SIADH, leading to water retention, dilutional hyponatremia, and elevated urine osmolality despite low serum osmolality. This condition is common in patients on medications such as antiepileptics, antidepressants, and certain antipsychotics.

Psychogenic polydipsia (**A**) leads to hyponatremia with low urine osmolality. Diuretic use (**C**) can cause hypovolemic hyponatremia. Hypothyroidism (**D**) can cause hyponatremia but is associated with other systemic symptoms. Cerebral salt wasting (**E**) results in hypovolemic hyponatremia and typically follows CNS injuries.

▸▸ Question 3

A 55-year-old male with a history of chronic alcohol abuse presents with weakness, tremors, and confusion. His laboratory results show a serum magnesium level of 0.6 mg/dL (normal: 1.7–2.2 mg/dL) and a serum calcium level of 7.8 mg/dL (normal: 8.5–10.2 mg/dL). Which of the following treatments is most appropriate?

- A. Oral magnesium oxide
- B. Intravenous magnesium sulfate
- C. Oral calcium carbonate
- D. Intravenous potassium chloride
- E. Oral vitamin D

Correct answer is B

Chronic alcohol abuse often leads to significant hypomagnesemia, which can cause symptoms such as weakness, tremors, and confusion. Hypomagnesemia is frequently associated with other electrolyte disturbances, such as hypocalcemia. Intravenous magnesium sulfate is the treatment of choice for symptomatic hypomagnesemia, as it rapidly corrects the magnesium deficit and alleviates symptoms.

Oral magnesium oxide (**A**) is appropriate for mild, asymptomatic cases. Oral calcium carbonate (**C**) and intravenous potassium chloride (**D**) do not

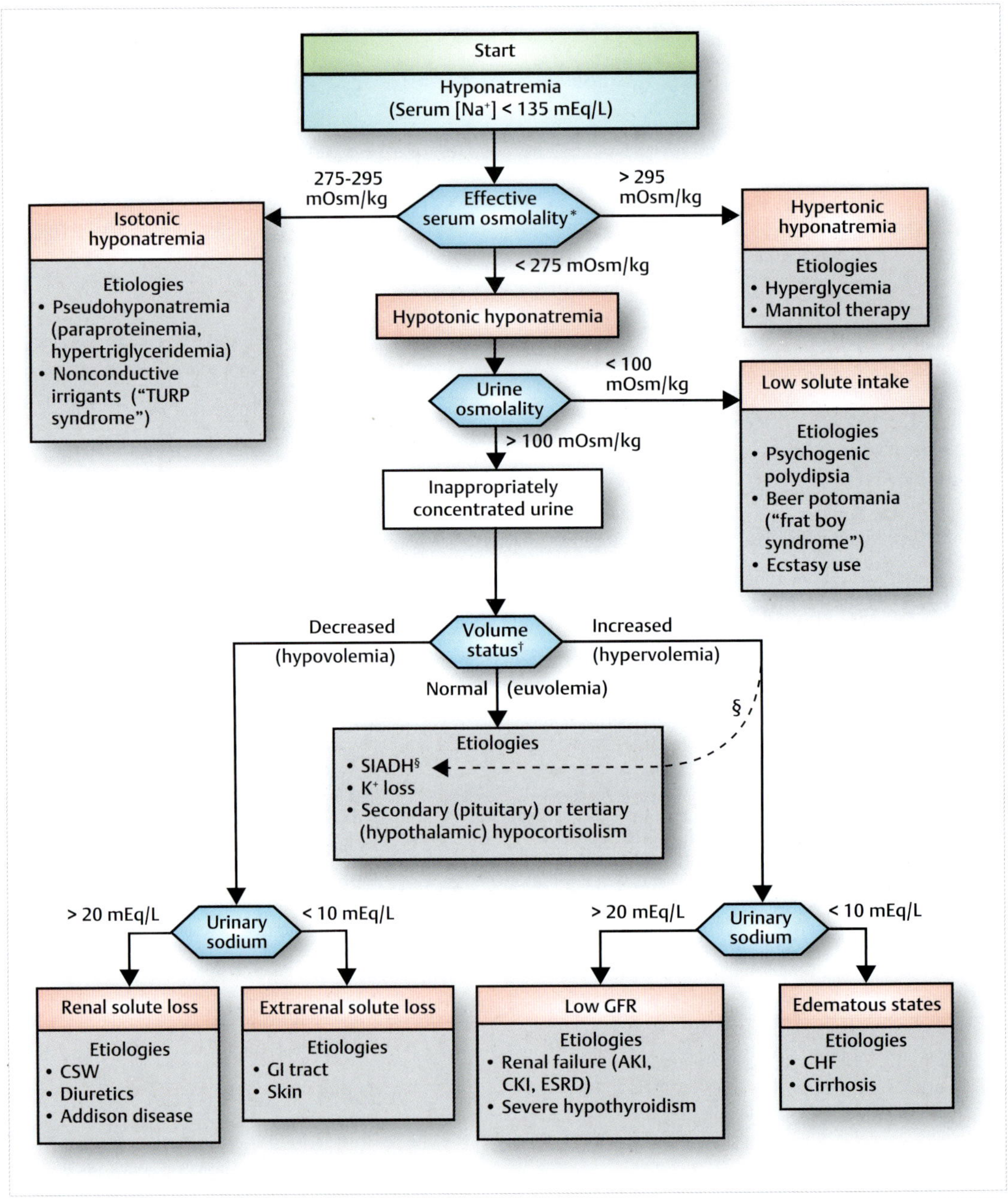

Fig. 6.1 *Effective serum osmolality = measured osmolality – [blood urea nitrogen]/2.8 (see formula in text).
†Volume status is usually assessed clinically, but this may be insensitive to volume depletion.
§SIADH may be associated with euvolemia or hypervolemia.
AKI, acute kidney injury; CHF, congestive heart failure; CKI, chronic kidney injury; CSW, cerebral salt wasting; [Na+] urine, urinary concentration of sodium; SIADH, syndrome of inappropriate antidiuretic hormone secretion.
(Source: Reproduced from Evaluation of hyponatremia. In: Greenberg M, ed. Greenberg's Handbook of Neurosurgery. 10th ed. New York: Thieme; 2023.)

address the magnesium deficiency. Oral vitamin D (**E**) is not relevant to the immediate correction of hypomagnesemia.

▸▸ Question 4

A 60-year-old male presents with hypotension, tachycardia, and cold, clammy skin. He has a history of myocardial infarction. His jugular venous pressure is elevated, and his lungs are clear on auscultation. Which of the following is the most likely type of shock?

- A. Hypovolemic shock
- B. Cardiogenic shock
- C. Septic shock
- D. Neurogenic shock
- E. Anaphylactic shock

Correct answer is B

Cardiogenic shock is characterized by inadequate cardiac output due to heart failure, often following myocardial infarction. The clinical presentation includes hypotension, tachycardia, cold and clammy skin, elevated jugular venous pressure, and clear lungs. Hypovolemic shock (**A**) presents with low jugular venous pressure and signs of fluid loss. Septic shock (**C**) typically shows warm skin due to vasodilation and is often associated with fever and signs of infection. Neurogenic shock (**D**) results from spinal cord injury and presents with hypotension and uniquely, bradycardia. Anaphylactic shock (**E**) involves a severe allergic reaction with hypotension, tachycardia, and respiratory symptoms.[1]

▸▸ Question 5

A 45-year-old female is brought to the emergency department after a motor vehicle accident. She is hypotensive, with a heart rate of 130 bpm, and has distended neck veins. There is no external bleeding. What is the most likely type of shock, and what is the initial management?

- A. Hypovolemic shock; intravenous fluids
- B. Cardiogenic shock; inotropes
- C. Neurogenic shock; vasopressors
- D. Obstructive shock; relieve the obstruction
- E. Septic shock; antibiotics

Correct answer is D

Obstructive shock is caused by physical obstruction to blood flow, such as tension pneumothorax, cardiac tamponade, or pulmonary embolism. The presence of hypotension, tachycardia, and distended neck veins without external bleeding suggests a mechanical obstruction. Initial management involves identifying and relieving the obstruction. For example, tension pneumothorax requires needle decompression, and cardiac tamponade requires pericardiocentesis.

Hypovolemic shock (**A**) would present with hypotension, tachycardia, and flat neck veins due to fluid loss. Cardiogenic shock (**B**) is managed with inotropes but is characterized by primary cardiac dysfunction. Neurogenic shock (**C**) involves hypotension and bradycardia due to spinal injury. Septic shock (**E**) requires antibiotics and presents with signs of infection and vasodilation.[2]

▸▸ Question 6

A 55-year-old woman is admitted to the intensive care unit with septic shock. Despite aggressive fluid resuscitation with 30 mL/kg, her blood pressure remains low. Which of the following is the next best step in management?

- A. Increase fluid resuscitation
- B. Administer norepinephrine
- C. Administer dopamine
- D. Administer hydrocortisone
- E. Administer broad-spectrum antibiotics

Correct answer is B

In septic shock, if hypotension persists despite adequate fluid resuscitation, the next step is to administer vasopressors, with norepinephrine being the first-line agent. Norepinephrine effectively increases vascular tone and blood pressure. Additional fluid resuscitation (**A**) may not be beneficial once adequate volume status is achieved. Dopamine (**C**) is less favored due to higher rates of arrhythmias and less predictable effects. Hydrocortisone (**D**) can be considered for refractory septic shock but is not the initial choice. Broad-spectrum antibiotics (**E**) are crucial but should already have been administered early in the treatment.[3]

▸▸ Question 7

A 67-year-old male with a history of chronic atrial fibrillation and hypertension presents with palpitations and shortness of breath. His ECG shows an irregularly irregular rhythm without distinct P waves. Which of the following is the most appropriate initial management?

- A. Immediate cardioversion
- B. Rate control with beta-blockers
- C. Rhythm control with antiarrhythmic drugs
- D. Anticoagulation therapy
- E. Implantable cardioverter-defibrillator (ICD) placement

Correct answer is B

The primary goal in the acute management of atrial fibrillation (AF) is to control the ventricular rate, which can be achieved with beta-blockers or calcium channel blockers. Immediate cardioversion (**A**) may be considered in hemodynamically unstable patients, but this patient is stable. Rhythm control (**C**) may be considered after rate control and anticoagulation have been initiated. Anticoagulation (**D**) is important for stroke prevention but is not the immediate priority. ICD placement (**E**) is not indicated for AF.

▸▸ Question 8

A 60-year-old male with a history of thyrotoxicosis presents with new-onset atrial fibrillation. What is the most appropriate initial treatment to control his heart rate?

- A. Digoxin
- B. Beta-blockers
- C. Calcium channel blockers
- D. Amiodarone
- E. Antithyroid medications

Correct answer is B

Beta-blockers are the first-line treatment for controlling heart rate in patients with atrial fibrillation associated with thyrotoxicosis. They not only control the heart rate but also mitigate the symptoms of thyrotoxicosis by blocking sympathetic activity. Digoxin (**A**) is less effective in hyperthyroid states. Calcium channel blockers (**C**) can be used but are not as effective as beta-blockers in this context. Amiodarone (**D**) is primarily used for rhythm control, and antithyroid medications (**E**) address the underlying cause but do not provide immediate rate control.

▸▸ Question 9

A 58-year-old male with a history of ischemic cardiomyopathy presents with acute decompensated heart failure. He has a blood pressure of 90/60 mm Hg, a heart rate of 110 bpm, and severe dyspnea. Which of the following is the most appropriate initial treatment?

- A. Intravenous beta-blockers
- B. Intravenous diuretics
- C. Intravenous inotropes
- D. Oral angiotensin-converting enzyme (ACE) inhibitors
- E. Oral digoxin

Correct answer is C

In patients with acute decompensated heart failure and low blood pressure, intravenous inotropes (e.g., dobutamine or milrinone) are indicated to improve cardiac output and hemodynamic stability. Intravenous diuretics (**B**) are also important to relieve congestion but should be used cautiously if hypotension is present. Beta-blockers (**A**) are generally avoided in the acute setting of decompensation due to their negative inotropic effects. Oral ACE inhibitors (**D**) and digoxin (**E**) are not immediate treatments in this scenario.

▸▸ Question 10

A 70-year-old male presents to the emergency department with sudden-onset chest pain and palpitations. His ECG shows ventricular fibrillation. What is the most appropriate immediate intervention?

- A. Administration of intravenous amiodarone
- B. Administration of intravenous lidocaine
- C. Cardiopulmonary resuscitation (CPR) and defibrillation
- D. Administration of beta-blockers
- E. Administration of intravenous magnesium sulfate

Correct answer is C

Ventricular fibrillation is a life-threatening arrhythmia that requires immediate **CPR** and defibrillation to restore a perfusing rhythm. Intravenous amiodarone (**A**) or lidocaine (**B**) may be used after defibrillation if the rhythm persists. Beta-blockers (**D**) and magnesium sulfate (**E**) are not indicated in the initial management of ventricular fibrillation.

▸▸ Question 11

A 35-year-old male presents to the emergency department after a motor vehicle accident with a Glasgow coma scale (GCS) score of 6, hypertension, and a fixed, dilated pupil on the left. What is the most likely diagnosis, and what is the immediate management?

- A. Epidural hematoma (EDH); urgent craniotomy
- B. Subdural hematoma (SDH); monitoring and observation
- C. Diffuse axonal injury; supportive care
- D. Intracerebral hemorrhage; administration of antihypertensives
- E. Skull fracture; administration of antibiotics

Correct answer is A

The presence of a fixed, dilated pupil suggests a transtentorial herniation, often caused by an EDH. This condition requires urgent surgical intervention with a craniotomy to evacuate the hematoma and relieve intracranial pressure. Subdural hematomas (**B**) typically present with a slower onset of symptoms and may require monitoring or surgery depending on the size and symptoms. Diffuse axonal injury (**C**) is managed with supportive care and monitoring. Intracerebral hemorrhage (**D**) management includes controlling blood pressure, but urgent surgery is required for EDH. Skull fractures (**E**) may require antibiotics but do not address the acute life-threatening issue in this case. ▸ Fig. 6.2 shows a coronal CT illustrating an EDH (*yellow arrowheads*) crossing the tentorium (*white arrow*), which, in addition to its biconvex shape, helps distinguish this from an SDH.

▸▸ Question 12

A 50-year-old male with a history of epilepsy is brought to the emergency department after a head injury. He is having continuous tonic-clonic seizures. What is the most appropriate initial treatment?

- A. Intravenous fosphenytoin
- B. Intravenous diazepam
- C. Oral carbamazepine
- D. Intramuscular midazolam
- E. Oral valproate

Correct answer is B

Status epilepticus, characterized by continuous or recurrent seizures without recovery between episodes, is a medical emergency requiring prompt treatment. Intravenous diazepam or lorazepam is the initial treatment of choice due to their rapid onset of action. Intravenous fosphenytoin (**A**) is used for ongoing management after initial seizure control. Oral medications (**C and E**) are not appropriate for immediate management. Intramuscular midazolam (**D**) can be used if intravenous access is not available.[4]

▸▸ Question 13

A 45-year-old male involved in a high-speed motor vehicle accident is brought to the emergency department with hypotension, bradycardia, and warm extremities. He has a complete T6 spinal cord injury. What is the most likely type of shock, and what is the primary treatment?

- A. Hypovolemic shock; intravenous fluids
- B. Cardiogenic shock; inotropes
- C. Septic shock; antibiotics
- D. Neurogenic shock; vasopressors and fluids
- E. Anaphylactic shock; epinephrine

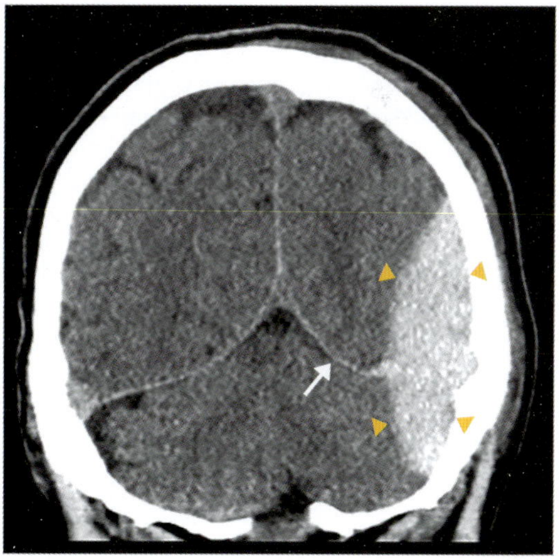

Fig. 6.2 (Source: Reproduced from CT scan in EDH. In: Greenberg M, ed. Greenberg's Handbook of Neurosurgery. 10th ed. New York: Thieme; 2023.)

Correct answer is D

Neurogenic shock occurs due to the loss of sympathetic tone following a spinal cord injury, leading to hypotension, bradycardia, and warm extremities. The primary treatment includes vasopressors to restore vascular tone, fluids to maintain adequate blood pressure, and atropine to manage bradycardia. Hypovolemic shock (**A**) would present with tachycardia and cold extremities. Cardiogenic shock (**B**) results from heart failure and is treated with inotropes. Septic shock (**C**) presents with fever and infection signs. Anaphylactic shock (**E**) involves an allergic reaction and is treated with epinephrine.[5]

▸▸ Question 14

A 25-year-old male is admitted to the ICU with multiple traumatic injuries, including a severe traumatic brain injury. Over the next few days, he develops a high urine output, low serum sodium level of 125 mEq/L, high urine osmolality, and elevated urine sodium. What is the most likely cause of his hyponatremia?

- A. Syndrome of inappropriate antidiuretic hormone (SIADH)
- B. Cerebral salt wasting
- C. Hypovolemia
- D. Renal failure
- E. Adrenal insufficiency

Correct answer is B

Cerebral salt wasting is characterized by hyponatremia, high urine osmolality, and elevated urine sodium in the context of brain injury. It is due to the renal loss of sodium leading to hypovolemia. SIADH (**A**) also presents with hyponatremia and high urine osmolality, but patients are usually euvolemic or slightly hypervolemic, not hypovolemic. Hypovolemia (**C**) alone would not cause high urine sodium. Renal failure (**D**) and adrenal insufficiency (**E**) present differently.[6]

▸▸ Question 15

A 72-year-old female with atrial fibrillation is started on dabigatran for stroke prevention. She presents to the emergency department with severe gastrointestinal bleeding. What is the most appropriate reversal agent?

- A. Fresh frozen plasma (FFP)
- B. Vitamin K
- C. Prothrombin complex concentrate (PCC)
- D. Idarucizumab
- E. Desmopressin (DDAVP)

Correct answer is D

Idarucizumab is a specific reversal agent for dabigatran, providing rapid reversal of its anticoagulant effects. Fresh frozen plasma (FFP) (**A**) and prothrombin complex concentrate (PCC) (**C**) are not effective for dabigatran reversal but can be used for coumadin reversal. Vitamin K (**B**) is used for reversing warfarin but not dabigatran. Desmopressin (DDAVP) (**E**) is not indicated for anticoagulant reversal (▸ Table 6.1).[7]

▸▸ Question 16

A 58-year-old male with a history of mechanical heart valve replacement is on long-term warfarin therapy. He presents with a large subdural hematoma. His INR is 3.8. What is the most appropriate management to reverse the anticoagulation?

- A. Fresh frozen plasma (FFP)
- B. Vitamin K
- C. Prothrombin complex concentrate (PCC) and vitamin K
- D. Desmopressin (DDAVP)
- E. Platelet transfusion

Correct answer is C

The combination of PCC and vitamin K is recommended for the rapid and effective reversal of warfarin anticoagulation in patients with life-threatening bleeding, such as a subdural hematoma. PCC provides immediate reversal, while vitamin K ensures sustained correction of the INR. Fresh frozen plasma (FFP) (**A**) is less effective and slower. Desmopressin (DDAVP) (**D**) and platelet transfusion (**E**) are not appropriate for warfarin reversal.[8]

▸▸ Question 17

A 50-year-old female presents with easy bruising and prolonged bleeding after minor injuries. Her laboratory results show a normal platelet count, prolonged bleeding time, and a prolonged activated partial thromboplastin time (aPTT). What is the most likely diagnosis?

- A. Hemophilia A
- B. von Willebrand disease
- C. Disseminated intravascular coagulation (DIC)

Table 6.1 Anticoagulants

Drug name (brand)	Administration	Mechanism	Monitoring	Metabolism	Reversal strategy	Hold time[a]	Comments
Unfractionated heparin	IV for therapeutic anticoagulation; SQ for prophylaxis	Binds antithrombin III. Inhibits conversion of prothrombin → thrombin and fibrinogen → fibrin	aPTT, ACT, or antifactor Xa	Liver; excreted in urine; T1/2 60–90 min	1 mg protamine sulfate/100 units of heparin administered	Full anticoagulation 4–6 h, consider repeat aPTT; SQ "mini-dose" 12 h	Heparin produced since 2009 is 10% less potent; incidence of HIT is variable and reportedly 1–2%; "heparin rebound" may occur 8–9 h after protamine infusion
Enoxaparin (Lovenox, Sanofi Aventis) (an LMWH)	SQ for DVT prophylaxis and therapeutic anticoagulation	Binds antithrombin III and accelerates activity; inhibits thrombin and factor Xa	Antifactor Xa (therapeutic level 0.4–0.8 units/mL)	Liver; renal clearance, caution in patients with CrCl < 30 mL/min	protamine sulfate (1 mg/1 mg enoxaparin given in last 8 h); will only partially reverse effects (60%)	12 h after prophylactic dose; 24 h after therapeutic dose	more selective inhibitor of factor Xa than thrombin
Fondaparinux (Arixtra, GlaskoSmithKline)	SQ for DVT prophylaxis and therapeutic anticoagulation	Inhibits factor Xa	Antifactor Xa Prophylactic dose (0.4–0.5 mg/L) Therapeutic dose (1.2–1.26 mg/L)	Unknown; excreted in urine; T1/2 17–21 h	No approved antidote; consider rVIIa, but no studies examining the role of rVIIa in reversing fondaparinux in the setting of bleeding, hemodialysis reduces ≈ 20%	2–4 d in patients with normal renal function	Does not cause HIT, useful in patients with HIT; recommend 50% dose reduction if CrCl 30–50, contraindicated if CrCl < 30

(*continued*)

Table 6.1 Anticoagulants (*continued*)

Drug name (brand)	Administration	Mechanism	Monitoring	Metabolism	Reversal strategy	Hold time[a]	Comments
Warfarin (Coumadin, Bristol-Myers Squibb)	PO	Vitamin K antagonist (vitamin K-dependent factors are II, VII, IX, X, proteins C and S)	PT; INR (goal varies with indication)	Liver; excreted in urine ≈ 92%, bile; T1/2 20–60 h (highly variable)	Vitamin K 10 mg IV × 3 d and/or PCC (25–100 UI/kg) or FFP (15 mL/kg)[b]	5 d	Consider decreasing dose with hepatic impairment
Argatroban (GlaskoSmithKline)	IV for prophylaxis and treatment of thrombosis in patients with HIT	Direct thrombin inhibitor	aPTT (goal 1.5–3 × normal); ACT	Liver; excreted in feces ≈ 65% and urine ≈ 22%; T1/2 39–51 min	No reversal agent; supportive care; hemodialysis can remove some drug from the bloodstream, but unknown effect on bleeding, consider FFP or cryoprecipitate	2–4 h	Liver disease; consider decreasing the starting dose and titrating slowly
Dabigatran (Pradaxa, Boehringer Ingelheim)	PO, BID dosing	Direct thrombin inhibitor, reversible	No routine monitoring; normal aPTT implies no effect	Liver; renal clearance in urine; T1/2 12–17 h	Idarucizumab (Praxbind) (see text below)	1–2 d, longer if renal CrCl < 50 mL/min	For the prevention of stroke with afib; PCC has been shown to be most effective but unproven in human studies
Rivaroxaban (Xarelto, Bayer HealthCare)	PO daily dosing	Factor Xa inhibitor	No routine monitoring; normal antifactor Xa indicates no effect	Liver; renal clearance ≈ 66%, feces ≈ 28%; T1/25–9 h	Andexxa. If not available, consider rVIIa (partial reversal in animals	24 h	For prevention of stroke in afib and DVT treatment; caution: use with CrCl 15–50; CrCl < 30 avoid use. Not dialyzable

(*continued*)

Table 6.1 Anticoagulants (*continued*)

Drug name (brand)	Administration	Mechanism	Monitoring	Metabolism	Reversal strategy	Hold time[a]	Comments
Apixaban (Elliquis, Bristol-Myers Squibb)	PO, BID dosing	Factor Xa inhibitor	No routine monitoring; normal antifactor Xa indicates no effect	Liver ≈ 75% renal clearance ≈ 25%; T1/2 12 h	Andexxa. If not available, consider PCC, or rVIIa. rVIIa decreases bleeding time in animal model but does not reverse the anticoagulant effect.	48 h	For prevention of stroke in afib and DVT prophylaxis after orthopedic surgery. Decrease dose if Cr > 1.5; do not use with severe hepatic impairment. Not dialyzable
Edoxaban (Savaysa, Daiichi Sankyo Co.)	PO, daily dosing. Do not use if CrCl > 95 mL/min	Factor Xa inhibitor	No routine monitoring. Changes in PT and INRs are small and not useful. Normal antifactor Xa indicates no effect	Renal ≈ 50% (unchanged drug). Remainder: biliary/ intestinal excretion and minimal metabolism. T1/2 10–14 h	No specific antagonist	48 h	For DVT and PE after 5–10 d of parenteral anticoagulant; to reduce the risk of stroke and embolism in nonvalvular afib
Antithrombin, recombinant (ATryn, Lundbeck)	IV	Inhibits thrombin and factor Xa	AT levels	T1/2 11.6–17.7 h			For thromboembolism prophylaxis in hereditary antithrombin deficiency
Antithrombin III (Thrombate III, Grifols)	IV	Forms a bond with thrombin	AT levels	T1/2 2–3 d			For thromboembolism prophylaxis in hereditary antithrombin deficiency

(*continued*)

Table 6.1 Anticoagulants (*continued*)

Drug name (brand)	Administration	Mechanism	Monitoring	Metabolism	Reversal strategy	Hold time[a]	Comments
Dalteparin (Fragmin, Eisai)	SQ for DVT prophylaxis and therapeutic anticoagulation	Accelerates the activity of antithrombin III (inhibits thrombin and factor Xa)		Liver, urine; T1/ 23–5 h (longer with renal impairment)			Caution when use with CrCl < 30; caution with hepatic impairment
Bivalirudin (Angiomax, The Medicines Company)	IV	Direct thrombin inhibitor (reversible)	ACT	Plasma; excreted in urine; T1/ 225 min (longer with renal impairment)	None		Caution when use with CrCl < 30
Desidurin (Iprivask, Canyon)	SC	Direct thrombin inhibitor (selectively inhibits free and clot-bound thrombin	aPTT	Kidney; excreted in urine; T1/2 2 h (longer with renal impairment)	None		CrCl < 60 use caution, decrease initial dose

Abbreviations: ACT, activated clotting time; afib, atrial fibrillation; aPTT, partial thromboplastin time; AT, antithrombin; CrCl, creatinine clearance; DVT, deep venous thrombosis; HIT, heparin-induced thrombocytopenia; IV, intravenous; LMWH, low-molecular-weight heparin; PCC, prothrombin complex concentrate; SQ, subcutaneous.

Source: Reproduced from Management of anticoagulants prior to neurosurgical procedures. In: Greenberg M, ed. Greenberg's Handbook of Neurosurgery. 10th ed. New York: Thieme; 2023.

[a]Hold time is the recommended time to wait after discontinuing the drug before doing an elective operation in order to eliminate the effects of the drug.

[b]Intravenous vitamin K has a more rapid onset than subcutaneous vitamin K and current formulations, made with micelles of lecithin and glycol, seem to have a lower complication profile than older formulations containing polyethylated castor oil.

- D. Vitamin K deficiency
- E. Thrombocytopenia

Correct answer is B

von Willebrand disease (VWD) is the most common inherited bleeding disorder, characterized by a deficiency or dysfunction of von Willebrand factor (vWF). This results in prolonged bleeding time and a prolonged aPTT due to the associated reduction in factor VIII levels. Hemophilia A (**A**) causes a prolonged aPTT but normal bleeding time. DIC (**C**) typically presents with abnormalities in multiple coagulation parameters. Vitamin K deficiency (**D**) affects PT primarily. Thrombocytopenia (**E**) presents with a low platelet count.

▸▸ Question 18

A 70-year-old male with a history of chronic obstructive pulmonary disease (COPD) is admitted to the ICU with acute respiratory distress syndrome (ARDS) following severe pneumonia. Which of the following ventilatory strategies is most appropriate for managing his condition?

- A. High tidal volume ventilation
- B. Low tidal volume ventilation
- C. High-frequency oscillatory ventilation
- D. Noninvasive ventilation
- E. Pressure-controlled ventilation

Correct answer is B

Low tidal volume ventilation (4–6 mL/kg of predicted body weight) is the recommended strategy for managing ARDS as it minimizes ventilator-induced lung injury by reducing overdistension of the alveoli and preventing barotrauma. High tidal volume ventilation (**A**) can exacerbate lung injury. High-frequency oscillatory ventilation (**C**) is not commonly used due to a lack of demonstrated benefit over conventional ventilation. Noninvasive ventilation (**D**) is generally not suitable for severe ARDS. Pressure-controlled ventilation (**E**) can be used, but low tidal volumes must be ensured to avoid lung injury.

▸▸ Question 19

A 60-year-old female presents with fever, cough, and progressive shortness of breath. She is diagnosed with ventilator-associated pneumonia (VAP). Which of the following is the most important initial step in her management?

- A. Start broad-spectrum antibiotics
- B. Increase ventilator settings
- C. Administer bronchodilators
- D. Perform bronchoscopy
- E. Initiate noninvasive ventilation

Correct answer is A

The most important initial step in the management of VAP is to start broad-spectrum antibiotics to cover the likely pathogens, including gram-negative bacteria and MRSA. Timely antibiotic therapy is crucial to improve outcomes. Increasing ventilator settings (**B**) is not indicated without assessing the underlying cause. Bronchodilators (**C**) may be used for bronchospasm but are not the primary treatment. Bronchoscopy (**D**) can be considered for diagnostic purposes but is not an initial step. Noninvasive ventilation (**E**) is not suitable for patients already on mechanical ventilation.

▸▸ Question 20

A 45-year-old male is admitted with acute respiratory distress syndrome (ARDS) following severe trauma. He is on mechanical ventilation with high positive end-expiratory pressure (PEEP) settings. What is the primary rationale for using high PEEP in ARDS?

- A. To increase cardiac output
- B. To improve oxygenation
- C. To prevent atelectasis
- D. To reduce work of breathing
- E. To decrease respiratory rate

Correct answer is B

The primary rationale for using high PEEP in ARDS is to improve oxygenation by keeping alveoli open at the end of expiration, thereby enhancing gas exchange and reducing shunt. High PEEP helps prevent alveolar collapse (atelectasis) (**C**) and improves oxygenation. While PEEP can have an impact on other factors, such as reducing work of breathing (**D**) and affecting cardiac output (**A**), its primary use in ARDS is to improve oxygenation.

▸▸ Question 21

A 38-year-old male with Guillain-Barré syndrome develops respiratory failure and is intubated. Which of the following ventilatory support modes is most appropriate for this patient?

- A. Noninvasive positive pressure ventilation (NIPPV)
- B. Pressure support ventilation (PSV)
- C. Synchronized intermittent mandatory ventilation (SIMV)

- D. Volume-controlled ventilation (VCV)
- E. Continuous positive airway pressure (CPAP)

Correct answer is D

VCV is appropriate for patients with Guillain-Barré syndrome who develop respiratory failure because it ensures a consistent tidal volume, which is critical in patients with muscle weakness and compromised respiratory mechanics. NIPPV (**A**) is unsuitable once the patient is intubated and can be used prior to intubation. PSV (**B**) may not provide adequate support in severe cases. SIMV (**C**) can be used but may not guarantee consistent tidal volumes. CPAP (**E**) is primarily used for sleep apnea and is unsuitable for ventilatory support in this context.

▸▸ Question 22

A 55-year-old female with a history of severe asthma presents with respiratory distress and is intubated. What is the most appropriate ventilation strategy for this patient?

- A. High tidal volume and low respiratory rate
- B. Low tidal volume and high respiratory rate
- C. High tidal volume and high respiratory rate
- D. Low tidal volume and prolonged expiratory time
- E. Volume-controlled ventilation with high positive end-expiratory pressure (PEEP)

Correct answer is D

In patients with severe asthma, the goal is to avoid air trapping and dynamic hyperinflation. Therefore, a ventilation strategy with low tidal volume and prolonged expiratory time is most appropriate to allow for adequate exhalation and prevent high intrinsic PEEP. High tidal volume (**A and C**) can exacerbate air trapping. High respiratory rates (**B**) reduce the time for expiration. Volume-controlled ventilation with high PEEP (**E**) is not ideal for asthma management.

▸▸ Question 23

A 60-year-old male presents with fatigue, muscle weakness, and hypertension. Laboratory tests show hypokalemia and metabolic alkalosis. A CT scan reveals a 3-cm adrenal mass. What is the most likely diagnosis?

- A. Cushing syndrome
- B. Addison disease
- C. Pheochromocytoma
- D. Primary aldosteronism
- E. Secondary hyperaldosteronism

Correct answer is D

Primary aldosteronism, also known as Conn syndrome, is characterized by excessive production of aldosterone from the adrenal glands, leading to hypertension, hypokalemia, and metabolic alkalosis. The presence of an adrenal mass on a CT scan supports the diagnosis. Cushing syndrome (**A**) involves hypercortisolism and presents with different clinical features. Addison disease (**B**) involves adrenal insufficiency with hyperkalemia and hypotension. Pheochromocytoma (**C**) presents with episodic hypertension and catecholamine excess symptoms. Secondary hyperaldosteronism (**E**) is due to increased renin production, often from renal artery stenosis or heart failure.

▸▸ Question 24

A 35-year-old female with a history of recent thyroidectomy for papillary thyroid carcinoma presents with perioral tingling and muscle cramps. Her laboratory tests reveal hypocalcemia and hyperphosphatemia. What is the most appropriate initial management?

- A. Oral calcium carbonate
- B. Intravenous calcium gluconate
- C. Oral vitamin D
- D. Intravenous magnesium sulfate
- E. Oral phosphate binders

Correct answer is B

The patient presents with signs of hypocalcemia, likely due to hypoparathyroidism following thyroidectomy. Intravenous calcium gluconate is the most appropriate initial treatment for symptomatic hypocalcemia to rapidly increase serum calcium levels. Oral calcium carbonate (**A**) and vitamin D (**C**) are used for maintenance therapy. Intravenous magnesium sulfate (**D**) is used for hypomagnesemia. Oral phosphate binders (**E**) are not indicated in this acute setting.

▸▸ Question 25

A 50-year-old female presents with severe headache, sweating, and palpitations. Laboratory results reveal elevated metanephrines. A CT scan shows a 4-cm adrenal mass. What is the most likely diagnosis and the appropriate preoperative management?

- A. Cushing syndrome; hydrocortisone
- B. Addison disease; fludrocortisone
- C. Pheochromocytoma; alpha-blockers followed by beta-blockers
- D. Primary aldosteronism; spironolactone
- E. Hyperthyroidism; propylthiouracil

Correct answer is C

Pheochromocytoma is a catecholamine-secreting tumor that presents with episodic hypertension, severe headache, sweating, and palpitations. Elevated metanephrines and the presence of an adrenal mass support the diagnosis. Preoperative management includes alpha-blockers to control blood pressure and prevent catecholamine-induced crises, followed by beta-blockers to manage tachycardia. Cushing syndrome (**A**) involves hypercortisolism. Addison disease (**B**) involves adrenal insufficiency and requires fludrocortisone. Primary aldosteronism (**D**) is treated with spironolactone. Hyperthyroidism (**E**) requires antithyroid medications like propylthiouracil.

▸▸ Question 26

A 65-year-old male with a history of chronic nonsteroidal anti-inflammatory drug (NSAID) use presents with severe epigastric pain, hematemesis, and melena. His blood pressure is 90/60 mm Hg and heart rate is 120 bpm. What is the most likely diagnosis, and what is the initial management?

- A. Acute gastritis; oral proton pump inhibitor (PPI)
- B. Acute upper gastrointestinal bleeding; intravenous PPI and endoscopy
- C. Mallory-Weiss tear; antiemetics and observation
- D. Esophageal varices; intravenous octreotide and endoscopic banding
- E. Duodenal ulcer; oral antacids

Correct answer is B

The patient's presentation suggests acute upper gastrointestinal bleeding, likely from a peptic ulcer, given his history of chronic NSAID use. Initial management includes intravenous PPIs to reduce gastric acid secretion and stabilize the clot, followed by urgent endoscopy to identify and treat the bleeding source. Acute gastritis (**A**) typically presents with milder symptoms. Mallory-Weiss tear (**C**) involves mucosal lacerations usually after severe vomiting. Esophageal varices (**D**) are more common in patients with liver cirrhosis. Duodenal ulcer (**E**) can cause upper gastrointestinal bleeding but requires intravenous management in acute cases.

▸▸ Question 27

A 50-year-old female presents with a sudden-onset of severe abdominal pain radiating to the back. She has a history of gallstones. Laboratory results show elevated serum amylase and lipase. What is the most likely diagnosis, and what is the initial management?

- A. Acute cholecystitis; laparoscopic cholecystectomy
- B. Acute pancreatitis; intravenous fluids and pain management
- C. Peptic ulcer disease; oral proton pump inhibitors
- D. Acute hepatitis; supportive care
- E. Biliary colic; analgesics and observation

Correct answer is B

The patient's presentation and laboratory results suggest acute pancreatitis, likely secondary to gallstones. Initial management includes aggressive intravenous fluid resuscitation and pain control. Acute cholecystitis (**A**) presents with right upper quadrant pain and requires cholecystectomy. Peptic ulcer disease (**C**) typically presents with epigastric pain and usually does not cause elevated amylase and lipase. Acute hepatitis (**D**) presents with jaundice and elevated liver enzymes. Biliary colic (**E**) causes intermittent right upper quadrant pain without the significant enzyme elevation seen in pancreatitis.

▸▸ Question 28

A 45-year-old male with a history of heavy alcohol use presents with hematemesis and signs of hypovolemic shock. An urgent endoscopy reveals esophageal varices. What is the most appropriate initial treatment?

- A. Intravenous proton pump inhibitors (PPIs)
- B. Endoscopic sclerotherapy
- C. Intravenous octreotide and endoscopic band ligation
- D. Blood transfusion and observation
- E. Oral beta-blockers

Correct answer is C

Esophageal varices are a common complication of chronic liver disease and portal hypertension. The most appropriate initial treatment includes intravenous octreotide to reduce portal pressure and endoscopic band ligation to control the bleeding. Intravenous PPIs (**A**) are used for peptic ulcer bleeding. Endoscopic sclerotherapy (**B**) is less preferred due to higher complication rates. Blood transfusion (**D**) is necessary to stabilize the patient, but it is not a definitive treatment. Oral beta-blockers (**E**) are used for secondary prevention but not for acute bleeding.

▸▸ Question 29

A 40-year-old male presents with severe abdominal pain, fever, and rebound tenderness in the right lower quadrant. Laboratory results show an elevated white blood cell count. What is the most likely diagnosis, and what is the initial management?

- A. Acute pancreatitis; intravenous fluids and pain management
- B. Acute cholecystitis; intravenous antibiotics and cholecystectomy
- C. Acute appendicitis; intravenous antibiotics and appendectomy
- D. Perforated peptic ulcer; intravenous proton pump inhibitors and surgery
- E. Diverticulitis; oral antibiotics and observation

Correct answer is C

The patient's presentation suggests acute appendicitis, characterized by severe abdominal pain, fever, rebound tenderness in the right lower quadrant, and elevated white blood cell count. The initial management involves intravenous antibiotics and surgical removal of the appendix (appendectomy). Acute pancreatitis (**A**) presents with epigastric pain and elevated pancreatic enzymes. Acute cholecystitis (**B**) involves right upper quadrant pain and often requires cholecystectomy. Perforated peptic ulcer (**D**) presents with sudden-onset severe epigastric pain and requires surgical intervention. Diverticulitis (**E**) typically presents with left lower quadrant pain.

▸▸ Question 30

A 65-year-old male with a history of diabetes presents with decreased urine output, swelling in the legs, and fatigue. Laboratory results reveal elevated serum creatinine and blood urea nitrogen (BUN). Urinalysis shows muddy brown granular casts. What is the most likely diagnosis?

- A. Acute tubular necrosis
- B. Acute interstitial nephritis
- C. Postrenal azotemia
- D. Prerenal azotemia
- E. Glomerulonephritis

Correct answer is A

Acute tubular necrosis is characterized by acute kidney injury with elevated serum creatinine and BUN, decreased urine output, and the presence of muddy brown granular casts in the urine. It often results from ischemic or nephrotoxic injury to the renal tubules. Acute interstitial nephritis (**B**) typically presents with pyuria and eosinophils in the urine. Postrenal azotemia (**C**) is caused by urinary tract obstruction. Prerenal azotemia (**D**) is due to decreased renal perfusion and usually shows bland urine sediment. Glomerulonephritis (**E**) presents with hematuria, proteinuria, and red blood cell casts.[9]

▸▸ Question 31

A 55-year-old male presents with a sudden onset of severe right flank pain radiating to the groin, along with nausea and vomiting. His urine dipstick is positive for blood. What is the most likely diagnosis, and what is the next step in management?

- A. Acute pyelonephritis; intravenous antibiotics
- B. Acute glomerulonephritis; corticosteroids
- C. Nephrolithiasis; noncontrast CT scan of the abdomen
- D. Urinary tract infection; oral antibiotics
- E. Bladder cancer; cystoscopy

Correct answer is C

The patient presents with classic symptoms of nephrolithiasis (kidney stones), including severe flank pain radiating to the groin and hematuria. The next step in management is to confirm the diagnosis with a noncontrast CT scan of the abdomen, which is the gold standard for detecting kidney stones. Acute pyelonephritis (**A**) presents with fever, chills, and costovertebral angle tenderness. Acute glomerulonephritis (**B**) involves hematuria, proteinuria, and hypertension. Urinary tract infection (**D**) typically causes dysuria and urinary frequency. Bladder cancer (**E**) can present with hematuria but requires cystoscopy for diagnosis.

▸▸ Question 32

A 50-year-old male with a history of benign prostatic hyperplasia (BPH) presents with acute urinary retention. He is unable to void and has lower abdominal pain. What is the most appropriate initial management?

- A. Oral alpha-blockers
- B. Intravenous antibiotics
- C. Urinary catheterization
- D. Transurethral resection of the prostate (TURP)
- E. Oral 5-alpha reductase inhibitors

Correct answer is C

The most appropriate initial management for acute urinary retention, especially in a patient with BPH, is urinary catheterization to relieve the obstruction and decompress the bladder. Oral alpha-blockers (**A**) and 5-alpha reductase inhibitors (**E**) are used for long-term management of BPH but do not provide immediate relief. Intravenous antibiotics (**B**) are indicated if there is a concurrent infection. TURP (**D**) is a surgical treatment for BPH but is not an initial management step.

▸▸ Question 33

A 45-year-old female presents with fever, flank pain, and dysuria. She has a history of recurrent urinary tract infections. Physical examination reveals costovertebral angle tenderness. Urinalysis shows pyuria and bacteriuria. What is the most likely diagnosis, and what is the next step in management?

- A. Acute pyelonephritis; intravenous antibiotics
- B. Acute cystitis; oral antibiotics
- C. Interstitial cystitis; pain management
- D. Urethritis; oral antibiotics
- E. Glomerulonephritis; corticosteroids

Correct answer is A

The patient presents with classic symptoms of acute pyelonephritis, including fever, flank pain, dysuria, and costovertebral angle tenderness, along with pyuria and bacteriuria on urinalysis. The next step in management is to start intravenous antibiotics to treat the infection and prevent complications. Acute cystitis (**B**) presents with dysuria and urinary frequency without systemic symptoms. Interstitial cystitis (**C**) causes chronic pelvic pain and bladder pressure. Urethritis (**D**) presents with dysuria and urethral discharge. Glomerulonephritis (**E**) involves hematuria and proteinuria.

▸▸ Question 34

A 60-year-old female with a history of epilepsy presents with confusion, tremors, and ataxia. She is taking phenytoin for seizure control. Her serum phenytoin level is 25 µg/mL (therapeutic range: 10–20 µg/mL). What is the most appropriate management?

- A. Increase the dose of phenytoin
- B. Discontinue phenytoin and switch to levetiracetam
- C. Administer activated charcoal
- D. Decrease the dose of phenytoin
- E. Start intravenous diazepam

Correct answer is D

The patient presents with symptoms of phenytoin toxicity, indicated by a serum phenytoin level above the therapeutic range. The appropriate management is to decrease the dose of phenytoin to reduce the serum concentration to a therapeutic level. Increasing the dose (**A**) would worsen toxicity. Discontinuing phenytoin and switching to another antiepileptic drug (**B**) may be considered in cases of severe toxicity or intolerance but is not the immediate step. Activated charcoal (**C**) is used for acute overdose but not for chronic toxicity. Intravenous diazepam (**E**) is used for acute seizure control, not for phenytoin toxicity.[10]

▸▸ Question 35

A 45-year-old male with severe hepatic failure is being treated with lorazepam for agitation. He develops profound sedation and respiratory depression. Which of the following is the most appropriate antidote?

- A. Flumazenil
- B. Naloxone
- C. Physostigmine
- D. Activated charcoal
- E. Atropine

Correct answer is A

Flumazenil is a benzodiazepine receptor antagonist and is the appropriate antidote for benzodiazepine overdose, such as lorazepam, which can cause profound sedation and respiratory depression. Naloxone (**B**) is used for opioid overdose. Physostigmine (**C**) is used for anticholinergic toxicity. Activated charcoal (**D**) is used for gastrointestinal decontamination in certain poisonings. Atropine (**E**) is used for organophosphate poisoning and bradycardia.[11]

▸▸ Question 36

A 70-year-old man with Parkinson disease presents with severe nausea and vomiting. Which of the following antiemetic medications should be avoided due to the risk of significantly worsening his Parkinsonian symptoms?

- A. Ondansetron
- B. Metoclopramide
- C. Prochlorperazine
- D. Promethazine
- E. Domperidone

Correct answer is B

Patients with Parkinson disease have decreased central dopamine activity. Antiemetics that act centrally as dopamine receptor antagonists (such as metoclopramide, prochlorperazine, and promethazine) can exacerbate motor symptoms like rigidity, tremor, and bradykinesia. Among these, metoclopramide is commonly used as an antiemetic and prokinetic agent, posing a particularly high risk in clinical practice.

Ondansetron, a serotonin (5-HT3) receptor antagonist, does not antagonize dopamine receptors and thus is safe in patients with Parkinson disease.

Domperidone is a peripheral dopamine antagonist that does not cross the blood–brain barrier significantly, making it safe for patients with Parkinson disease requiring dopamine-sparing antiemetic treatment.

Thus, metoclopramide (option **B**) should be strictly avoided due to the significant risk of worsening Parkinsonian symptoms.[12]

▸▸ Question 37

A 40-year-old male with a history of bipolar disorder presents with tremors, confusion, and polyuria. He is on long-term lithium therapy. His serum lithium level is 2.0 mEq/L (therapeutic range: 0.6–1.2 mEq/L). What is the most appropriate initial management?

- A. Increase the dose of lithium
- B. Discontinue lithium and start hemodialysis
- C. Administer intravenous sodium bicarbonate
- D. Reduce the dose of lithium and monitor closely
- E. Start antipsychotic medication

Correct answer is D

The patient presents with symptoms of lithium toxicity, indicated by a serum lithium level above the therapeutic range. The appropriate initial management is to reduce the dose of lithium and monitor the patient closely. Discontinuing lithium and starting hemodialysis (**B**) is reserved for severe toxicity or renal failure. Increasing the dose (**A**) would worsen toxicity. Intravenous sodium bicarbonate (**C**) is not indicated for lithium toxicity. Starting an antipsychotic medication (**E**) is not appropriate for managing lithium toxicity.[13]

▸▸ Question 38

A 75-year-old male with a history of chronic obstructive pulmonary disease (COPD) presents with fever, cough, and purulent sputum. He is diagnosed with community-acquired pneumonia (CAP). Which of the following is the most appropriate initial antibiotic therapy?

- A. Amoxicillin
- B. Azithromycin
- C. Levofloxacin
- D. Ceftriaxone
- E. Doxycycline

Correct answer is C

In patients with COPD and CAP, levofloxacin is an appropriate choice because it covers both typical and atypical pathogens and provides good coverage for potential drug-resistant *Streptococcus pneumoniae*. Amoxicillin (**A**) is often used for mild cases without comorbidities. Azithromycin (**B**) and doxycycline (**E**) are also options but may not provide as broad coverage. Ceftriaxone (**D**) is used in hospitalized patients but may not cover atypical pathogens.

▸▸ Question 39

A 50-year-old male with a history of intravenous drug use presents with fever, night sweats, weight loss, and cough. A chest X-ray shows cavitary lesions in the upper lobes. What is the most likely diagnosis, and what is the initial treatment?

- A. Bacterial pneumonia; intravenous ceftriaxone
- B. Lung abscess; clindamycin
- C. Tuberculosis; rifampin, isoniazid, rifampin, pyrazinamide, and ethambutol (RIPE)
- D. Fungal infection; amphotericin B
- E. Lung cancer; chemotherapy

Correct answer is C

The patient's symptoms and chest X-ray findings are highly suggestive of tuberculosis (TB), particularly in a patient with a history of intravenous drug use, which is a risk factor. The initial treatment for active TB includes the RIPE regimen: isoniazid, rifampin, pyrazinamide, and ethambutol. Bacterial pneumonia (**A**) and lung abscess (**B**) present with different radiographic and clinical findings. Fungal infection (**D**) may present similarly but requires specific diagnostic tests. Lung cancer (**E**) requires tissue biopsy for diagnosis.

▸▸ Question 40

A 28-year-old female presents with fever, sore throat, and a sandpaper-like rash. Physical examination reveals a strawberry tongue and cervical lymphadenopathy. What is the most likely diagnosis, and what is the first-line treatment?

- A. Infectious mononucleosis; corticosteroids
- B. Scarlet fever; penicillin
- C. Rubella; supportive care
- D. Kawasaki disease; intravenous immunoglobulin
- E. Measles; vitamin A

Correct answer is B

Scarlet fever is caused by group A Streptococcus and presents with fever, sore throat, a sandpaper-like rash, strawberry tongue, and cervical lymphadenopathy. The first-line treatment is penicillin to eradicate the infection and prevent complications. Infectious mononucleosis (**A**) presents with pharyngitis, lymphadenopathy, and fatigue but not a sandpaper-like rash. Rubella (**C**) presents with a maculopapular rash and lymphadenopathy. Kawasaki disease (**D**) presents with fever, rash, conjunctivitis, and mucosal changes but affects younger children. Measles (**E**) presents with a maculopapular rash and Koplik spots.

▸▸ Question 41

A 35-year-old male presents with fever, severe headache, photophobia, and a petechial rash. Lumbar puncture reveals elevated white blood cell count, low glucose, and high protein levels in the cerebrospinal fluid (CSF). What is the most likely diagnosis, and what is the appropriate initial management?

- A. Viral meningitis; acyclovir
- B. Bacterial meningitis; intravenous ceftriaxone and vancomycin
- C. Fungal meningitis; amphotericin B
- D. Tuberculous meningitis; isoniazid, rifampin, pyrazinamide, and ethambutol
- E. Encephalitis; intravenous immunoglobulin

Correct answer is B

The patient's presentation and lumbar puncture findings (elevated white blood cell count, low glucose, and high protein levels in the CSF) are indicative of bacterial meningitis. The appropriate initial management includes broad-spectrum antibiotics such as intravenous ceftriaxone and vancomycin to cover common bacterial pathogens, including *Streptococcus pneumoniae* and *Neisseria meningitidis*. Viral meningitis (**A**) presents with normal glucose levels and is treated with supportive care or acyclovir for herpes simplex virus. Fungal meningitis (**C**) typically occurs in immunocompromised patients. Tuberculous meningitis (**D**) has a more chronic course. Encephalitis (**E**) presents with altered mental status and requires specific antiviral or immunologic treatments.

▸▸ Question 42

A 40-year-old female presents with agitation, mydriasis, hyperthermia, and tachycardia after ingesting an unknown substance. She is suspected of having serotonin syndrome. What is the most appropriate initial management?

- A. Benzodiazepines
- B. Cyproheptadine
- C. Activated charcoal
- D. Intravenous fluids
- E. Beta-blockers

Correct answer is A

The patient's presentation suggests serotonin syndrome, which is characterized by agitation, mydriasis, hyperthermia, and tachycardia. The initial management includes supportive care with benzodiazepines to reduce agitation and hyperthermia. Cyproheptadine (**B**) is a serotonin antagonist used in severe cases but is not the first step. Activated charcoal (**C**) is useful if ingestion is recent but is not a specific treatment for serotonin syndrome. Intravenous fluids (**D**) are supportive but not the primary treatment. Beta-blockers (**E**) are generally avoided as they can worsen hyperthermia.[14]

▸▸ Question 43

A 25-year-old male is found unconscious with pinpoint pupils and respiratory depression. A syringe is found next to him. What is the most appropriate immediate intervention?

- A. Intravenous naloxone
- B. Intravenous flumazenil
- C. Intravenous glucose
- D. Intravenous thiamine
- E. Activated charcoal

Correct answer is A

The patient's presentation of unconsciousness, pinpoint pupils, and respiratory depression suggests opioid overdose. The most appropriate immediate intervention is the administration of intravenous naloxone, an opioid antagonist. Intravenous flumazenil (**B**) is used for benzodiazepine overdose. Intravenous glucose (**C**) and thiamine (**D**) are used for hypoglycemia and Wernicke encephalopathy, respectively. Activated charcoal (**E**) is used for gastrointestinal decontamination but is not the first step in managing opioid overdose.[15]

▸▸ Question 44

A 30-year-old male presents with abdominal pain, vomiting, and confusion after ingesting antifreeze. Laboratory tests reveal metabolic acidosis with an elevated anion gap and calcium oxalate crystals in the urine. What is the most appropriate antidote?

- A. Ethanol
- B. Fomepizole
- C. Activated charcoal
- D. Intravenous sodium bicarbonate
- E. Intravenous calcium gluconate

Correct answer is B

The patient's presentation and laboratory findings suggest ethylene glycol poisoning, commonly found in antifreeze. The presence of metabolic acidosis with an elevated anion gap and calcium oxalate crystals in the urine further supports this diagnosis. The most appropriate antidote is fomepizole, which inhibits alcohol dehydrogenase and prevents the metabolism of ethylene glycol to toxic metabolites. Ethanol (**A**) is an alternative antidote but is not preferred. Activated charcoal (**C**) is not effective for ethylene glycol. Intravenous sodium bicarbonate (**D**) can be used to correct acidosis but is not the primary treatment. Intravenous calcium gluconate (**E**) is used to treat hypocalcemia.[16]

▸▸ Question 45

A 50-year-old female presents with nausea, vomiting, and abdominal pain after ingesting a large number of acetaminophen tablets. Her serum acetaminophen level is significantly elevated. What is the most appropriate antidote?

- A. Activated charcoal
- B. Intravenous N-acetylcysteine
- C. Intravenous sodium bicarbonate
- D. Intravenous naloxone
- E. Intravenous glucose

Correct answer is B

The patient's presentation and elevated serum acetaminophen level suggest acetaminophen overdose. The most appropriate antidote is intravenous N-acetylcysteine, which replenishes glutathione stores and prevents liver damage. Activated charcoal (**A**) can be used for gastrointestinal decontamination if administered within a few hours of ingestion. Intravenous sodium bicarbonate (**C**) is not indicated for acetaminophen overdose. Intravenous naloxone (**D**) is used for opioid overdose. Intravenous glucose (**E**) is not specific for acetaminophen toxicity.

▸▸ Question 46

A 65-year-old male with diabetes presents with a nonhealing foot ulcer. The ulcer has been present for several months despite local wound care. What is the most likely contributing factor to the delayed healing?

- A. Bacterial infection
- B. Poor glycemic control
- C. Inadequate protein intake
- D. Peripheral arterial disease
- E. All of the above

Correct answer is E

Delayed wound healing in a diabetic patient can be attributed to multiple factors, including bacterial infection, poor glycemic control, inadequate protein intake, and peripheral arterial disease. These factors can impair the body's ability to repair tissue and fight infection. Addressing each contributing factor is essential for promoting wound healing.

▸▸ Question 47

A 45-year-old female presents with a surgical wound that is not healing properly. She is a smoker and has a history of peripheral vascular disease. What is the most important factor contributing to her impaired wound healing?

- A. Smoking
- B. Age
- C. Gender
- D. Surgical technique
- E. Type of sutures used

Correct answer is A

Smoking is a significant risk factor for impaired wound healing due to its effects on blood flow and oxygen delivery to tissues. Nicotine causes vasoconstriction, reducing blood supply to the wound, while carbon monoxide decreases oxygen-carrying capacity. Age (**B**), gender (**C**), surgical technique (**D**), and type of sutures (**E**) also affect wound healing, but smoking has a more profound impact.

▸▸ Question 48

A 70-year-old female presents with a chronic venous leg ulcer. What is the primary underlying pathophysiology of this type of ulcer?

- A. Arterial insufficiency
- B. Venous hypertension
- C. Diabetic neuropathy
- D. Pressure necrosis
- E. Trauma

Correct answer is B

Chronic venous leg ulcers are primarily caused by venous hypertension, which results from chronic venous insufficiency. This condition leads to increased pressure in the veins, resulting in leakage of fluid and proteins into the surrounding tissues, causing edema, inflammation, and eventually ulceration. Arterial insufficiency (**A**) leads to arterial ulcers. Diabetic neuropathy (**C**) causes diabetic foot ulcers. Pressure necrosis (**D**) leads to pressure ulcers. Trauma (**E**) can cause acute wounds, but it is not the underlying cause of chronic venous ulcers.

▸▸ Question 49

A 45-year-old male undergoing elective surgery develops malignant hyperthermia shortly after induction with succinylcholine and sevoflurane. What is the most appropriate immediate treatment?

- A. Intravenous dantrolene
- B. Intravenous atropine
- C. Intravenous sodium bicarbonate
- D. Intravenous lidocaine
- E. Intravenous diazepam

Correct answer is A

Malignant hyperthermia is a life-threatening condition triggered by certain anesthetic agents like succinylcholine and sevoflurane. It is characterized by the rapid onset of hyperthermia, muscle rigidity, and acidosis. The most appropriate immediate treatment is intravenous dantrolene, a muscle relaxant that inhibits calcium release from the sarcoplasmic reticulum. Atropine (**B**) is used for bradycardia. Sodium bicarbonate (**C**) can be used to treat acidosis, but it is not the primary treatment. Lidocaine (**D**) is used for arrhythmias. Diazepam (**E**) is used for muscle spasms but not for malignant hyperthermia.[17]

▸▸ Question 50

A 60-year-old female with a history of hypertension and asthma presents for elective surgery. Which of the following anesthetic agents should be avoided due to her asthma?

- A. Propofol
- B. Sevoflurane
- C. Isoflurane
- D. Ketamine
- E. Etomidate

Correct answer is C

Isoflurane should be avoided in patients with asthma because it can cause airway irritation and bronchospasm. Propofol (**A**) is safe and commonly used. Sevoflurane (**B**) is preferred for inhalation induction in asthmatic patients due to its bronchodilatory properties. Ketamine (**D**) is also safe and provides bronchodilation. Etomidate (**E**) is safe but does not provide bronchodilation.

▸▸ **Question 51**

A 30-year-old female undergoing surgery is given an inhalational anesthetic. Shortly after induction, she develops tachycardia, hyperthermia, and muscle rigidity. What genetic mutation is most likely responsible for her condition?
- A. RYR1
- B. SCN5A
- C. CACNA1C
- D. KCNQ1
- E. CFTR

Correct answer is A
Malignant hyperthermia is most commonly associated with mutations in the *RYR1* gene, which encodes the ryanodine receptor, a calcium release channel in skeletal muscle. These mutations lead to excessive calcium release and sustained muscle contraction in response to certain anesthetics. SCN5A (**B**) is associated with cardiac arrhythmias. CACNA1C (**C**) is linked to Timothy syndrome. KCNQ1 (**D**) is associated with long QT syndrome. CFTR (**E**) is related to cystic fibrosis.[18]

▸▸ **Question 52**

A 50-year-old male with chronic liver disease requires surgery. Which of the following anesthetic agents is most appropriate given his condition?
- A. Halothane
- B. Sevoflurane
- C. Isoflurane
- D. Enflurane
- E. Desflurane

Correct answer is B
Sevoflurane is the most appropriate inhalational anesthetic for patients with chronic liver disease because it has minimal hepatic metabolism and a lower potential for hepatotoxicity compared to other agents. Halothane (**A**) is known for its hepatotoxicity. Isoflurane (**C**) and enflurane (**D**) have more hepatic metabolism than sevoflurane. Desflurane (**E**) is safe but can cause airway irritation.

▸▸ **Question 53**

A 55-year-old male presents with a sudden severe headache, photophobia, and neck stiffness. A CT scan shows subarachnoid hemorrhage (SAH). Which of the following is a common metabolic complication associated with SAH?
- A. Hypernatremia
- B. Hyponatremia
- C. Hyperkalemia
- D. Hypokalemia
- E. Hypercalcemia

Correct answer is B
Hyponatremia is a common metabolic complication associated with subarachnoid hemorrhage (SAH), often due to the syndrome of inappropriate antidiuretic hormone secretion or cerebral salt wasting. Hypernatremia (**A**) and hyperkalemia (**C**) are less common. Hypokalemia (**D**) and hypercalcemia (**E**) are not typically associated with SAH.

▸▸ **Question 54**

A 60-year-old male with a history of hypertension presents with a sudden onset of hemiparesis and is diagnosed with an ischemic stroke. What metabolic disturbance is commonly seen in the acute phase of ischemic stroke?
- A. Hyperglycemia
- B. Hypoglycemia
- C. Hypercalcemia
- D. Hyponatremia
- E. Hypokalemia

Correct answer is A
Hyperglycemia is commonly seen in the acute phase of ischemic stroke and is associated with worse outcomes. It can result from the stress response and the release of stress hormones. Hypoglycemia (**B**) is less common and can mimic stroke symptoms. Hypercalcemia (**C**), hyponatremia (**D**), and hypokalemia (**E**) are not typically associated with acute ischemic stroke.

▸▸ **Question 55**

A 45-year-old male with a history of epilepsy presents with new-onset confusion and an elevated serum ammonia level. Which antiepileptic drug is most likely responsible for this condition?
- A. Phenytoin
- B. Valproic acid
- C. Carbamazepine
- D. Lamotrigine
- E. Levetiracetam

Correct answer is B

Valproic acid is known to cause hyperammonemia, which can lead to encephalopathy and confusion. This condition is due to the inhibition of the urea cycle by valproic acid. Phenytoin (**A**), carbamazepine (**C**), lamotrigine (**D**), and levetiracetam (**E**) are less likely to cause hyperammonemia.

▸▸ Question 56

A 30-year-old female presents with a history of severe headaches, and a recent MRI reveals a brain tumor in the pituitary region. She is noted to have polyuria and polydipsia. Which of the following metabolic disturbances is most likely present?

- A. Hypercalcemia
- B. Hyponatremia
- C. Hyperkalemia
- D. Hypernatremia
- E. Hypokalemia

Correct answer is D

Hypernatremia is most likely present in this patient, suggesting diabetes insipidus (DI), which can occur with pituitary tumors. DI leads to decreased antidiuretic hormone (ADH) production, resulting in excessive water loss and increased serum sodium levels. Hypercalcemia (**A**), hyponatremia (**B**), hyperkalemia (**C**), and hypokalemia (**E**) are less commonly associated with pituitary tumors causing DI.

▸▸ Question 57

A 70-year-old female with a history of atrial fibrillation presents with a sudden onset of left-sided weakness and is diagnosed with a cardioembolic stroke. Which metabolic intervention has been shown to improve outcomes if administered within the appropriate time window?

- A. Intravenous glucose
- B. Intravenous insulin
- C. Intravenous sodium bicarbonate
- D. Intravenous tissue plasminogen activator (tPA)
- E. Intravenous mannitol

Correct answer is D

Intravenous tPA is a metabolic intervention that has been shown to improve outcomes in patients with acute ischemic stroke if administered within the appropriate time window (generally within 3 to 4.5 hours from symptom onset). It works by dissolving the thrombus causing the stroke, thereby restoring blood flow. Intravenous glucose (**A**) and insulin (**B**) are used for managing blood sugar levels but are not specific treatments for stroke. Intravenous sodium bicarbonate (**C**) and mannitol (**E**) are used for specific indications but not for acute stroke thrombolysis.

▸▸ Question 58

A 30-year-old man is stabilized after a penetrating brain injury due to a gunshot wound to the head. Imaging reveals diffuse cerebral edema and herniation. Examination shows coma, brainstem areflexia, and a lack of respiratory drive. There is suspicion that the patient has progressed to brain death (death by neurologic criteria). What is the most appropriate next step?

- A. Ensure all possible confounders are ruled out and prepare for apnea testing
- B. Skip apnea testing and obtain an ancillary study
- C. Declare brain death based on the mechanism of injury without additional testing
- D. Administer steroids
- E. Proceed with withdrawal of life-sustaining therapy

Correct answer is A

In the appropriate clinical context after a catastrophic neurologic injury, the declaration of brain death or death by neurologic criteria is performed after ruling out possible confounders (metabolic, residual sedation/analgesia/paralytics, toxic, hypotension, hypothermia, etc.), and if the patient demonstrates coma, brainstem areflexia, and the absence of a respiratory drive. Apnea testing will be performed by credentialed providers to demonstrate hypercarbia and acidemia following recommended guidelines. Skipping apnea testing (**B**) must not be done unless the patient has a contraindication to apnea testing, such as hemodynamic instability or hypoxemia-prohibiting testing. Steroids (**D**) have no role in traumatic brain injury. Declaration of brain death without complete testing (**C**) or withdrawal of life-sustaining therapy (**E**) without goals of care conversations with the family would be inappropriate.[19]

▸▸ Question 59

A patient undergoes apnea testing and meets criteria for brain death. The only confounder to the examination is a penetrating injury through the right eye, prohibiting the complete assessment of brainstem reflexes. Which of the following can be obtained as an ancillary test for the declaration of brain death?

- A. CT angiography of the brain
- B. Electroencephalogram (EEG) monitoring
- C. MR angiography of the brain
- D. Radionuclide cerebral scintigraphy
- E. Auditory evoked potentials (AEPs) and somatosensory evoked potentials (SEPs)

Correct answer is D

If any portion of the brain death examination or apnea testing cannot be completed, an ancillary test should be obtained in addition to all parts of the examination that can be completed to the fullest extent possible. CT angiography (**A**), MR angiography (**C**), and neurophysiologic testing (**B**) and EEG, AEP, and SEP (**E**) are not recommended as ancillary tests for brain death. Conventional four-vessel catheter angiography, radionuclide perfusion scintigraphy and transcranial Doppler ultrasonography may be used as ancillary tests to aid in the diagnosis of brain death in adult patients.[19]

References

[1] Thiele H, Ohman EM, deWaha-Thiele S, Zeymer U, Desch S. Management of cardiogenic shock complicating myocardial infarction: an update 2019. Eur Heart J 2019;40(32):2671–2683

[2] Cecconi M, De Backer D, Antonelli M, et al. Consensus on circulatory shock and hemodynamic monitoring. Task force of the European Society of Intensive Care Medicine. Intensive Care Med 2014;40(12):1795–1815

[3] Evans L, Rhodes A, Alhazzani W, et al. Surviving sepsis campaign: international guidelines for management of sepsis and septic shock 2021. Intensive Care Med 2021;47(11):1181–1247

[4] Trinka E, Cock H, Hesdorffer D, et al. A definition and classification of status epilepticus – report of the ILAE Task Force on Classification of Status Epilepticus. Epilepsia 2015;56(10):1515–1523

[5] Dave S, Dahlstrom JJ, Weisbrod LJ. Neurogenic shock. 2023 Oct 29. In: StatPearls [Internet]. Treasure Island, FL: StatPearls Publishing; 2025

[6] Sterns RH, Silver SM. Cerebral salt wasting versus SIADH: what difference? J Am Soc Nephrol 2008;19(2):194–196

[7] Pollack CV Jr., Reilly PA, van Ryn J, et al. Idarucizumab for dabigatran reversal - full cohort analysis. N Engl J Med 2017;377(5):431–441

[8] Frontera JA, Lewin JJ III, Rabinstein AA, et al. Guideline for reversal of antithrombotics in intracranial hemorrhage: a statement for healthcare professionals from the Neurocritical Care Society and Society of Critical Care Medicine. Neurocrit Care 2016;24(1):6–46

[9] Schrier RW, Wang W, Poole B, Mitra A. Acute renal failure: definitions, diagnosis, pathogenesis, and therapy. J Clin Invest 2004;114(1):5–14 [Erratum in: J Clin Invest. 2004;114(4):598]

[10] Patsalos PN, Berry DJ, Bourgeois BF, et al. Antiepileptic drugs–best practice guidelines for therapeutic drug monitoring: a position paper by the Subcommission on Therapeutic Drug Monitoring, ILAE Commission on Therapeutic Strategies. Epilepsia 2008;49(7):1239–1276

[11] Hoffman EJ, Warren EW. Flumazenil: a benzodiazepine antagonist. Clin Pharm 1993;12(9):641–656; quiz 699–701 [Erratum in: Clin Pharm 1993;12(11):803. PMID: 8306565]

[12] Seppi K, Ray Chaudhuri K, Coelho M, et al. The collaborators of the Parkinson's Disease Update on Non-Motor Symptoms Study Group on behalf of the Movement Disorders Society Evidence-Based Medicine Committee. Update on treatments for nonmotor symptoms of Parkinson's disease - an evidence-based medicine review. Mov Disord 2019;34(2):180–198 [Erratum in: Mov Disord. 2019 May;34(5):765]

[13] McKnight RF, Adida M, Budge K, Stockton S, Goodwin GM, Geddes JR. Lithium toxicity profile: a systematic review and meta-analysis. Lancet 2012;379(9817):721–728

[14] Boyer EW, Shannon M. The serotonin syndrome. N Engl J Med 2005;352(11):1112–1120 [Erratum in: N Engl J Med. 2007;356(23):2437. Erratum in: N Engl J Med. 2009;361(17):1714. PMID: 15784664]

[15] Kim HK, Nelson LS. Reducing the harm of opioid overdose with the safe use of naloxone: a pharmacologic review. Expert Opin Drug Saf 2015;14(7):1137–1146

[16] Barceloux DG, Krenzelok EP, Olson K, Watson W. American Academy of Clinical Toxicology Practice Guidelines on the Treatment of Ethylene Glycol Poisoning. Ad Hoc Committee. J Toxicol Clin Toxicol 1999;37(5):537–560

[17] Rosenberg H, Pollock N, Schiemann A, Bulger T, Stowell K. Malignant hyperthermia: a review. Orphanet J Rare Dis 2015;10:93

[18] Maclennan DH, Zvaritch E. Mechanistic models for muscle diseases and disorders originating in the sarcoplasmic reticulum. Biochim Biophys Acta 2011;1813(5):948–964

[19] Greer DM, Kirschen MP, Lewis A, et al. Pediatric and adult brain death/death by Neurologic Criteria Consensus Guideline. Neurology 2023;101(24):1112–1132 [Erratum in: Neurology 2024;102(3):e208108]

7 Peripheral Nerve

Syed I. Khalid, Zachary A. Pennington, Aladine Elsamadicy, Robert J. Spinner

▸▸ Question 1

Which nerve transfer for elbow flexion is most appropriate in a patient with a complete brachial plexus injury?

- A. Ulnar nerve to the biceps motor branch
- B. Median nerve to the brachialis motor branch
- C. Spinal accessory nerve to the suprascapular nerve
- D. Intercostal nerves to the musculocutaneous nerve
- E. Phrenic nerve to suprascapular nerve

Correct answer is D

The intercostal nerve to the musculocutaneous nerve is a common nerve transfer used for biceps reinnervation in patients with brachial plexus injuries. This transfer helps restore elbow flexion, which is crucial for upper limb function. Ulnar and median nerve fascicular transfers are being used for elbow flexion restoration but can only be performed when the donors are functioning (such as in patients with C5, C6 injuries); in this case with a complete paralysis (flail limb), ulnar and median nerves would not be functioning and could not be used as a donor for a nerve transfer. The spinal accessory nerve to the suprascapular nerve is a common nerve transfer designed to provide shoulder stabilization. The phrenic nerve is also used by some surgeons to target the suprascapular nerve for shoulder stabilization; it is also used for other purposes, including biceps reinnervation. Each transfer is selected based on the specific functional loss and anatomical considerations. Additionally, for motor function restoration, donor nerves should be (1) purely motor, (2) allow for tension-free transfer to recipient nerve without the need for an intervening cable graft, (3) have multiple motor axons, (4) be functionally redundant (so its use does not compromise another function), and (5) have a normal role synergistic with that performed by the injured recipient.[1,2,3]

▸▸ Question 2

Which nerve transfer is commonly used to restore shoulder abduction in patients with upper brachial plexus injuries?

- A. Ulnar nerve to axillary nerve
- B. Radial nerve to suprascapular nerve
- C. Spinal accessory nerve to suprascapular nerve
- D. Median nerve to axillary nerve
- E. Phrenic nerve to axillary nerve

Correct answer is C

The spinal accessory nerve to the suprascapular nerve transfer is commonly used to restore shoulder stability and function (abduction and external rotation) in patients with upper brachial plexus injuries. The spinal accessory nerve is chosen due to its motor function and proximity to the suprascapular nerve. Typically, the proximal branch to the trapezius muscle is maintained in this nerve transfer to preserve some trapezius function, and the distal portion of the nerve is transferred. Radial nerve branches to the triceps are also commonly transferred to the anterior portion of the axillary nerve to restore deltoid function; these triceps branches are not used as a transfer to the suprascapular nerve. Ulnar and median nerve transfers are typically used for elbow flexion restoration. The phrenic nerve is used as a nerve transfer by some surgeons, but the donor morbidity from the diaphragmatic paralysis has limited its routine use by many surgeons.[4]

▸▸ Question 3

Which nerve is typically used as a nerve transfer to restore wrist extension in a patient with radial nerve palsy?

- A. Ulnar nerve
- B. Anterior interosseous nerve
- C. Intercostal nerves
- D. Spinal accessory nerve
- E. Pronator teres branch of the median nerve

Correct answer is E

Restoration of distal radial nerve function (e.g., wrist/finger extension) following proximal injury requires the use of donor nerves close to the motor endplate of the denervated muscle. Donors very proximal to the muscle may require so long to regenerate axons as to preclude effective endplate targeting. In patients with radial nerve palsy, distal function (wrist and finger extension) can be restored, transferring expendable branches of the median nerve (such as a pronator teres branch or a flexor digitorum superficialis branch) to the extensor carpi radialis branch and posterior interosseous nerve. This transfer effectively reinnervates wrist and finger extension. Ulnar and anterior interosseous nerve transfers are used for different reinnervation purposes, often targeting hand muscles. Intercostal and spinal accessory nerves are less commonly used for wrist extension but may be considered for other reinnervation strategies of proximal recipients. This targeted approach helps address the specific deficit caused by radial nerve injury.[5]

▸▸ Question 4

A 39-year-old man requires lower leg fasciotomy for impending compartment syndrome after sustaining a crush injury. To maximize the chances of preserving foot eversion, which of the following compartments is most appropriate to open?

- A. Anterior compartment
- B. Lateral compartment
- C. Superficial posterior compartment
- D. Deep posterior compartment
- E. Medial compartment

Correct answer is B

The lateral compartment contains the superficial peroneal nerve, which innervates the peroneus longus and brevis muscles responsible for foot eversion. In compartment syndrome or crush injuries, opening the lateral compartment can help relieve pressure and preserve the function of these muscles. The anterior compartment contains muscles responsible for dorsiflexion, the superficial posterior compartment contains the gastrocnemius and soleus muscles for plantarflexion, and the deep posterior compartment contains muscles for toe flexion and inversion. The medial compartment of the thigh is not typically involved in lower leg fasciotomies.[6,7]

▸▸ Question 5

A 17-year-old boy is stabbed in the arm and loses function of the radial nerve. After surgical nerve repair, which of the following is the most likely rate of nerve regeneration?

- A. 1 mm/day
- B. 5 mm/day
- C. 10 mm/day
- D. 2 cm/day
- E. 5 cm/day

Correct answer is A

The typical rate of peripheral nerve regeneration is approximately 1 mm/day or about 1 inch/month. This rate can vary based on factors such as the age of the patient, the location of the injury, and the extent of the damage. Attempts to speed nerve recovery have been a source of much research; suffice it to say that faster rates like 5 mm/day or 1 cm/day are not realistic for peripheral nerves at this time. Proper postoperative care and rehabilitation are crucial to optimizing recovery and function after nerve repair. The slow process of axonal regeneration underlies the choice of donor fascicle in nerve transfers (thus the popularity of distal nerve transfers). The donor must be close enough to the motor endplate of the target muscle so as to allow for full axonal regeneration prior to irreversible endplate degradation.[8,9]

▸▸ Question 6

A 72-year-old man is evaluated because of intractable facial pain caused by trigeminal neuralgia that has not responded to medical management. Triggers for the pain include laughing and brushing his teeth. Neurological examination shows no abnormalities. Stereotactic radiosurgery is suggested, and he is counseled regarding the risks and benefits. This patient should be informed that the most likely adverse effect of this treatment is which of the following?

- A. Hearing loss
- B. Sensory loss
- C. Dysphagia
- D. Diplopia
- E. Facial weakness

Correct answer is B

Sensory loss is the most common adverse effect of stereotactic radiosurgery for trigeminal neuralgia. This can occur because the procedure targets the trigeminal nerve to disrupt pain pathways; this same nerve provides somatosensory inputs from the face. Hearing loss, dysphagia, diplopia, and facial weakness are less common side effects but can occur depending on the precise location and extent of the treatment. In rare cases, the patient can also develop painful numbness or hyperesthesia known as anesthesia dolorosa.[10]

▸▸ Question 7

Which of the following features best differentiates between Becker and Duchenne muscular dystrophies?

- A. Age of onset
- B. Presence of calf pseudohypertrophy
- C. Respiratory involvement
- D. Cardiac involvement
- E. Rate of progression

Correct answer is A

The primary differences between Becker muscular dystrophy and Duchenne muscular dystrophy (DMD) are the age of onset and severity of symptomatology. DMD typically presents in early childhood (before the age of 5) with rapid progression, while Becker muscular dystrophy has a later onset (usually after the age of 5) and a slower progression. Both conditions can present with calf pseudohypertrophy, cardiac involvement, and respiratory issues, but these features do not differentiate between the two. The rate of progression is also significantly faster in DMD compared to Becker muscular dystrophy, as the former results from a nonsense or frameshift mutation that produces nonfunctional or unstable dystrophin protein, whereas Becker muscular dystrophy results from short deletions that produce some partially functional protein.[11]

▸▸ Question 8

A 65-year-old man has had proximal leg and arm weakness for 3 months. He also reports having a dry mouth and the inability to maintain an erection. He has smoked two packs of cigarettes daily for 35 years. He says the weakness resolves temporarily once he starts moving. On examination, he has areflexia, a waddling gait, and difficulty raising his arms. There is no ptosis. On electromyography of the deltoid muscle, repetitive stimulation (20–50 Hz) causes the compound muscle action potential to double in size. Which of the following is the most likely diagnosis?

- A. Myasthenia gravis
- B. Amyotrophic lateral sclerosis
- C. Lambert–Eaton myasthenic syndrome (LEMS)
- D. Guillain–Barré syndrome
- E. Polymyositis

Correct answer is C

LEMS is characterized by proximal muscle weakness, autonomic symptoms (such as dry mouth and erectile dysfunction, especially in small cell lung cancer–associated cases), and improvement of muscle strength with repeated use (due to increasing Ca^{2+} concentrations in the synaptic cleft with repetitive stimulation). It is caused by autoantibodies against P/Q-type calcium channels in the presynaptic terminal, and electromyography showing increased muscle action potentials with repetitive stimulation indicates LEMS. It is often associated with small-cell lung carcinoma, especially in heavy smokers. Myasthenia gravis typically presents with fluctuating muscle weakness without autonomic involvement; ptosis is also characteristic. Symptoms usually worsen throughout the day and with repetitive activation due to progressive depletion of presynaptic acetylcholine stores. Classically, the edrophonium (Tensilon test)—observation of symptom improvement following administration of the acetylcholinesterase inhibitor edrophonium —was used to help with diagnosis. Amyotrophic lateral sclerosis presents with both upper and lower motor neuron signs. Guillain–Barré syndrome typically presents with ascending paralysis and areflexia. Polymyositis involves proximal muscle weakness but lacks the autonomic and EMG findings seen in LEMS.

▸▸ Question 9

Two days after digging post holes, a 30-year-old man awakens with severe left shoulder pain, which results in an emergency department visit. Ten days later, he noticed weakness of the left shoulder girdle muscles and biceps. By 3 weeks, there is obvious atrophy of the involved muscles. Little or no change in sensory function is noted on follow-up examination. Which of the following is the most likely diagnosis?

- A. Cervical radiculopathy
- B. Brachial plexitis
- C. Rotator cuff tear
- D. Thoracic outlet syndrome
- E. Myasthenia gravis

Correct answer is B

Brachial plexitis, also known as Parsonage–Turner syndrome, affects 3 to 100 per 100,000 persons annually, typically presenting with a sudden onset of severe shoulder/arm pain followed by weakness and atrophy of the shoulder girdle and proximal arm muscles. Sensory changes are usually minimal or absent. This condition often follows triggers such as physical exertion, surgery, or viral illness. Cervical radiculopathy would present with sensory changes and specific nerve root distribution weakness; here, C5 or C6 radiculopathy would need to be excluded. Rotator cuff tear presents with shoulder pain and weakness but lacks the sudden onset, and atrophy would only be expected at a very late stage with chronic limb disuse. Thoracic outlet syndrome involves compression of the brachial plexus (usually with arm elevation) and subclavian vessels, leading to symptoms in the arm and hand. Myasthenia gravis (MG) presents with fluctuating muscle weakness without the acute pain or progressive atrophy seen in brachial plexitis. Weakness in MG is also commonly bilateral.

▸▸ Question 10

A 37-year-old man has severe medication-resistant pain 2 years after a traumatic brachial plexus avulsion. There is no evidence of the return of function. Which of the following surgical interventions is most appropriate for the management of this patient's pain?

- A. Peripheral nerve grafting
- B. Spinal cord stimulation
- C. Motor cortex stimulation
- D. Dorsal root entry zone lesioning
- E. Intrathecal baclofen pump

Correct answer is D

Dorsal root entry zone lesioning is a surgical technique used to manage intractable pain following preganglionic brachial plexus avulsion. It involves creating dorsal root entry zone lesions to disrupt pain pathways. This procedure is particularly effective for deafferentation pain resulting from nerve root avulsions. Peripheral nerve grafting is not indicated in cases with no potential for functional recovery (i.e., 2 years after injury); it would also not treat the patient's pain. Spinal cord stimulation and motor cortex stimulation are options for chronic pain but are not as effective for deafferentation pain. Intrathecal baclofen is used for spasticity rather than pain management.[12]

▸▸ Question 11

A 27-year-old man is evaluated because of muscular dystrophy. Examination shows greater distal than proximal weakness in the extremities. Which of the following types of muscular dystrophy is most likely in this patient?

- A. Duchenne muscular dystrophy
- B. Becker muscular dystrophy
- C. Myotonic dystrophy
- D. Limb-girdle muscular dystrophy
- E. Facioscapulohumeral muscular dystrophy

Correct answer is C

Myotonic dystrophy is a disease caused by CTG trinucleotide expansion of the dystrophia myotonic protein kinase (*DMPK*) gene and is characterized by greater distal than proximal weakness and myotonia (delayed relaxation after muscle contraction). It is a multisystem disorder that can also present with cataracts, cardiac arrhythmias, and endocrine abnormalities. Duchenne and Becker muscular dystrophies primarily affect proximal muscles and are present earlier in life. Limb-girdle muscular dystrophy involves proximal muscles, particularly around the hips and shoulders. Facioscapulohumeral muscular dystrophy typically affects facial and shoulder muscles.

▸▸ Question 12

A 45-year-old man presents with new-onset right forearm pain and slowly progressive weakness in his right hand. Physical examination shows mild wrist extension weakness with radial deviation, severe weakness of finger and thumb extension, and weakness of thumb abduction. Findings on sensory examination are normal. Spurling's sign is absent. Deltoid, biceps, triceps, and brachioradialis strength is normal. Which of the following is the most likely diagnosis?

- A. Cubital tunnel syndrome
- B. Carpal tunnel syndrome

- C. Posterior interosseous nerve (PIN) syndrome
- D. C6 radiculopathy
- E. Thoracic outlet syndrome

Correct answer is C

PIN syndrome, a form of radial nerve entrapment (usually at the arcade of Frohse), typically presents with weakness in finger and thumb extension and wrist extension with radial deviation. Sensory examination is normal because the PIN is a motor nerve. Radial tunnel syndrome also involves radial nerve entrapment at the radial tunnel (proximal forearm) but usually presents with pain rather than motor weakness. Carpal tunnel syndrome affects the median nerve, causing sensory and motor deficits in the hand. C6 radiculopathy and thoracic outlet syndrome would present with different patterns of weakness and sensory loss (▶ Fig. 7.1).

▸▸ Question 13

A 45-year-old male laborer is evaluated for a 3-month history of progressive numbness of the ring and little fingers and dorsomedial aspect of the left hand. He has no history of serious illness and takes no medication. Physical examination shows weakness of the interossei muscles of the hand. Compression in which of the following structures is most likely?

- A. Carpal tunnel
- B. Cubital tunnel
- C. Guyon canal
- D. Thoracic outlet
- E. Spinal groove

Correct answer is B

Cubital tunnel syndrome results from ulnar nerve compression at the elbow. It presents with numbness in the ring and little fingers and weakness predominantly of the intrinsic hand muscles, such as the interossei and the adductor pollicis. Compression at Guyon canal (compression of the ulnar nerve at the wrist) is less common than cubital tunnel syndrome. Compression of the ulnar nerve at Guyon canal also frequently results in interossei weakness, but sensation on the dorsum of the wrist would be normal (note, the dorsal cutaneous branch of the ulnar nerve originates about 6–8 cm above the wrist). Carpal tunnel syndrome involves the median nerve at the wrist and would produce sensory loss in the radial 3½ digits and, in severe cases, weakness in the abductor pollicis brevis (not the interossei). Thoracic outlet syndrome and radial nerve compression at the spiral groove involve different sensory and motor deficit patterns (▶ Fig. 7.2).

▸▸ Question 14

A 27-year-old woman undergoes placement of a right ventriculoperitoneal shunt. The catheter track passes through the right posterior triangle of the neck. Postoperatively, she is unable to lift the right arm more than 45 degrees. Injury to which of the following nerves is the most likely cause of this weakness?

- A. Phrenic nerve
- B. Spinal accessory nerve
- C. Brachial plexus
- D. Long thoracic nerve
- E. Dorsal scapular nerve

Correct answer is B

The spinal accessory nerve innervates the sternocleidomastoid and trapezius muscles. In the posterior triangle, the accessory nerve innervation to the trapezius is at risk. Injury to this nerve during surgery in the posterior triangle of the neck is well known from procedures such as lymph node biopsies but also can occur with shunt tunneling. Spinal accessory nerve dysfunction leads to loss of scapular stability, which manifests itself with difficulty lifting the arm (despite abductors (deltoid and supraspinatus muscles) and a winged scapula. The other nerves listed would affect different muscle groups and functions (▶ Fig. 7.3).

▸▸ Question 15

Which of the following muscles is most likely to compress the posterior interosseous nerve in the proximal forearm?

- A. Brachioradialis
- B. Supinator
- C. Pronator teres
- D. Flexor carpi radialis
- E. Palmaris longus

Correct answer is B

The supinator arch (arcade of Frohse) is a fibrous band connecting the two heads of the supinator muscle and can compress the radial nerve in the proximal forearm, leading to radial tunnel

Cardinal features

- Inability to extend fingers at metacarpophalangeal joints
- No wrist drop (but radial deviation on wrist extension due to involvement of extensor carpi ulnaris and sparing of extensor carpi radialis)
- Sensation normal

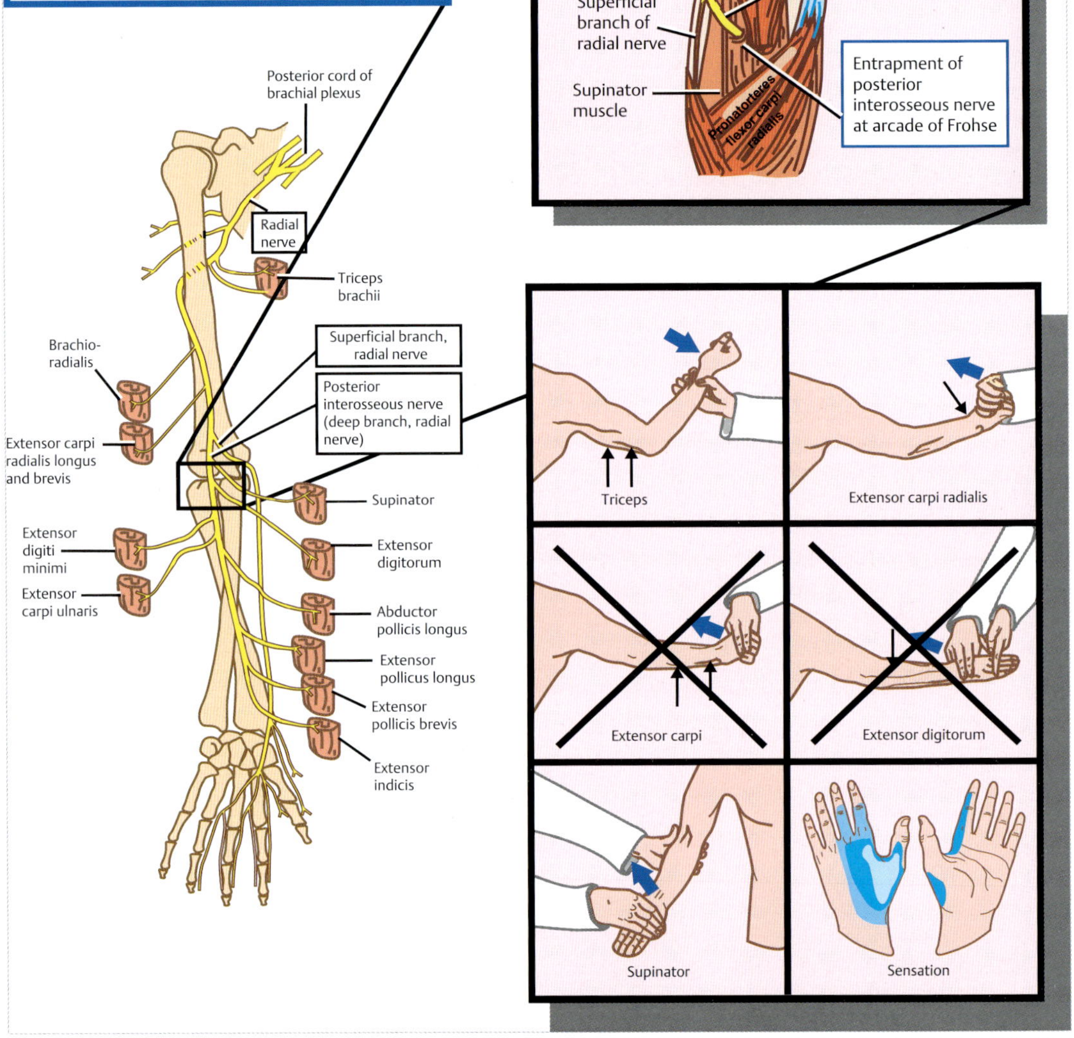

Fig. 7.1 (Source: Reproduced from Posterior interosseous nerve syndrome. In: Alberstone C, Benzel E, Jones S, Wang Z, Steinmetz M, eds. Anatomic Basis of Neurologic Diagnosis. 2nd ed. New York: Thieme; 2023.)

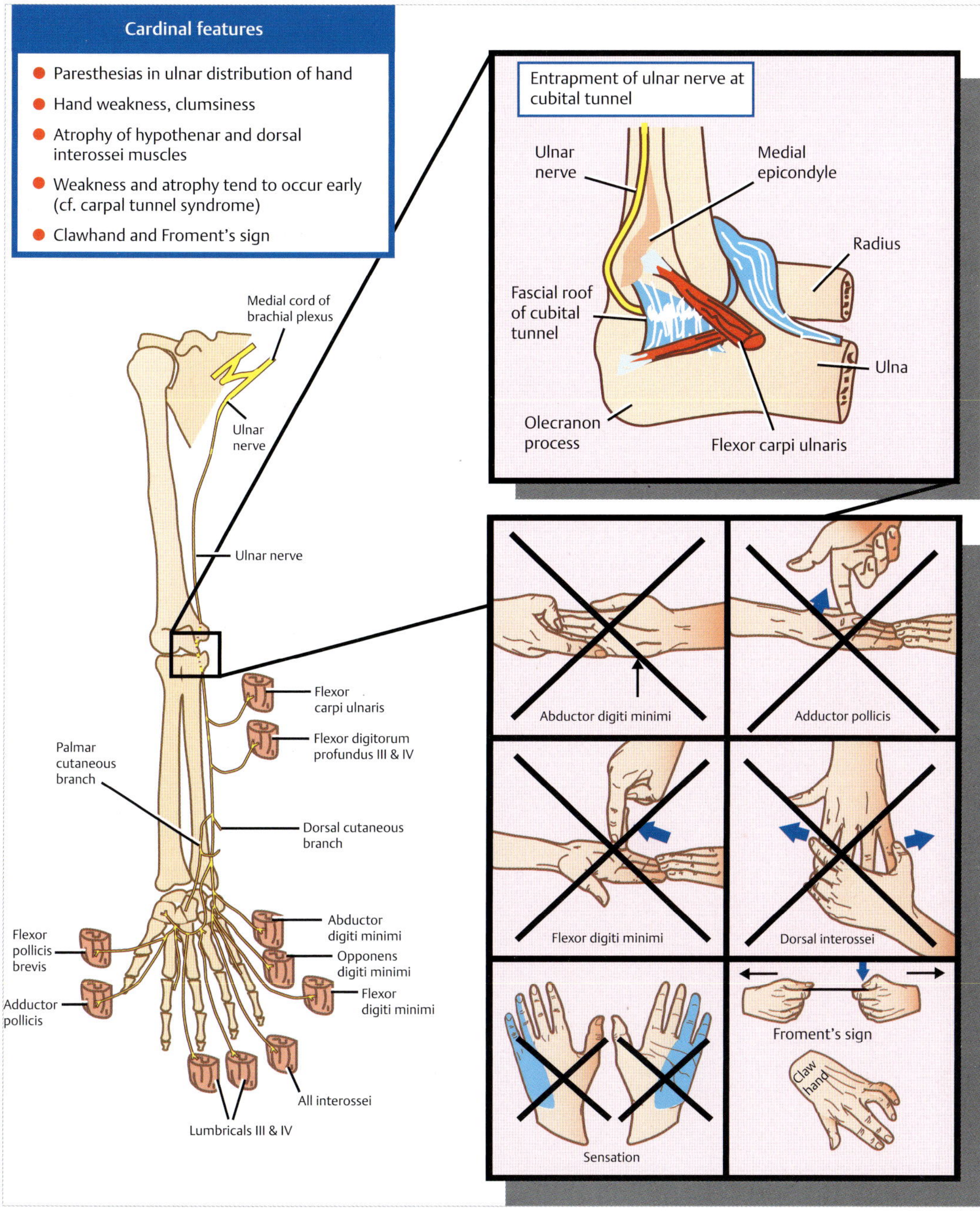

Fig. 7.2 (Source: Reproduced from Cubital tunnel syndrome. In: Alberstone C, Benzel E, Jones S, Wang Z, Steinmetz M, eds. Anatomic Basis of Neurologic Diagnosis. 2nd ed. New York: Thieme; 2023.)

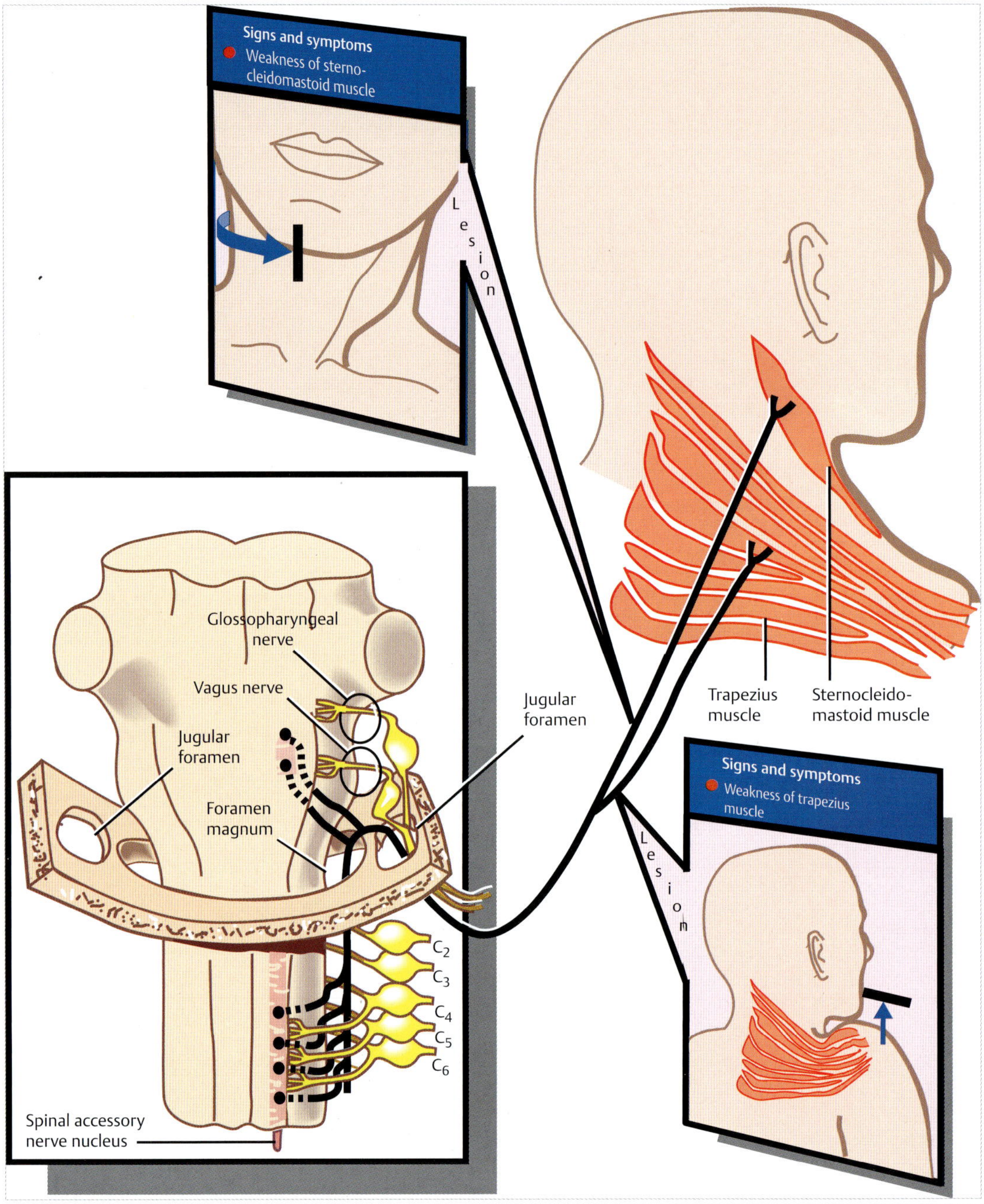

Fig. 7.3 (Source: Reproduced from The accessory nerve. In: Alberstone C, Benzel E, Jones S, Wang Z, Steinmetz M, eds. Anatomic Basis of Neurologic Diagnosis. 2nd ed. New York: Thieme; 2023.)

syndrome or posterior interosseous nerve syndrome. Compression of the posterior interosseous nerve (PIN) may result in pain and/or weakness in the posterior interosseous nerve distribution. The other muscles listed are not typically involved in PIN compression.

▸▸ Question 16

A 75-year-old woman presents with wrist and finger drop immediately after a fall on an outstretched arm and mid-shaft humeral fracture. Sensory examination reveals hypesthesia to light touch on the dorsal forearm and wrist. Spurling's sign is absent. Strength of the deltoid, biceps, and triceps is normal. Which of the following is the most likely diagnosis?
- A. Radial nerve injury
- B. Posterior interosseous nerve syndrome
- C. C6 radiculopathy
- D. Radial tunnel syndrome
- E. Thoracic outlet syndrome

Correct answer is A

Radial nerve injury is well known after arm trauma, such as humeral fractures; injury may occur where the radial nerve is vulnerable near the spiral groove. Radial nerve lesions can also occur from "Saturday night palsy" or compression of the arm (such as from prolonged pressure on it with alcohol or drug use). Radial nerve compression results in weakness or paralysis of the wrist and finger extensors. Triceps innervation is more proximal (axilla) and is normal in cases of arm-level compression. Posterior interosseous nerve syndrome presents with motor deficits in the distribution of the posterior interosseous nerve, including weakness of finger and thumb extension, wrist extension, and thumb abduction without sensory loss. Wrist extension is in radial deviation, as classically the nerve to the extensor carpi radialis longus (which arises proximal to the arcade of Frohse) is preserved and the nerve to the extensor carpi ulnaris is affected (it arises distal to the arcade of Frohse [point of compression in PIN]). Radial tunnel syndrome is described as a pain syndrome affecting the posterior interosseous nerve without motor deficits. C6 radiculopathy and thoracic outlet syndrome would present with different patterns of sensory and motor deficits (▸ Fig. 7.4).[13]

▸▸ Question 17

A 47-year-old man rides his bicycle 180 miles during a 2-day race. After the race, he complains that his right hand feels weak, and his fifth finger is abducted, as shown in the photograph. Dysfunction of which of the following nerves is present in this patient?
- A. Median nerve
- B. Radial nerve
- C. Ulnar nerve
- D. Musculocutaneous nerve
- E. Axillary nerve

Correct answer is C

The ulnar nerve is responsible for the innervation of the intrinsic hand muscles, including those controlling the fifth finger. Prolonged compression of the ulnar nerve during activities such as long-distance cycling can lead to ulnar neuropathy from compression of the nerve at Guyon canal, commonly known as ulnar tunnel syndrome or "handlebar palsy." This condition is characterized by ulnar-innervated muscle weakness in the hand, typically also with numbness in the ulnar 1½ digits on the palmar side. Dorsal sensation on the wrist/hand would be intact due to preservation of the dorsal cutaneous nerve. Cubital tunnel syndrome typically has sensory loss on the dorsoulnar aspect of the hand as well. Other nerves listed have different patterns of loss (▸ Fig. 7.5).

▸▸ Question 18

In patients with Duchenne muscular dystrophy, pseudohypertrophy of which of the following is the most common finding?
- A. Biceps
- B. Calves
- C. Thighs
- D. Deltoids
- E. Forearms

Correct answer is B

Pseudohypertrophy of the calves is a hallmark finding in Duchenne muscular dystrophy, resulting from the replacement of muscle tissue with fat and fibrous tissue. This gives the calves a bulky appearance despite muscle weakness. Pseudohypertrophy can occasionally be seen in other muscle groups but is most pronounced in the calves.

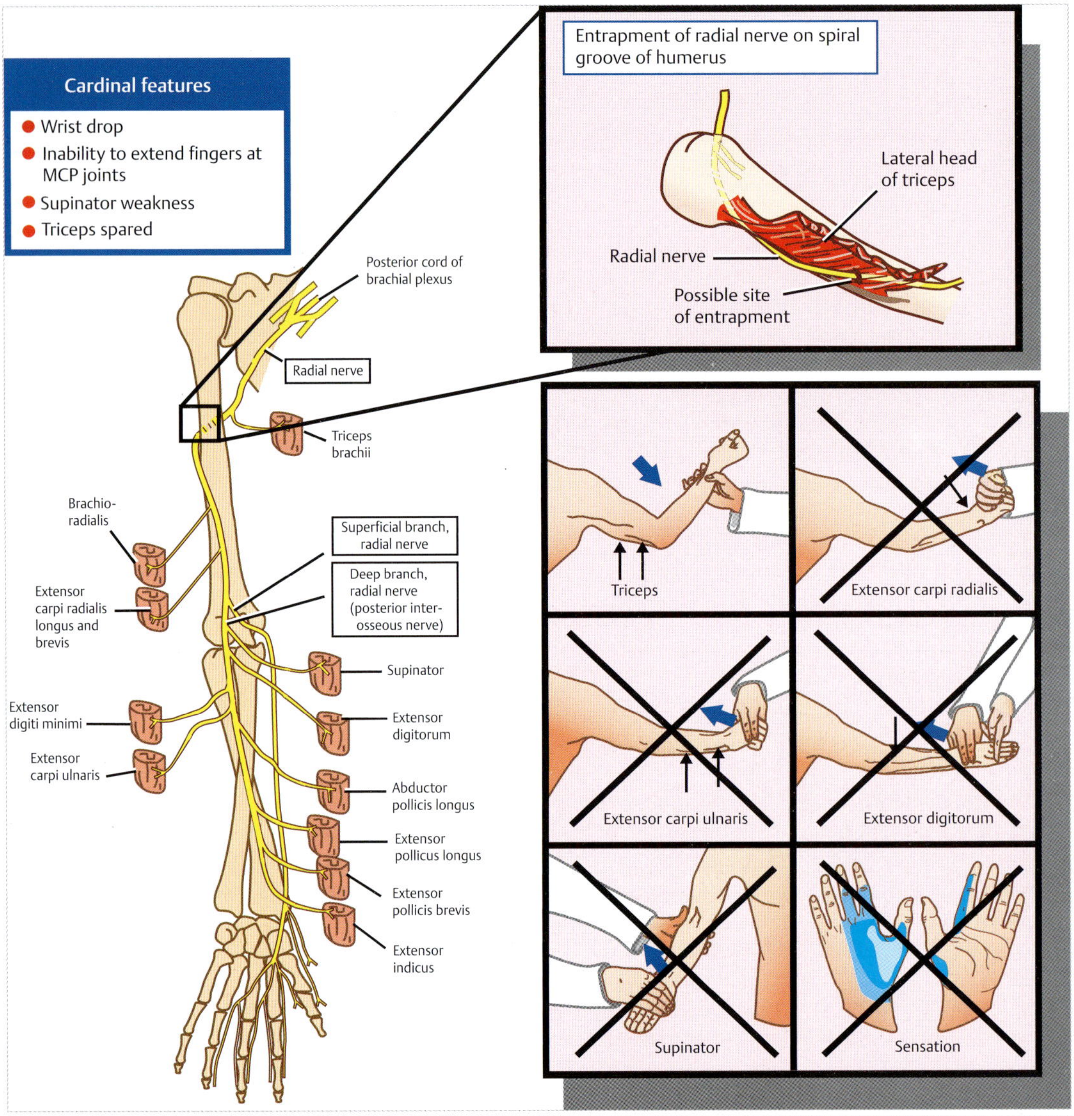

Fig. 7.4 (Source: Reproduced from Radial nerve palsy. In: Alberstone C, Benzel E, Jones S, Wang Z, Steinmetz M, eds. Anatomic Basis of Neurologic Diagnosis. 2nd ed. New York: Thieme; 2023.)

▸▸ Question 19

A patient presents with loss of thumb abduction/opposition and thenar muscle atrophy. Compression of which nerve is most likely responsible?

- A. Radial nerve
- B. Ulnar nerve
- C. Median nerve
- D. Axillary nerve
- E. Musculocutaneous nerve

Correct answer is C

Compression of the median nerve can lead to loss of thumb abduction and opposition and atrophy of the thenar muscles. Compression most commonly occurs at the carpal tunnel, the anatomical thoroughfare roofed by the transverse

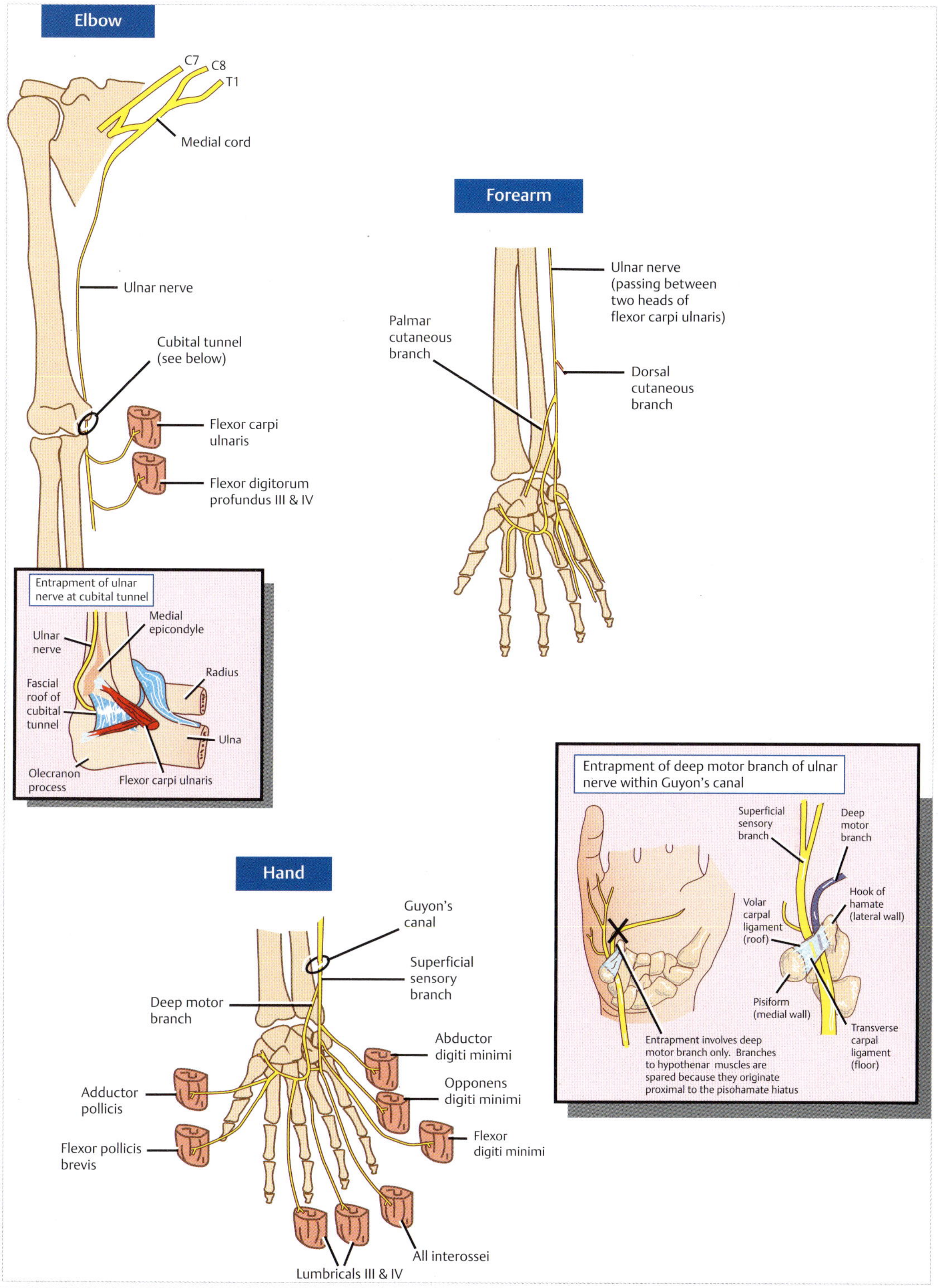

Fig. 7.5 (Source: Reproduced from Anatomy. In: Alberstone C, Benzel E, Jones S, Wang Z, Steinmetz M, eds. Anatomic Basis of Neurologic Diagnosis. 2nd ed. New York: Thieme; 2023.)

carpal ligament. This condition is known as carpal tunnel syndrome and treatment is initially nonoperative with a wrist orthosis, but in refractory cases is treated with release of the transverse carpal ligament. The median nerve innervates the thenar muscles, which are responsible for thumb abduction (abductor pollicis brevis) and opposition (opponens pollicis). Radial nerve compression affects the wrist and finger extensor muscles as well as the abductor pollicis longus but not intrinsic muscles, including the thenar muscles. The ulnar nerve innervates the intrinsic hand muscles, excluding the thenar muscles; the axillary nerve innervates the deltoid muscle, and the musculocutaneous nerve, the biceps. ▶ Fig. 7.6 demonstrates Carpal tunnel syndrome. Functions or

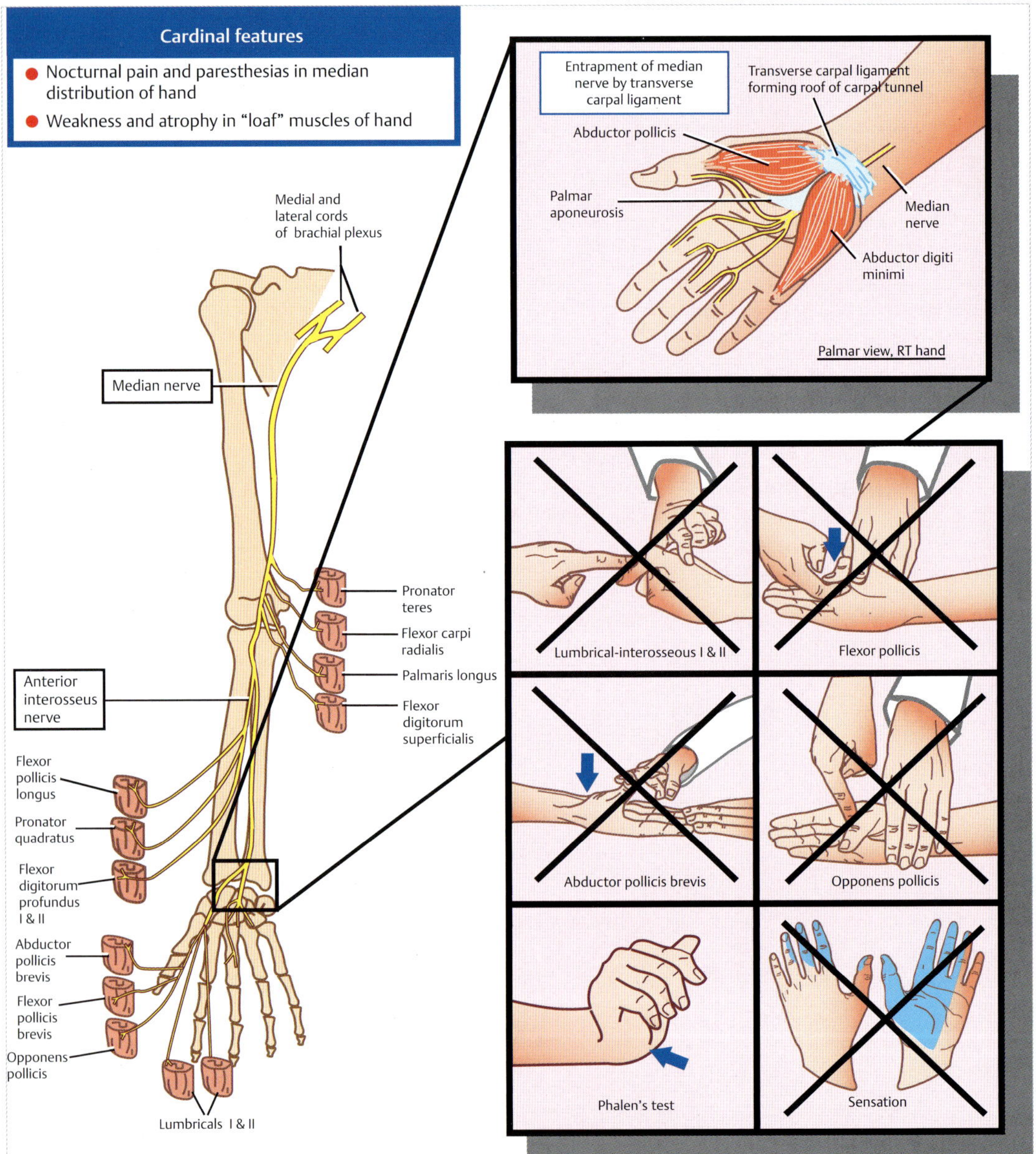

Fig. 7.6 (Source: Reproduced from Carpal tunnel syndrome. In: Alberstone C, Benzel E, Jones S, Wang Z, Steinmetz M, eds. Anatomic Basis of Neurologic Diagnosis. 2nd ed. New York: Thieme; 2023.)

responses marked with an "X" are impaired or absent.

▸▸ Question 20

What is the most common physical examination finding in patients with carpal tunnel syndrome?
- A. Positive elbow flexion test
- B. Positive Phalen's test
- C. Thenar atrophy
- D. Decreased grip strength
- E. Sensory loss in the little finger

Correct answer is B

A positive Phalen's test is one of the most common physical examination findings in patients with carpal tunnel syndrome, though its diagnostic utility is weak, with a sensitivity of 50% and specificity of 33%. This test involves flexing the wrist maximally and holding the position for 60 seconds, which often reproduces the symptoms of carpal tunnel syndrome, such as tingling or numbness in the median nerve distribution. Tinel sign is also commonly positive. Thenar atrophy and decreased grip strength can occur in more advanced cases. Elbow flexion is a provocative test for ulnar nerve compression at the elbow. Sensory loss in the little finger suggests ulnar nerve involvement rather than the median nerve.

▸▸ Question 21

Which of the following muscles is most likely to exhibit weakness following an upper trunk avulsion injury?
- A. Deltoid
- B. Triceps
- C. Latissimus dorsi
- D. Extensor digitorum
- E. Pronator teres

Correct answer is A

An upper trunk avulsion injury of the brachial plexus typically affects the C5 and C6 nerve roots, leading to weakness in muscles innervated by these roots, such as the deltoid, biceps, and infraspinatus. The C7 nerve root innervates the triceps and latissimus dorsi, with lesser contributions from C6 and C8, while the C6 and C7 root contributions to the median nerve are responsible for pronator teres activation. The extensor digitorum is primarily innervated by the C7 nerve root via the posterior interosseous branch of the radial nerve. Brachialis and brachioradialis weakness are also seen in upper trunk injuries (▸ Fig. 7.7).

▸▸ Question 22

A 45-year-old man presents with finger flexion weakness after an elbow dislocation. Which nerve is most likely injured?
- A. Median nerve
- B. Ulnar nerve
- C. Radial nerve
- D. Axillary nerve
- E. Musculocutaneous nerve

Correct answer is A

Different nerves may be injured with elbow dislocations or fractures. Median nerve injuries affect finger flexion and thumb opposition. Radial nerve injury is commonly associated with humeral fractures and can lead to wrist drop and an inability to extend the fingers. The radial nerve innervates the extensor muscles of the forearm and hand and can be injured in the spiral groove following humeral fractures. Ulnar nerve injuries affect the intrinsic hand muscles. Shoulder trauma may result in axillary nerve injuries (to the deltoid muscle) and musculocutaneous nerve injuries (to the biceps).

▸▸ Question 23

Which clinical feature helps differentiate common peroneal neuropathy from L5-radiculopathy?
- A. Ankle dorsiflexion weakness
- B. Foot eversion weakness
- C. Toe extensor weakness
- D. Inversion weakness of the foot
- E. Absence of ankle reflex

Correct answer is D

Inversion weakness of the foot tested in plantar flexion is provided by the posterior tibialis muscle (which is L5 and tibial innervated). Ankle dorsiflexion, toe extension, and foot eversion weakness can occur in both L5 radiculopathy and common peroneal neuropathy. The ankle reflex tests the S1 nerve. ▸ Fig. 7.8 demonstrates common peroneal nerve syndrome. Functions or responses marked with an "X" are impaired or absent.

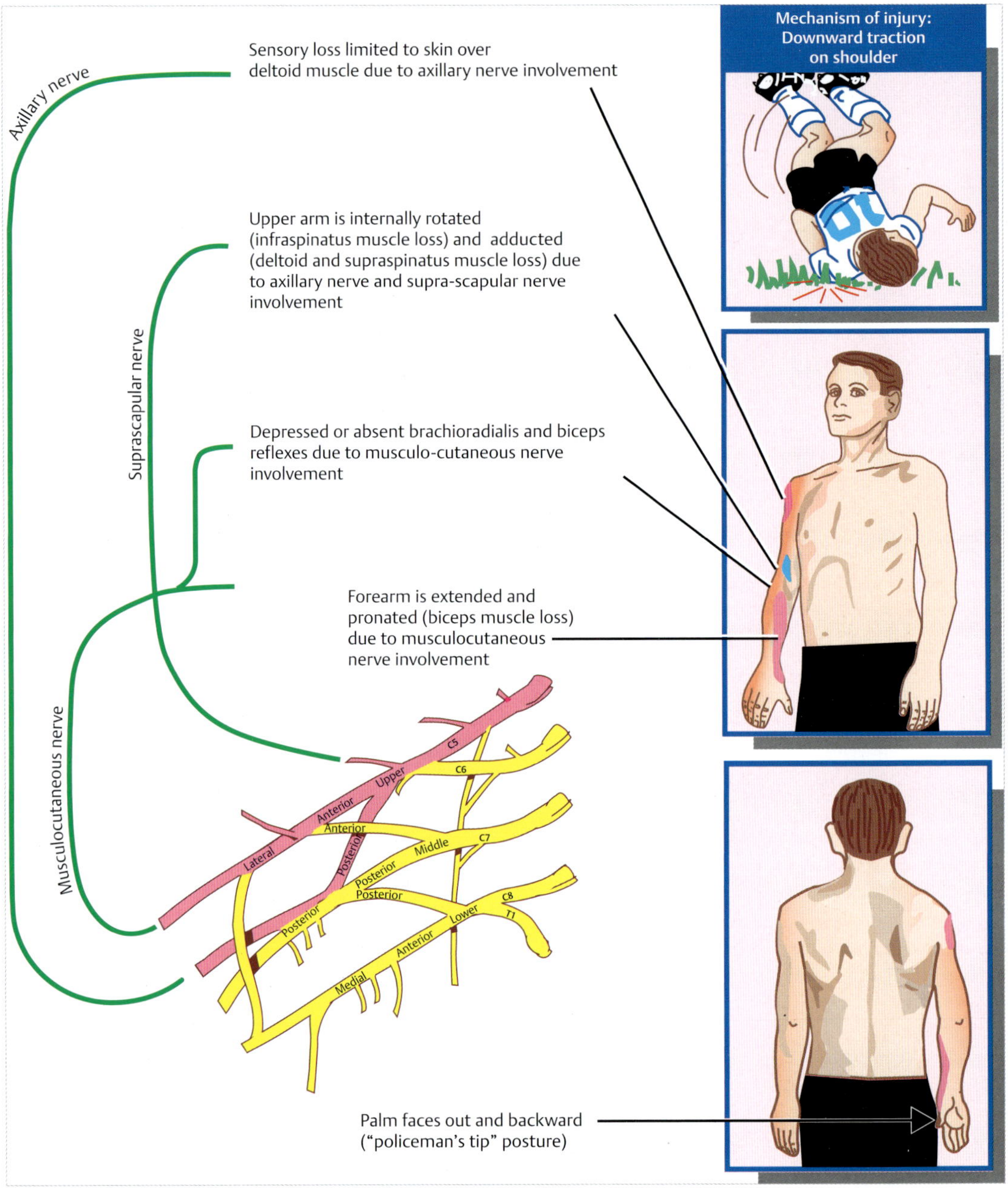

Fig. 7.7 (Source: Reproduced from Lesions of the upper brachial plexus (Erb-Duchenne type). In: Alberstone C, Benzel E, Jones S, Wang Z, Steinmetz M, eds. Anatomic Basis of Neurologic Diagnosis. 2nd ed. New York: Thieme; 2023.)

Cardinal features

- Weakness in foot eversion and dorsiflexion of foot and toes
- Sensory loss involving the lateral lower leg and the dorsum of the foot and toes

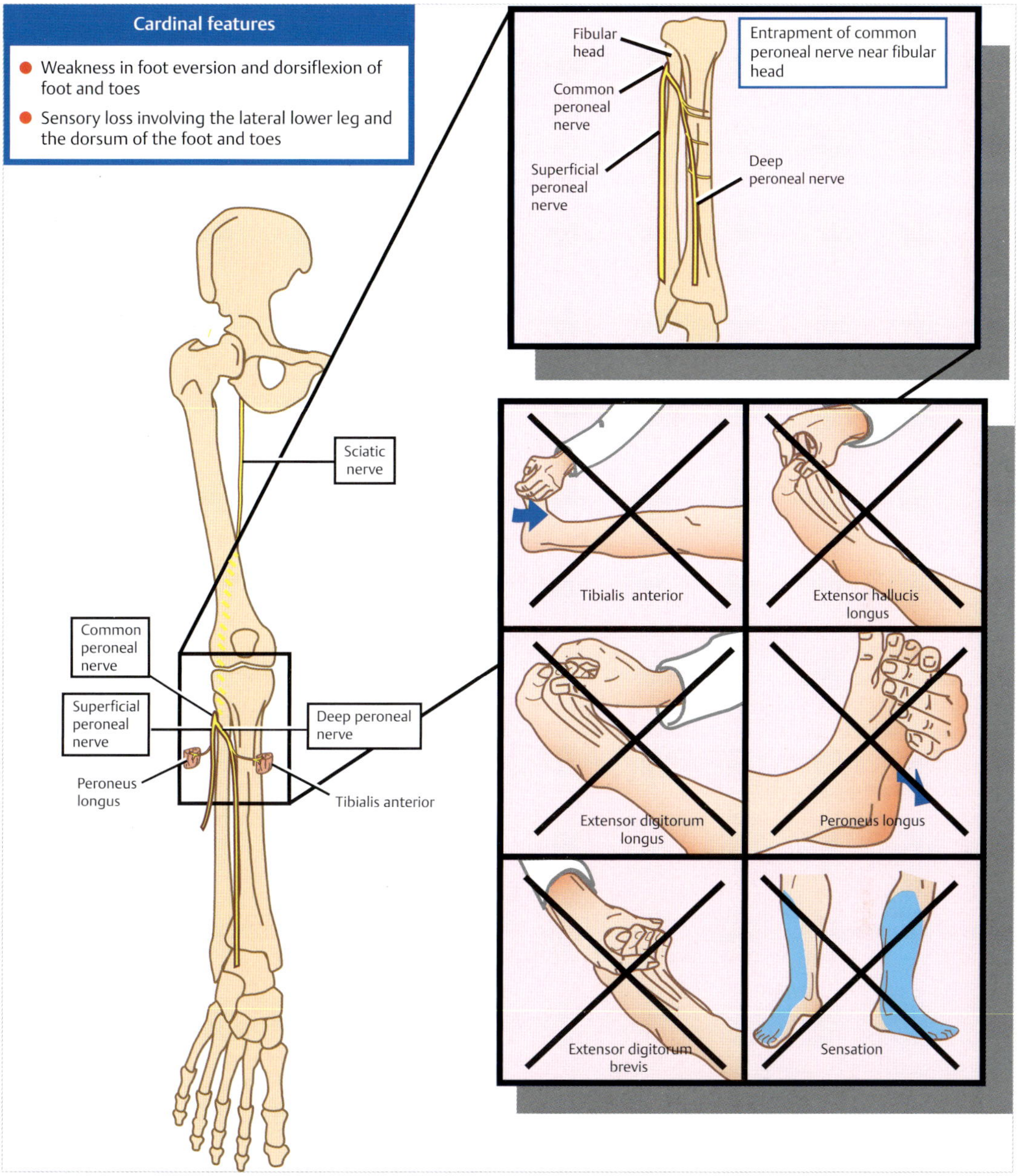

Fig. 7.8 (Source: Reproduced from Peroneal nerve syndrome. In: Alberstone C, Benzel E, Najm I, Steinmetz M, eds. Anatomic basis of neurologic diagnosis. 1st ed. New York: Thieme; 2009.)

▸▸ Question 24

What is the most common presenting symptom of Guillain–Barré syndrome in children?

- A. Proximal muscle weakness
- B. Distal sensory loss
- C. Back pain
- D. Facial paralysis
- E. Ascending muscle weakness

Correct answer is E

The most common presenting symptom of Guillain–Barré syndrome in children is ascending muscle weakness. This typically starts in the lower extremities and progresses upwards. Distal sensory loss, back pain, and facial paralysis can also occur but are less common as initial symptoms. Proximal muscle weakness is seen in later stages as the condition progresses.

▸▸ Question 25

A patient presents with weakness in the deltoid and biceps muscles following a motorcycle collision. MRI reveals an avulsion of the C5 nerve root. Which other muscle is most likely to be weak in this patient?

- A. Triceps
- B. Brachioradialis
- C. Pronator teres
- D. Flexor carpi ulnaris
- E. Palmaris longus

Correct answer is B

In a C5 nerve root avulsion, muscles innervated by the C5 nerve root will be affected. These include the deltoid, supraspinatus, infraspinatus, biceps, and brachioradialis muscles. The C7 nerve root primarily innervates the triceps. The median nerve from the C6 and C7 roots innervates the pronator teres. Flexor carpi ulnaris is innervated by the ulnar nerve (C8–T1), and palmaris longus is innervated by the median nerve (C7–C8). Coronal T2-weighted maximum intensity projection MRI image shows two right cervical nerve root avulsions (see *arrows* in ▸ Fig. 7.9).

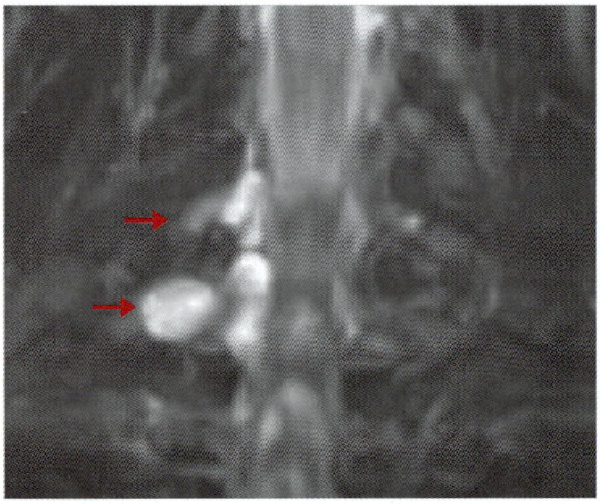

Fig. 7.9 (Source: Reproduced from Cervical nerve root avulsion. In: Alberstone C, Benzel E, Jones S, Wang Z, Steinmetz M, eds. Anatomic Basis of Neurologic Diagnosis. 2nd ed. New York: Thieme; 2023.)

▸▸ Question 26

Which muscle most likely exhibits atrophy following a median nerve injury at the wrist?

- A. Abductor pollicis brevis
- B. Adductor pollicis
- C. Flexor digitorum profundus
- D. Flexor carpi ulnaris
- E. Extensor pollicis longus

Correct answer is A

The abductor pollicis brevis muscle, innervated by the median nerve, is located in the thenar eminence of the hand. Median nerve injury at the wrist, such as in severe carpal tunnel syndrome, leads to atrophy of the thenar muscles. The adductor pollicis is innervated by the ulnar nerve. Flexor digitorum profundus has dual innervation in the proximal forearm from the median and ulnar nerves, while flexor carpi ulnaris and extensor pollicis longus are innervated by the ulnar and radial nerves, respectively.

▸▸ Question 27

A patient has a documented radial nerve injury. Which of the following patterns of weakness is expected?

- A. Weakness in finger abduction
- B. Weakness in thumb opposition
- C. Weakness in elbow flexion
- D. Weakness in wrist extension
- E. Weakness in shoulder abduction

Correct answer is D

Radial nerve injury typically results in wrist extension (wrist drop) and finger extension weakness. Finger abduction is controlled by the ulnar nerve, thumb opposition by the median nerve, elbow flexion by the musculocutaneous nerve, and shoulder abduction by the axillary nerve.

▸▸ Question 28

Which of the following clinical findings would most likely indicate an ulnar nerve injury at the elbow?

- A. Weakness in forearm supination
- B. Weakness in wrist flexion
- C. Atrophy of the hypothenar eminence
- D. Loss of sensation in the thumb
- E. Weakness in elbow extension

Correct answer is C

Ulnar nerve injury at the elbow often results in atrophy of the hypothenar eminence, which is innervated by the ulnar nerve. The radial nerve (supinator) and musculocutaneous nerve (biceps brachii) control forearm supination, wrist flexion is primarily controlled by the median nerve (though flexor carpi ulnaris is innervated by the ulnar nerve), the median nerve provides sensation in the thumb, and the radial nerve controls elbow extension. ▸ Fig. 7.10 shows a Gilliatt-Sumner hand. Note the atrophy of the thenar and the hypothenar eminences of the right hand.

▸▸ Question 29

A 50-year-old woman presents with a history of difficulty with fastening buttons, handwriting, and other fine motor movements in her right hand. Physical examination reveals clawing of the ring and little fingers and atrophy of the first dorsal interosseous muscle. Which nerve is most likely affected?

- A. Median nerve
- B. Ulnar nerve
- C. Radial nerve
- D. Musculocutaneous nerve
- E. Axillary nerve

Correct answer is B

Clawing of the ring, little fingers, and atrophy of the first dorsal interosseous muscle are classic signs of ulnar nerve injury. The ulnar nerve innervates the intrinsic muscles of the hand, which are responsible for fine motor movements (such as buttoning or pinching). The median nerve innervates the thenar muscles, the radial nerve innervates the extensor muscles, the musculocutaneous nerve innervates the biceps, and the axillary nerve innervates the deltoid.[14]

▸▸ Question 30

A patient develops difficulty lifting the arm following a neck dissection surgery; physical examination shows lateral displacement of their shoulder blade. Which nerve is likely damaged?

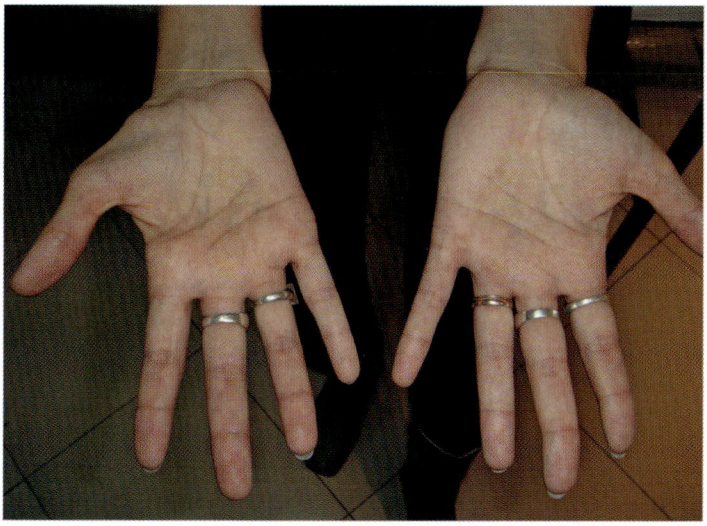

Fig. 7.10 (Source: Reproduced from Important concepts regarding TOS. In: Socolovsky M, Rasulic L, Midha R, Garozzo D, eds. Manual of Peripheral Nerve Surgery: From the Basics to Complex Procedures. 1st ed. Stuttgart: Thieme; 2017.)

- A. Long thoracic nerve
- B. Spinal accessory nerve
- C. Dorsal scapular nerve
- D. Axillary nerve
- E. Suprascapular nerve

Correct answer is B

The spinal accessory nerve, when damaged, can lead to lateral scapular winging and difficulty lifting the arm and elevating the shoulder due to the paralysis of the trapezius muscle. The spinal accessory nerve is at risk when doing lymph node dissections or biopsies in the neck. A long thoracic nerve injury causes medial scapular winging by affecting the serratus anterior muscle. The dorsal scapular, axillary, and suprascapular nerves do not cause scapular winging but affect other shoulder muscles.[15]

▸▸ Question 31

In patients with myotonic dystrophy, which endocrine abnormality is commonly observed?

- A. Hypothyroidism
- B. Hyperthyroidism
- C. Diabetes mellitus
- D. Addison disease
- E. Hyperparathyroidism

Correct answer is C

Diabetes mellitus is a common endocrine abnormality in patients with myotonic dystrophy. This condition is characterized by insulin resistance, leading to diabetes. Other endocrine abnormalities like hypothyroidism, hyperthyroidism, Addison disease, and hyperparathyroidism are less commonly associated with myotonic dystrophy.

▸▸ Question 32

Which genetic mutation is responsible for Duchenne muscular dystrophy?

- A. *DMD* gene deletion
- B. *SMN1* gene deletion
- C. *NF1* gene mutation
- D. GAA trinucleotide repeat expansion
- E. *PMP22* gene duplication

Correct answer is A

Duchenne muscular dystrophy is caused by nonsense or frameshift mutations in the *DMD* gene, leading to a nonfunctional form of the protein dystrophin with resultant muscle degeneration and weakness. *SMN1* gene deletion is associated with spinal muscular atrophy, *NF1* gene mutation with neurofibromatosis type 1, GAA trinucleotide repeat expansion with Friedreich's ataxia, and *PMP22* gene duplication with Charcot–Marie–Tooth disease type 1A.

▸▸ Question 33

A 62-year-old woman presents with progressive weakness in the legs and arms, areflexia, and sensory loss in a stocking-glove distribution. What is the most likely diagnosis?

- A. Myasthenia gravis
- B. Guillain–Barré syndrome (GBS)
- C. Multiple sclerosis
- D. Amyotrophic lateral sclerosis
- E. Chronic inflammatory demyelinating polyneuropathy (CIDP)

Correct answer is B

GBS is characterized by acute, progressive weakness, areflexia, and sensory loss in a stocking-glove distribution. It is an autoimmune disorder often triggered by an infection. Myasthenia gravis presents with fluctuating muscle weakness, multiple sclerosis with central nervous system lesions (leading to upper motor neuron findings, including hyperreflexia), amyotrophic lateral sclerosis with both upper and lower motor neuron signs, and CIDP with a chronic course.

▸▸ Question 34

A 34-year-old woman presents with numbness and tingling in her right hand, affecting the thumb, index, and middle fingers. Which nerve is most likely compressed?

- A. Radial nerve
- B. Ulnar nerve
- C. Median nerve
- D. Axillary nerve
- E. Musculocutaneous nerve

Correct answer is C

Compression of the median nerve, particularly in the carpal tunnel, leads to numbness and tingling in the thumb, index, and middle, and half of the ring fingers. This is characteristic of carpal tunnel syndrome. Radial nerve compression affects the dorsal hand, ulnar nerve compression affects half of the ring and little fingers, and the axillary and musculocutaneous nerves are associated with sensory loss in the lateral shoulder and lateral forearm, respectively.

▸▸ Question 35

A 45-year-old man presents with a right foot drop and numbness over the dorsal foot following a car accident during which the vehicle in which she was a passenger was T-boned on the front passenger side. What is the most likely diagnosis?

- A. L4 radiculopathy
- B. L5 radiculopathy
- C. Sciatic nerve injury
- D. Common peroneal nerve injury
- E. Tarsal tunnel syndrome

Correct answer is D

Common peroneal nerve injury, often caused by trauma near the fibular head or knee (e.g., due to impaction of the lateral knee/leg against a car door during a motor vehicle accident), leads to foot drop and numbness over the dorsal foot. L4 radiculopathy affects the anteromedial shin; L5 radiculopathy can cause similar symptoms as peroneal nerve injury but includes back pain and inversion weakness. Sciatic nerve injury typically affects the entire leg—with ankle and foot dorsiflexion/plantarflexion, toe extension and flexion, and eversion/inversion weakness, as well as numbness below the knee (except for the medial leg/foot from the saphenous nerve). Tarsal tunnel syndrome causes sensory symptoms in the plantar foot.

▸▸ Question 36

A 50-year-old woman presents with progressive weakness and atrophy of the intrinsic hand muscles and hyperreflexia in the lower extremities. Which diagnosis is most likely?

- A. Carpal tunnel syndrome
- B. Amyotrophic lateral sclerosis (ALS)
- C. Cervical spondylotic myelopathy
- D. Multiple sclerosis
- E. Guillain–Barré syndrome

Correct answer is B

ALS is characterized by progressive weakness with a mixture of upper and lower motor neuron findings, e.g., intrinsic hand muscle atrophy (lower motor neuron finding) and hyperreflexia upper motor neuron finding) without sensory symptoms. Carpal tunnel syndrome typically produces sensory symptoms in the thumb, index, middle, and the radial side of the ring finger and affects the median nerve intrinsic muscles (including abductor pollicis brevis) without hyperreflexia. Cervical spondylotic myelopathy presents with more diffuse myelopathic signs, including sensory symptoms. Multiple sclerosis has central nervous system lesions with varying symptoms, and Guillain–Barré syndrome causes areflexia rather than hyperreflexia.

▸▸ Question 37

Which procedure is most effective for relieving intractable cancer-related pain in patients with a life expectancy of less than 3 months?

- A. Intrathecal morphine pump implantation
- B. Spinal cord stimulation
- C. Dorsal root entry zone lesioning
- D. Percutaneous cordotomy
- E. Epidural steroid injection

Correct answer is D

Percutaneous cordotomy is a procedure that can effectively relieve intractable cancer-related pain, particularly in patients with a limited life expectancy. It involves the targeted destruction of pain-conducting pathways in the spinal cord. Intrathecal morphine pumps and spinal cord stimulation are effective for chronic pain management but are less suited for end-of-life care. Dorsal root entry zone lesioning is used for specific types of pain, such as brachial plexus avulsion. Epidural steroid injections are generally used for inflammatory pain but are not effective for cancer-related pain.

▸▸ Question 38

Which patient is most likely to benefit from dorsal column spinal cord stimulation?

- A. A patient with intractable cancer pain
- B. A patient with complex regional pain syndrome (CRPS)
- C. A patient with radicular pain due to lumbar disk herniation
- D. A patient with chronic migraine
- E. A patient with diabetic neuropathy

Correct answer is B

Dorsal column spinal cord stimulation is most effective in treating CRPS and failed back surgery syndrome. It provides significant relief by modulating pain signals at the spinal cord level. While it can be used for radicular pain and diabetic neuropathy, it is not typically the first choice for intractable cancer pain or chronic migraine. Importantly, spinal cord stimulation should not be used in the presence of a compressive lesion—such as spinal stenosis or foraminal narrowing—unless the underlying structural issue has first been adequately addressed, as ongoing compression may reduce efficacy and potentially worsen symptoms.[16]

▸▸ Question 39

Which of the following complications is most commonly associated with high-concentration intrathecal opioid administration?

- A. Granuloma formation
- B. Spinal cord injury
- C. Subdural hematoma
- D. Meningitis
- E. Epidural abscess

Correct answer is A

Granuloma formation is a known complication of long-term intrathecal opioid administration, particularly with high-dose therapy. These granulomas can cause neurological symptoms and require surgical intervention. Spinal cord injury, subdural hematoma, meningitis, and epidural abscess are less common but possible complications of intrathecal drug delivery systems. ▸ Fig. 7.11 shows (**a**) closure of the tip of a spinal catheter through intrathecal granuloma formation at T10 after continuous morphine application for 11 years and (**b**) intrathecal granuloma after 12-year intrathecal residence of a spinal catheter at T9.

▸▸ Question 40

Which of the following is the primary indication for dorsal root entry zone lesioning?

- A. Chronic lower back pain
- B. Cancer-related pain
- C. Phantom limb pain
- D. Pain from brachial plexus avulsion
- E. Post-herpetic neuralgia

Correct answer is D

Dorsal root entry zone lesioning is primarily indicated for treating intractable pain from brachial plexus avulsion injuries. It involves creating dorsal root entry zone lesions to disrupt pain pathways. It is less commonly used for chronic lower back pain, cancer-related pain, phantom limb pain, or post-herpetic neuralgia, for which other treatments are preferred.

▸▸ Question 41

Which test is most useful for confirming the diagnosis of carpal tunnel syndrome?

- A. MRI of the wrist
- B. Nerve conduction study
- C. Ultrasound of the median nerve
- D. Electromyography
- E. Blood tests for inflammation

Correct answer is B

A nerve conduction study is the most useful test for confirming the diagnosis of carpal tunnel syndrome. It measures the speed and amplitude of electrical conduction in the median nerve, identifying delays or blockages indicative of compression. MRI and ultrasound can be useful adjuncts, and EMG can help assess muscle involvement, but nerve conduction study remains the gold standard.

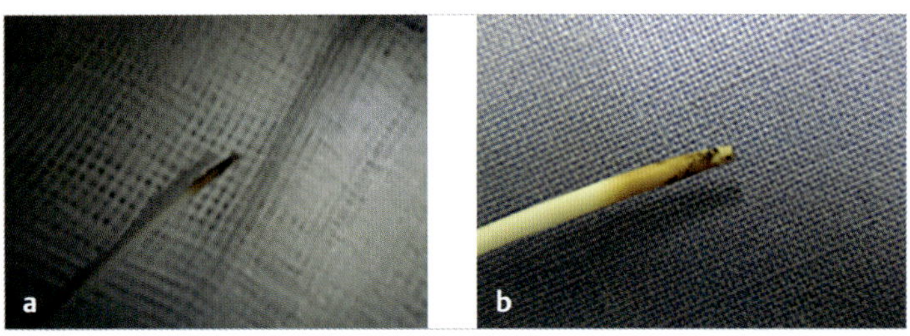

Fig. 7.11 (Source: Reproduced from Foreign body granuloma. In: Kim D, Abdi S, Schütze G, eds. Epiduroscopy: Atlas of Procedures. 1st ed. New York: Thieme; 2017.)

▸▸ **Question 42**

Which electrophysiological finding is most characteristic in patients with suspected Lambert–Eaton myasthenic syndrome (LEMS)?

- A. Decremental response on repetitive nerve stimulation at low frequencies
- B. Incremental response on repetitive nerve stimulation at high frequencies
- C. Prolonged distal motor latencies
- D. Reduced sensory nerve action potentials
- E. Continuous muscle fiber activity on EMG

Correct answer is B

LEMS is characterized by an incremental response to repetitive nerve stimulation at high frequencies due to increased acetylcholine release with repetitive stimulation. This is in contrast to myasthenia gravis, which shows a decremental response at low frequencies. In LEMS, which is characterized by decreased calcium current amplitudes at the presynaptic density due to anti-P/Q-type calcium channel antibodies, repetitive stimulation of the neuron leads to increases in Ca^{2+} in the synaptic button large enough to trigger vesicular fusion. This results in greater acetylcholine release and incremental response. Prolonged distal motor latencies and reduced sensory nerve action potentials are not typical findings in LEMS.

▸▸ **Question 43**

What is electromyography's primary role in evaluating peripheral neuropathies?

- A. Identify metabolic causes of neuropathy
- B. Assess the integrity of the central nervous system
- C. Evaluate muscle function and nerve integrity
- D. Diagnose autoimmune conditions
- E. Measure blood flow to nerves

Correct answer is C

Electromyography is used primarily to evaluate muscle function and nerve integrity in diagnosing peripheral neuropathies. It helps determine the location and extent of nerve damage and can differentiate between neuropathies and myopathies. It does not identify metabolic causes, diagnose autoimmune conditions, or measure blood flow.[17]

▸▸ **Question 44**

Which intraoperative diagnostic modality is most useful for deciding whether to proceed with excision of a neuroma-in-continuity and perform a graft repair?

- A. MRI
- B. Ultrasound
- C. Intraoperative nerve action potential recording
- D. IV fluorescein
- E. Fluoroscopy

Correct answer is C

Intraoperative nerve action potential recording is most useful for assessing the functional status of a neuroma-in-continuity and deciding whether to proceed with excision and graft repair. It provides real-time information on nerve conduction across the neuroma. MRI and ultrasound are useful for preoperative planning but not for intraoperative decision-making. Research is being done with intraoperative ultrasound to promote intraoperative decision-making and may be applicable in the future. IV fluorescein and fluoroscopy are not typically used for this purpose.

▸▸ **Question 45**

A 65-year-old man presents with new right-sided foot drop following an elective total knee arthroplasty. Examination shows weakness in foot dorsiflexion and eversion, and sensory loss on the lateral aspect of the lower leg and dorsum of the foot. On examination, ankle inversion is intact. What is the most likely diagnosis?

- A. L4 radiculopathy
- B. L5 radiculopathy
- C. Sciatic nerve injury
- D. Common peroneal nerve injury
- E. Tibial nerve injury

Correct answer is D

Common peroneal nerve injury occurs following approximately 0.4% of total knee arthroplasties and is characterized by weakness in foot dorsiflexion and eversion, along with sensory loss involving the lateral aspect of the lower leg and dorsum of the foot. Ankle inversion typically remains intact because the tibialis posterior muscle is innervated by the tibial nerve, which branches proximal to the common peroneal nerve injury site. In contrast, an L5 radiculopathy generally presents with weakness in foot dorsiflexion, inversion, and eversion, accompanied by sensory deficits along the lateral leg and dorsal aspect of the foot. The involvement of ankle inversion helps distinguish L5 radiculopathy from an isolated common peroneal nerve injury.

▸▸ Question 46

A 30-year-old baseball pitcher presents with shoulder pain and decreased throwing power. He notes his shoulder blade feels prominent on high-back chairs and examination shows winging of the scapula when pushing open doors. Which nerve is most likely injured if the medial border of the scapula is prominent?

- A. Long thoracic nerve
- B. Spinal accessory nerve
- C. Dorsal scapular nerve
- D. Axillary nerve
- E. Suprascapular nerve

Correct answer is A

Long thoracic neuropathy is often due to inflammatory causes, such as Parsonage–Turner syndrome. It results in winging of the scapula, which may be noted as a prominent medial scapular border when flexing the arm at the shoulder. This nerve innervates the serratus anterior muscle, which stabilizes the scapula against the thoracic wall. Injury to the spinal accessory nerve affects the trapezius muscle, leading to lateral scapular winging. Winged scapula can also occur from dorsal scapular neuropathy but is exceedingly rare. Suprascapular neuropathy results in atrophy of the supraspinatus and infraspinatus muscles, making the scapula more prominent; it does not produce a winged scapula.[15] ▸ Fig. 7.12 shows a lesion of the right long thoracic nerve. Weakness of the serratus anterior muscle causes winging of the scapula, which is particularly evident when the patient extends the arms forward and pushes against a wall.

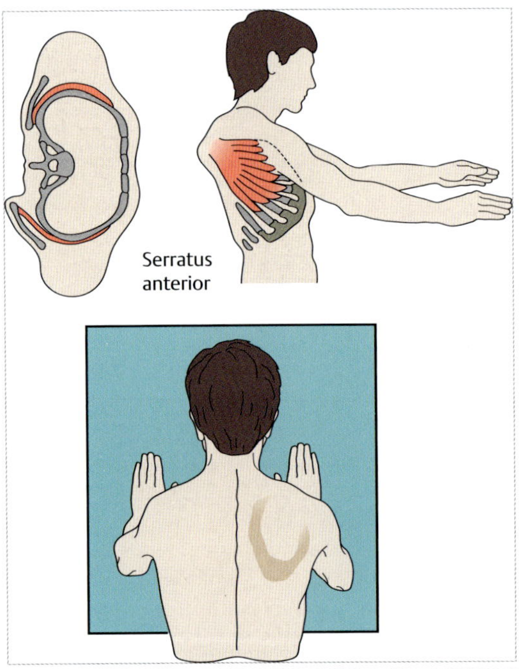

Fig. 7.12 (Source: Reproduced from Long thoracic nerve (C5–C7). In: Mattle H, Mumenthaler M, Taub E, eds. Fundamentals of Neurology: An Illustrated Guide. 2nd ed. Stuttgart: Thieme; 2016.)

▸▸ Question 47

A 45-year-old man presents with foot drop and sensory loss over the dorsum of the foot. Which of the following would differentiate L5 radiculopathy from peroneal nerve injury?

- A. Weakness in hip abduction
- B. Weakness in knee extension
- C. Weakness in foot inversion
- D. Sensory loss in the medial thigh
- E. Reflex changes in the Achilles tendon

Correct answer is C

Foot inversion weakness suggests L5 radiculopathy because the tibialis posterior muscle, responsible for inversion, is innervated by the tibial nerve (L5 contribution). In peroneal nerve injury, inversion is typically preserved because the tibial nerve is unaffected. Sensory loss over the dorsum of the foot and foot drop can be seen in both conditions.

▸▸ Question 48

A patient with Guillain–Barré syndrome (GBS) is most likely to have which of the following findings on nerve conduction studies?

- A. Decreased distal latency
- B. Increased conduction velocity
- C. Normal amplitude of sensory nerve action potentials
- D. Reduced or absent reflexes
- E. Presence of myotonic discharges

Correct answer is D

GBS typically presents with reduced or absent reflexes due to demyelination of peripheral nerves. Nerve conduction studies in GBS show prolonged distal latencies, decreased conduction velocities, and reduced sensory and motor nerve action potential amplitudes. Myotonic discharges are not a feature of GBS.[18]

▸▸ Question 49

A 60-year-old woman presents with swallowing difficulty, falls, and complaints of dropping objects. Examination shows atrophy of the quadriceps and forearms. Sensation is intact, and reflexes are normal. Which condition is most likely?
- A. Carpal tunnel syndrome
- B. Spinal muscular atrophy
- C. Inclusion body myositis (IBM)
- D. Peripheral neuropathy
- E. Myasthenia gravis

Correct answer is C

IBM is an inflammatory myopathy that presents with dysphagia (> 50% of patients) along with weakness and atrophy of the proximal and distal limb musculature, particularly in the quadriceps and long finger flexors (flexor digitorum superficialis and profundus muscles). At the same time, sensation remains intact, and reflexes are often normal or only mildly reduced. Carpal tunnel syndrome and peripheral neuropathy typically involve sensory changes. Spinal muscular atrophy primarily affects proximal muscles, and myasthenia gravis affects neuromuscular transmission without causing significant atrophy.[19]

▸▸ Question 50

A 35-year-old woman presents with progressive weakness in her upper arms and thighs. Laboratory tests show elevated creatine kinase levels. Which condition is most likely?
- A. Duchenne muscular dystrophy
- B. Myasthenia gravis
- C. Polymyositis
- D. Carpal tunnel syndrome
- E. Multiple sclerosis

Correct answer is C

Polymyositis is an inflammatory myopathy characterized by progressive weakness in the proximal limb muscles and elevated creatine kinase levels. Duchenne muscular dystrophy primarily affects males and presents in childhood; pseudohypertrophy of the calf muscles is noted. Myasthenia gravis affects neuromuscular transmission without causing elevated creatine kinase levels; symptoms are generally temporally dependent, being worse at the end of the day and with increased activity. Carpal tunnel syndrome is a compressive neuropathy and may produce thenar weakness. Multiple sclerosis affects the central nervous system.[20]

▸▸ Question 51

A 20-year-old male presents with difficulty walking, frequent falls, and atrophy of the calf muscles. On examination, he has an inverted champagne bottle appearance of the legs. What is the most likely diagnosis?
- A. Duchenne muscular dystrophy
- B. Charcot–Marie–Tooth (CMT) disease
- C. Myasthenia gravis
- D. Guillain–Barré syndrome
- E. Amyotrophic lateral sclerosis

Correct answer is B

The patient's distal extremity atrophy is most consistent with a peripheral neuropathy. Hyporeflexia, muscle atrophy, and fasciculations are all clinical signs consistent with lower motor neuron disease. CMT disease is a family of hereditary motor and sensory neuropathies characterized by distal muscle atrophy, particularly in the calves, leading to an inverted champagne bottle appearance. Duchenne muscular dystrophy presents in early childhood with proximal muscle weakness and calf pseudohypertrophy. Myasthenia gravis affects neuromuscular transmission and is not associated with atrophy. Guillain–Barré syndrome presents with ascending weakness, and amyotrophic lateral sclerosis affects both upper and lower motor neurons.[21]

▸▸ Question 52

A 50-year-old man presents with generalized muscle weakness, fatigue, and difficulty climbing stairs. On examination, he has ptosis and diplopia. His symptoms worsen with activity and improve with rest. Which condition is most likely?
- A. Guillain–Barré syndrome
- B. Multiple sclerosis

- C. Myasthenia gravis
- D. Lambert–Eaton myasthenic syndrome
- E. Muscular dystrophy

Correct answer is C

Myasthenia gravis is an autoimmune disorder characterized by muscle weakness that worsens with activity and improves with rest. Ptosis and diplopia are common findings. This condition is caused by antibodies against acetylcholine receptors at the neuromuscular junction; it is often associated with thymoma. Guillain–Barré syndrome presents with ascending weakness, multiple sclerosis with varied neurological deficits, Lambert–Eaton myasthenic syndrome with improvement in strength after exertion, and muscular dystrophies with progressive muscle weakness.[22]

▸▸ Question 53

A 38-year-old man experiences severe unilateral headache, nasal congestion, and tearing of the eye. The headache episodes occur several times a day and are associated with restlessness. What is the most likely diagnosis?

- A. Migraine
- B. Tension headache
- C. Cluster headache
- D. Trigeminal neuralgia
- E. Temporal arteritis

Correct answer is C

Cluster headache—a type of trigeminal autonomic cephalalgia—is characterized by excruciating, unilateral pain, often retro-orbital in location, accompanied by ipsilateral autonomic symptoms such as lacrimation, conjunctival injection, nasal congestion, rhinorrhea, ptosis, and miosis. Episodes occur in clusters that can last from 7 days to 1 year, with attack frequency ranging from one every other day to up to 8 per day. These are separated by remission periods of at least 3 months (episodic cluster headache). Nocturnal onset is common, and the pain is often described as the most severe a person can experience. Attacks are associated with restlessness or agitation (in contrast to migraine, where patients prefer to lie still). Acute treatment includes high-flow oxygen and subcutaneous or intranasal triptans(e.g., sumatriptan), while preventive therapy includes verapamil (first-line) or lithium, especially for chronic forms.

In contrast, migraines are typically longer-lasting (4–72 hours); may include nausea, photophobia, and phonophobia; are more common in women; and rarely feature autonomic symptoms. Tension-type headaches are typically bilateral, pressing or tightening in quality, and milder in severity. Trigeminal neuralgia presents as brief, electric shock-like pain in the distribution of the trigeminal nerve. Temporal arteritis (giant cell arteritis) often presents with new-onset headache in older adults, scalp tenderness, jaw claudication, and elevated erythrocyte sedimentation/C-reactive protein.[23,24]

▸▸ Question 54

A 65-year-old woman presents with a sudden onset of hemiparesis and hemisensory loss. She also has severe burning pain on the affected side. MRI reveals a lesion in the thalamus. Which syndrome is most likely?

- A. Brown-Sequard syndrome
- B. Dejerine–Roussy syndrome
- C. Wallenberg syndrome
- D. Horner syndrome
- E. Central cord syndrome

Correct answer is B

Dejerine–Roussy syndrome, also known as thalamic pain syndrome, occurs after a stroke in the thalamus. It is characterized by initial hemiparesis and hemisensory loss, followed by severe, chronic pain on the affected side. Brown-Sequard syndrome results from hemisection of the spinal cord (hemiparesis and hemianesthesia ipsilateral to the lesion; loss of nociceptive and thermal inputs contralateral to the lesion), Wallenberg syndrome from a lateral medullary infarction (tongue deviation ipsilateral to the lesion, dysarthria, hoarseness, dysphagia, loss of pain/temperature sensation ipsilateral to the lesion; loss of body sensory inputs contralateral to the lesion), Horner syndrome from disruption of the sympathetic outflow through the superior cervical ganglion, and central cord syndrome from injury to the central part of the spinal cord.

▸▸ Question 55

A 60-year-old man presents with chronic, severe burning pain in his feet, which has been unresponsive to oral medications. He has a history of

diabetes mellitus. Which treatment option is most appropriate for managing his peripheral neuropathic pain?
- A. Physical therapy
- B. Intrathecal morphine pump
- C. Spinal cord stimulation (SCS)
- D. Dorsal root entry zone lesioning
- E. Transcutaneous electrical nerve stimulation

Correct answer is C

SCS is an effective treatment for managing chronic peripheral neuropathic pain, particularly in patients with diabetic neuropathy. SCS delivers electrical impulses to the spinal cord, altering pain signals before they reach the brain. Recently, the SENZA-PDN randomized clinical trial showed that high-frequency (10 kHz) stimulation led to a significant increase in the proportion of patients experiencing ≥ 50% relief in their pain by 3-month follow-up (79 vs. 5%; $p < 0.001$). Physical therapy and transcutaneous electrical nerve stimulation can help manage pain but may be insufficient for severe cases. An intrathecal morphine pump is typically reserved for severe cancer pain, and surgical nerve decompression is not indicated for diffuse neuropathic pain.[25,26]

▸▸ Question 56

A 30-year-old woman with chronic migraine presents with pain radiating from the base of the skull up the posterior scalp to the crown of the head. It is exacerbated by neck movements and has proven refractory to multiple oral medications. Which procedure might provide significant pain relief?
- A. Occipital nerve block
- B. Carotid endarterectomy
- C. Trigeminal ganglion block
- D. Anterior cervical diskectomy
- E. Thoracic sympathectomy

Correct answer is A

Occipital nerve block can provide significant relief for patients with occipital neuralgia and chronic migraines that involve occipital pain. This procedure involves injecting a combination of local anesthetic and corticosteroid (commonly methylprednisolone or dexamethasone) around the occipital nerve, reducing pain and inflammation. Carotid endarterectomy and thoracic sympathectomy are not indicated for this type of pain. Trigeminal ganglion block is used for trigeminal neuralgia, and anterior cervical diskectomy is used for cervical radiculopathy.[27,28]

▸▸ Question 57

A 65-year-old man sustains a shoulder dislocation and presents with weak shoulder abduction and loss of sensation over the lateral shoulder. Which nerve is most likely injured?
- A. Suprascapular nerve
- B. Axillary nerve
- C. Radial nerve
- D. Long thoracic nerve
- E. Musculocutaneous nerve

Correct answer is B

Axillary nerve injury is the most common nerve injury associated with anterior shoulder dislocation. The axillary nerve innervates the deltoid and teres minor muscles and provides sensory innervation to the lateral aspect of the shoulder via the superior lateral cutaneous nerve. Injury to this nerve results in weakness or inability to abduct the shoulder beyond approximately 15 to 30 degrees (initial abduction to about 15 degrees is performed by the supraspinatus), decreased strength when resisting shoulder abduction, and loss of sensation over the lateral shoulder region.

In contrast, suprascapular nerve injury also impairs shoulder abduction (due to supraspinatus muscle dysfunction), but typically does not affect skin sensation. Radial nerve injury predominantly results in weakness of wrist and finger extension ("wrist drop") without directly affecting shoulder abduction or lateral shoulder sensation. Long thoracic nerve injury causes characteristic winging of the scapula due to weakness of the serratus anterior. Lastly, musculocutaneous nerve injury primarily leads to impaired elbow flexion and sensory loss along the lateral forearm, without directly affecting shoulder abduction.[29,30]

▸▸ Question 58

A 40-year-old man is brought to the emergency department after a motor vehicle collision. He cannot flex his elbow and has a loss of sensation over the lateral forearm. Which nerve is most likely injured?
- A. Radial nerve
- B. Ulnar nerve

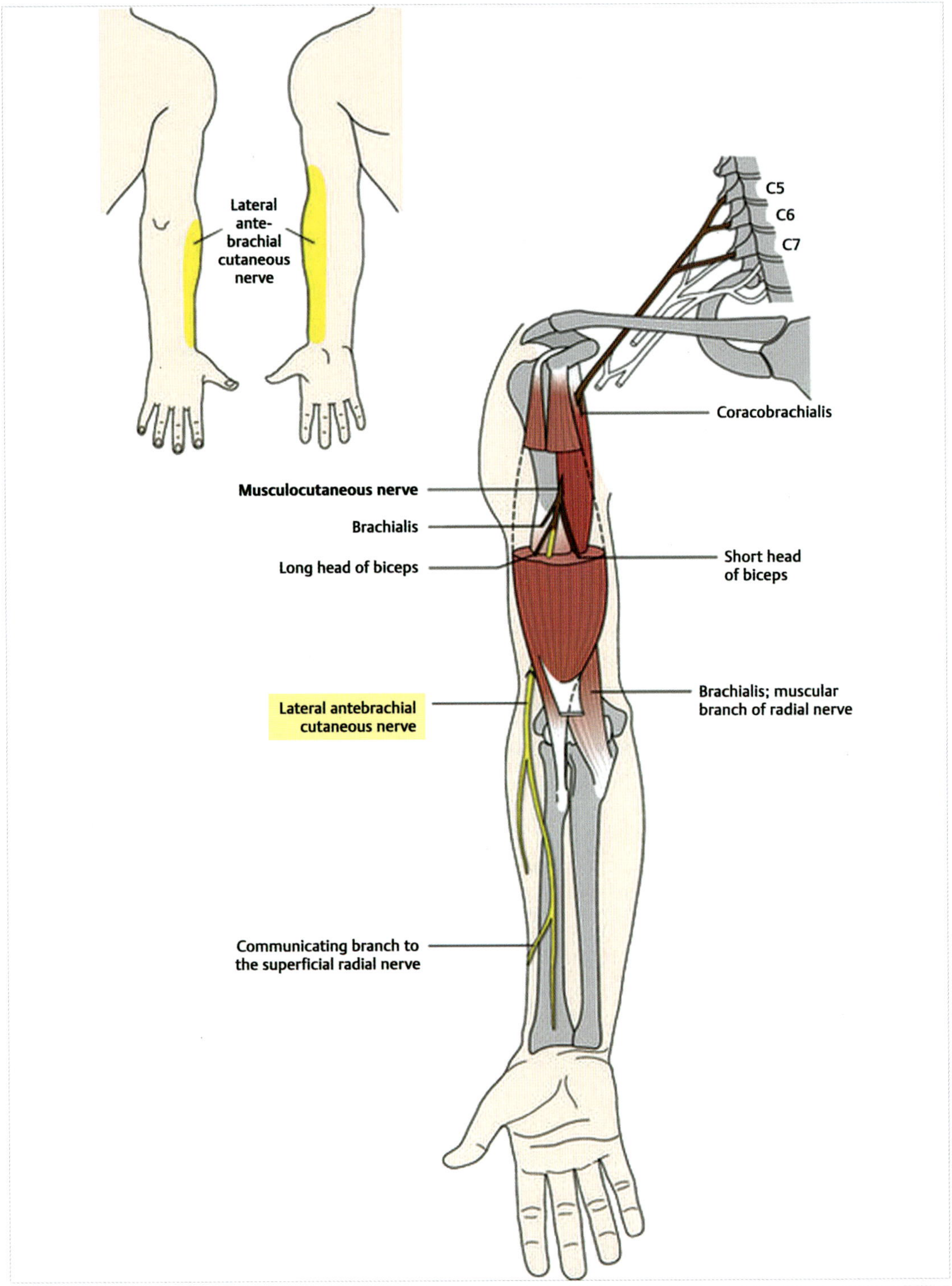

Fig. 7.13 (Source: Reproduced from Musculocutaneous nerve (C5–C7). In: Mattle H, Mumenthaler M, Taub E, eds. Fundamentals of Neurology: An Illustrated Guide. 2nd ed. Stuttgart: Thieme; 2016.)

- C. Median nerve
- D. Axillary nerve
- E. Musculocutaneous nerve

Correct answer is E

The musculocutaneous nerve innervates the biceps brachii and brachialis muscles, primarily responsible for elbow flexion, as well as the coracobrachialis, which contributes to shoulder flexion. It also provides sensory innervation to the lateral forearm via its terminal branch, the lateral cutaneous nerve of the forearm. Injury to the musculocutaneous nerve results in significant weakness or inability to flex the elbow and loss of sensation over the lateral forearm.

In contrast, axillary nerve injury causes weakness of the deltoid muscle, impairing shoulder abduction primarily, with secondary weakness in shoulder flexion and extension. Radial nerve injury typically presents with wrist drop due to impaired wrist and finger extension. Ulnar nerve injury predominantly affects intrinsic hand muscles, resulting in difficulty with fine hand movements and characteristic claw-hand deformity. Lastly, median nerve injury affects forearm pronators and flexors, as well as thumb opposition, causing impaired precision grip and sensory loss in the lateral palm and fingers (▶ Fig. 7.13).[31,32]

References

[1] Ray WZ, Chang J, Hawasli A, Wilson TJ, Yang L. Motor nerve transfers: a comprehensive review. Neurosurgery 2016;78 (1):1–26.

[2] Oberlin C, Béal D, Leechavengvongs S, Salon A, Dauge MC, Sarcy JJ. Nerve transfer to biceps muscle using a part of ulnar nerve for C5-C6 avulsion of the brachial plexus: anatomical study and report of four cases. Ann Plast Surg 1994;19(2):232–237

[3] Texakalidis P, Hardcastle N, Tora MS, Boulis NM. Functional restoration of elbow flexion in nonobstetric brachial plexus injuries: a meta-analysis of nerve transfers versus grafts. Microsurgery 2020;40(2):261–267

[4] Bertelli JA, Ghizoni MF. Results of spinal accessory to suprascapular nerve transfer in 110 patients with complete palsy of the brachial plexus. J Neurosurg Spine 2016;24(6):990–995

[5] Ray WZ, Mackinnon SE. Clinical outcomes following median to radial nerve transfers. J Hand Surg Am 2011;36 (2):201–208

[6] Shadgan B, Menon M, Sanders D, et al. Current thinking about acute compartment syndrome of the lower extremity. Can J Surg 2010;53(5):329–334

[7] Gulli B, Templeman D. Compartment syndrome of the lower extremity. Orthop Clin North Am 1994;25(4):677–684

[8] Seddon HJ, ed. Surgical Disorders of the Peripheral Nerves. 2nd ed. Edinburgh: Churchill Livingstone; 1972

[9] Fu SY, Gordon T. The cellular and molecular basis of peripheral nerve regeneration. Mol Neurobiol 1997;14(1–2):67–116

[10] Régis J, Metellus P, Hayashi M, Roussel P, Donnet A, Bille-Turc F. Prospective controlled trial of gamma knife surgery for essential trigeminal neuralgia. J Neurosurg 2006;104 (6):913–924

[11] Emery AE. The muscular dystrophies. Lancet 2002;359 (9307):687–695

[12] Gebreyohanes AMH, Ahmed AI, Choi D. Dorsal root entry zone lesioning for brachial plexus avulsion: a comprehensive literature review. Oper Neurosurg 2021;20(4):324–333

[13] Nader R, Sabbagh AJ, Elbabaa SK, et al. Neurosurgery Case Review: Questions and Answers. Section VII Peripheral Nerve Pathology: Case 143 Radial Nerve Injury. 2020. Doi: 10.1055/b-0040-175432

[14] Campbell WW. Evaluation and management of peripheral nerve injury. Clin Neurophysiol 2008;119(9):1951–1965

[15] Martin RM, Fish DE. Scapular winging: anatomical review, diagnosis, and treatments. Curr Rev Musculoskelet Med 2008;1(1):1–11

[16] Zhou M, Zhong H, Xing C, et al. Comparison of clinical outcomes associated with spinal cord stimulation (SCS) or conventional medical management (CMM) for chronic pain: a systematic review and meta-analysis. Eur Spine J 2023;32 (6):2029–2041

[17] Posuniak EA. Electrodiagnosis and nerve conduction studies. Clin Podiatry 1984;1(2):279–90

[18] van den Berg B, Walgaard C, Drenthen J, Fokke C, Jacobs BC, van Doorn PA. Guillain-Barré syndrome: pathogenesis, diagnosis, treatment and prognosis. Nat Rev Neurol 2014;10 (8):469–482

[19] Dalakas MC. Sporadic inclusion body myositis—diagnosis, pathogenesis and therapeutic strategies. Nat Clin Pract Neurol 2006;2(8):437–447

[20] Findlay AR, Goyal NA, Mozaffar T. An overview of polymyositis and dermatomyositis. Muscle Nerve 2015;51(5):638–656

[21] Okamoto Y, Takashima H. The current state of Charcot-Marie-Tooth disease treatment. Genes (Basel) 2023;14 (7):1391

[22] Lennon VA, Kryzer TJ, Griesmann GE, et al. Calcium-channel antibodies in the Lambert–Eaton syndrome and other paraneoplastic syndromes. N Engl J Med 1995;332(22):1467–1475

[23] Kudrow L. Cluster headache: diagnosis and management. Headache 1979;19(3):142–150

[24] Ekbom K, Hardebo JE. Cluster headache: aetiology, diagnosis and management. Drugs 2002;62(1):61–69

[25] Henson J V, Varhabhatla NC, Bebic Z, et al. Spinal cord stimulation for painful diabetic peripheral neuropathy: a systematic review. Pain Ther 2021;10(2):895–908

[26] Petersen EA, Stauss TG, Scowcroft JA, et al. Effect of high-frequency (10-kHz) spinal cord stimulation in patients with painful diabetic neuropathy. JAMA Neurol 2021;78(6):687

[27] Ashkenazi A, Blumenfeld A, Napchan U, et al. Peripheral nerve blocks and trigger point injections in headache management – a systematic review and suggestions for future research. Headache 2010;50(6):943–952
[28] Velásquez-Rimachi V, Chachaima-Mar J, Cárdenas-Baltazar EC, et al. Greater occipital nerve block for chronic migraine patients: a meta-analysis. Acta Neurol Scand 2022;146 (2):101–114
[29] Stecco C, Gagliano G, Lancerotto L, et al. Surgical anatomy of the axillary nerve and its implication in the transdeltoid approaches to the shoulder. J Shoulder Elbow Surg 2010;19 (8):1166–1174
[30] Gosk J, Urban M, Rutowski R. Entrapment of the suprascapular nerve: anatomy, etiology, diagnosis, treatment. Ortop Traumatol Rehabil 2007;9(1):68–74
[31] Omer GE Jr. Injuries to nerves of the upper extremity. J Bone Joint Surg Am 1974;56(8):1615–1624
[32] Drake RL, Vogl W, Mitchell AWM. Gray's Anatomy for Students. Elsevier Health Sciences; 2014

8 Core Competencies

Syed I. Khalid, Lei Liu, Mark Dapash, Aladine Elsamadicy, Yoon Soo Park, Sean Hogan

▸▸ Question 1

A 55-year-old man with limited English proficiency presents with symptoms of myelopathy. He is accompanied by his adult daughter, who offers to translate. The neurosurgeon needs to obtain informed consent for a surgical decompression. Which of the following is the most appropriate action to ensure valid informed consent?

- A. Use the daughter as an interpreter to obtain consent
- B. Proceed with consent using simplified English
- C. Utilize a professional medical interpreter
- D. Provide written materials in English
- E. Delay surgery until the patient learns English

Correct answer is C

Obtaining informed consent requires clear communication to ensure the patient understands the risks, benefits, and alternatives of the procedure. Using a professional medical interpreter ensures accurate and unbiased translation, maintains patient confidentiality, and reduces misunderstandings. Relying on family members may introduce bias and breaches of confidentiality.[1,2]

▸▸ Question 2

During a heated disagreement outside a patient's room, two residents raise their voices, causing distress to the patient and family. As their attending physician, which Accreditation Council for Graduate Medical Education (ACGME) core competency should you focus on to address this situation?

- A. Medical knowledge
- B. Professionalism
- C. Systems-based practice
- D. Practice-based learning
- E. Patient care

Correct answer is B

The residents' behavior reflects a lapse in professionalism, which encompasses respectful interactions, ethical behavior, and sensitivity to patient concerns. Addressing this competency involves teaching appropriate communication skills, conflict resolution, and maintaining a professional demeanor in all clinical settings.

▸▸ Question 3

A neurosurgeon is on call when a patient with a traumatic brain injury arrives at a nearby hospital that lacks neurosurgical services. The neurosurgeon refuses the transfer due to anticipated reimbursement issues. According to the Emergency Medical Treatment and Active Labor Act (EMTALA), which of the following best describes this situation?

- A. Acceptable if the neurosurgeon is not on-site
- B. Violation of EMTALA regulations
- C. Permissible if the hospital is at capacity
- D. Allowed if the patient is uninsured
- E. Legal if the neurosurgeon has scheduling conflicts

Correct answer is B

Under EMTALA, hospitals with specialized capabilities cannot refuse to accept appropriate transfers of unstable patients needing such services, regardless of the patient's ability to pay. Refusing a transfer due to reimbursement concerns is a violation, potentially resulting in penalties for both the physician and the hospital.[3,4]

▸▸ Question 4

A research study aims to evaluate the effectiveness of a new diagnostic tool for detecting cerebral aneurysms. The test has a sensitivity of 90% and a specificity of 85%. In a population where the prevalence of aneurysms is 10%, what is the positive predictive value (PPV) of the test?

- A. 40%
- B. 50%
- C. 60%
- D. 70%
- E. 80%

Correct answer is A

To calculate the PPV, we need to account for sensitivity, specificity, and disease prevalence. In this scenario, the sensitivity is 90%, the specificity is 85%, and the prevalence of aneurysms is 10%.

The PPV reflects the probability that a patient actually has an aneurysm when the test result is positive.

Here is how we calculate it:

1. Assume a population of 1,000 individuals:
   - **100 individuals** have aneurysms (10% prevalence).
   - **900 individuals** do not have aneurysms (90% nonprevalence).
2. Calculate true positives (TPs):
   - $TP = 0.9 \times 100 = 90$ $TP = 0.9 \times 100 = 90$
3. Calculate false positives (FPs):
   - $FP = 0.15 \times 900 = 135$ $FP = 0.15 \times 900 = 135$
4. Calculate PPV:
   - $PPV = TP/TP + FP = 90/225 \approx 40\%$

Thus, the PPV is **40%**, meaning that when the test is positive, there is a 40% chance that the patient actually has an aneurysm.

▸▸ Question 5

A neurosurgery resident exceeds the 80-hour workweek limit due to additional on-call duties. According to the Accreditation Council for Graduate Medical Education (ACGME) duty hour policies, which of the following actions should be taken?

- A. Report the violation to the program director and adjust the schedule
- B. Ignore the extra hours since patient care is paramount
- C. Exclude on-call hours from duty hour calculations
- D. Only report violations if they exceed 88 hours
- E. Compensate by reducing hours next month

Correct answer is A

ACGME duty-hour policies are designed to prevent resident fatigue and enhance patient safety. Residents must report duty hour violations so that the program can adjust schedules accordingly. The ACGME recognizes that urgent patient care matters arise, making it necessary for residents to occasionally devote more than 80 hours in a given week to clinical and educational activities. That is why the standard allows the 80 hours to be averaged over the course of a 4-week period. Keeping tabs on hours worked will allow the resident's schedule in the following weeks to be adjusted to remain true to the intent of the standard.[5,6,7,8]

▸▸ Question 6

A 60-year-old man is scheduled for deep brain stimulation surgery to treat Parkinson's disease. During the consent process, he appears confused and unable to repeat back the procedure details. His adult son insists on proceeding. Which ethical principle is at risk if the surgery moves forward without addressing the patient's confusion?

- A. Autonomy
- B. Beneficence
- C. Non-maleficence
- D. Justice
- E. Fidelity

Correct answer is A

Autonomy requires that patients make informed decisions about their care. If the patient lacks decision-making capacity, proceeding without proper consent violates this principle. In this case, the patient appears confused and unable to demonstrate understanding of the procedure, suggesting impaired capacity. If the son does not have a legally recognized authority (such as a power of attorney for healthcare) to make medical decisions, the neurosurgeon must follow legal and ethical guidelines by assessing the patient's capacity and, if necessary, identifying a legally authorized representative. Moving forward without addressing these concerns undermines the patient's autonomy and could lead to ethical and legal issues.

▸▸ Question 7

A physician receives a gift worth $15 from a pharmaceutical company representative. According to the Physician Payments Sunshine Act, which of the following is true regarding the reporting of this gift?

- A. It must be reported to the Centers for Medicare and Medicaid Services (CMS) and will be publicly available
- B. It does not need to be reported due to low value
- C. Reporting is optional for gifts under $20
- D. The physician is responsible for reporting the gift
- E. Such gifts are prohibited under the Act

Correct answer is A

The Physician Payments Sunshine Act requires healthcare companies to report any payments or transfers of value provided to physicians if they exceed $10 individually or $100 cumulatively per year. For instance, a single gift valued at $15 exceeds the individual threshold and therefore must be reported. It is important to note that these thresholds are adjusted annually for inflation; thus, reporting entities should verify the most current limits published by the Centers for Medicare and Medicaid Services. The primary aim of the Sunshine Act is to increase transparency in financial relationships between healthcare providers and companies. CMS maintains a publicly accessible database (open payments) to share this information with the public.[9,10,11]

▸▸ Question 8

A 52-year-old woman with a history of seizures is considering enrollment in a clinical trial for a new antiepileptic drug. She is concerned about potential side effects. Which ethical principle ensures she can withdraw from the study at any time without penalty?

- A. Beneficence
- B. Non-maleficence
- C. Justice
- D. Respect for persons
- E. Confidentiality

Correct answer is D

Respect for persons encompasses acknowledging a person's autonomy and the right to make decisions about their participation in research. It includes the ability to withdraw from a study at any time without penalty. This principle is a cornerstone of ethical research conduct.

▸▸ Question 9

In a randomized controlled trial, researchers conclude that a new surgical technique significantly reduces operative time compared to the standard method ($p = 0.04$). Which of the following best describes the likelihood of a Type I error in this study?

- A. 1%
- B. 4%
- C. 5%
- D. 10%
- E. 20%

Correct answer is B

A Type I error occurs when a true null hypothesis is incorrectly rejected. The *p*-value represents the probability of making a Type I error. In this study, with a *p*-value of 0.04, there is a 4% chance that the observed effect is due to chance, indicating the likelihood of a Type I error.

▸▸ Question 10

A hospital implements a new protocol to prevent wrong-site surgery, including mandatory time-outs and surgical site marking. This is an example of which quality improvement strategy?

- A. Root cause analysis
- B. Sentinel event reporting
- C. System-based practice
- D. Process improvement
- E. Risk management

Correct answer is D

Process improvement involves analyzing and modifying workflows to enhance outcomes and prevent errors. Implementing protocols like time-outs and site marking aims to standardize procedures and reduce the risk of wrong-site surgery, enhancing patient safety.[12,13,14]

▸▸ Question 11

A neurosurgeon publishes a study funded by a medical device company in which he holds stock options. According to ethical guidelines, which of the following must he ensure regarding his publication?

- A. Delay publication until stock is sold
- B. Disclose the financial conflict of interest in the publication
- C. Refrain from publishing due to bias
- D. Only disclose the conflict if asked by editors
- E. Transfer stock ownership to a family member

Correct answer is B

Transparency is essential in research. Disclosing financial conflicts of interest allows readers to assess potential biases. Ethical guidelines mandate disclosure of any financial relationships that could influence the research outcomes or interpretations.

▸▸ Question 12

A medical student witnesses a resident making derogatory comments about a patient's cultural background. Which of the following actions is most appropriate for the student to take?

- A. Ignore the comments to avoid conflict
- B. Report the incident to a supervising faculty member
- C. Confront the resident publicly
- D. Discuss the issue with other students
- E. Post about the incident on social media

Correct answer is B

Professionalism includes addressing unprofessional behavior. The student should report the incident to a supervisor who can handle the situation appropriately. This maintains a respectful environment and upholds ethical standards without causing public confrontation or violating confidentiality.[15,16]

▸▸ Question 13

A 70-year-old patient with a massive intracerebral hemorrhage is declared brain dead. The family consents to organ donation, but the patient's heart stops before organs can be harvested. Which organ is still viable for transplantation under Donation after Cardiac Death (DCD) protocols?

- A. Heart
- B. Lungs
- C. Kidneys
- D. Pancreas
- E. Small intestine

Correct answer is C

Under DCD protocols, organs that are more tolerant of warm ischemia, like the kidneys, can still be viable for transplantation after circulatory death. Organs requiring continuous perfusion, like the heart and lungs, are typically not suitable in this scenario.

▸▸ Question 14

A resident is concerned about potential HIPAA violations when discussing patient cases during teaching rounds. Which of the following practices helps ensure compliance with HIPAA regulations?

- A. Using patient's initials instead of full names during discussions
- B. Sharing patient details only with fellow residents
- C. Discussing cases in public areas for educational purposes
- D. Storing patient data on personal devices for convenience
- E. Accessing any patient records for learning opportunities

Correct answer is A

To maintain patient confidentiality, protected health information should be limited during discussions. Using patient initials or de-identified information minimizes the risk of unauthorized disclosure, aligning with HIPAA requirements.

▸▸ Question 15

In analyzing outcomes from a new surgical procedure, a researcher notes that the p-value is 0.20. Which of the following is the most appropriate conclusion?

- A. The results are statistically significant
- B. There is a 20% chance of Type I error
- C. The null hypothesis cannot be rejected
- D. The alternative hypothesis is accepted
- E. The study has high power

Correct answer is C

A p-value of 0.20 indicates that there is a 20% probability that the observed results are due to chance. This p-value is above the common significance level of 0.05, so the null hypothesis cannot be rejected, and no statistically significant difference is demonstrated.

Importantly, ***p*-values do not measure the probability that the hypothesis being tested is true** or the probability that the observed data arose purely by chance. According to the ASA, p-values must be interpreted with caution as they indicate only the compatibility of the data with the null hypothesis, rather than absolute evidence for or against it. Additionally, the p-value is not an indicator of effect size or study power and should always be interpreted in the broader context of the study design and prior evidence.[17]

▸▸ Question 16

A 58-year-old man develops a postoperative infection after spinal surgery. The hospital conducts

a root cause analysis. Which of the following is the primary goal of this process?
- A. Assign blame to the responsible individuals
- B. Determine legal liability
- C. Identify underlying system issues to prevent recurrence
- D. Document the event for accreditation purposes
- E. Report the incident to regulatory agencies

Correct answer is C

A root cause analysis is a structured method used to analyze serious adverse events. Its primary goal is to identify underlying problems that increase the likelihood of errors, focusing on systems and processes to implement changes and prevent future incidents.

▸▸ Question 17

A resident is asked to moonlight at an outside facility, potentially exceeding ACGME duty-hour limits. According to ACGME policies, which of the following is true regarding moonlighting?
- A. Moonlighting hours do not count toward duty-hour limits
- B. Residents are free to moonlight without restrictions
- C. Moonlighting is prohibited for PGY-1 residents
- D. Moonlighting requires the program director's approval but no hour limitations
- E. Moonlighting is encouraged to enhance clinical experience

Correct answer is C

According to ACGME regulations, PGY-1 residents are not permitted to moonlight. For residents at higher levels, moonlighting must be approved by the program director, and all hours worked must be counted toward the 80-hour weekly limit to ensure residents' well-being and patients' safety.

▸▸ Question 18

A neurosurgeon learns that a medical device used in several of her patients has been recalled due to safety concerns. Which of the following is her immediate ethical obligation?
- A. Wait for patients to report problems
- B. Inform affected patients promptly about the recall
- C. Remove the device from all patients immediately
- D. Contact legal counsel before taking action
- E. Notify the media about the recall

Correct answer is B

The neurosurgeon has an ethical duty to promptly inform patients about the recall, discussing potential risks and management options. This respects patient autonomy and promotes trust in the physician–patient relationship.

▸▸ Question 19

A 45-year-old woman presents with signs of increased intracranial pressure. Imaging reveals obstructive hydrocephalus due to a colloid cyst of the third ventricle. Emergency surgery is recommended, but the patient is unconscious and has no advance directive. Her estranged husband arrives and refuses consent. What is the most appropriate next step?
- A. Proceed with surgery under implied consent
- B. Delay surgery until consent is obtained
- C. Honor the husband's refusal
- D. Seek a court order
- E. Transfer the patient to another facility

Correct answer is A

In emergency situations where delaying treatment poses a threat to life or health, and the patient cannot consent, physicians may proceed under implied consent. Immediate surgery is justified to save the patient's life.

▸▸ Question 20

A patient inquires about accessing their electronic medical records (EMRs) through a patient portal. Under HIPAA regulations, which of the following statements is correct regarding patients' access to their health information?
- A. Patients have the right to access their EMRs and obtain copies.
- B. Access is granted only with the physician's approval.
- C. Patients have unrestricted access to psychotherapy notes.
- D. Patients may be charged unreasonable fees for digital records access.
- E. Access is limited only to billing information.

Correct answer is A

Under the Health Insurance Portability and Accountability Act (HIPAA), patients have the legal right to access and obtain copies of their protected health information, including electronic medical records. Although HIPAA allows certain exceptions—such as psychotherapy notes, which can legally be withheld—patients generally must be granted access without needing specific approval from a physician. Providers can charge a reasonable, cost-based fee for providing copies, but they cannot impose excessive or unreasonable charges. Additionally, patients' access extends well beyond billing data and includes clinical and medical records.

▸▸ Question 21

A new screening test for a neurological disease shows high sensitivity but low specificity. Which of the following is a likely consequence of using this test in the general population?

- A. High rate of false negatives
- B. High rate of false positives
- C. Accurate identification of all disease-free individuals
- D. Underestimation of disease prevalence
- E. Decreased need for confirmatory testing

Correct answer is B

A test with high sensitivity correctly identifies most individuals with the disease, but low specificity means it incorrectly labels many healthy individuals as positive, resulting in a high rate of false positives.

▸▸ Question 22

A neurosurgical team is developing a clinical practice guideline for managing traumatic brain injury. Which of the following levels of evidence provides the highest quality data for their guideline?

- A. Expert opinion
- B. Case series
- C. Randomized controlled trials (RCTs)
- D. Cohort studies
- E. Case–control studies

Correct answer is C

RCTs offer the highest level of evidence for clinical decision-making due to their design, which minimizes bias. They are considered the gold standard for evaluating the efficacy of interventions. However, **systematic reviews and meta-analyses of RCTs** provide an even more robust synthesis of data, demonstrating efficacy across multiple studies, locations, and time points. These reviews combine data from several RCTs, increasing generalizability and providing stronger guidance for clinical practice guidelines.

▸▸ Question 23

A neurosurgical team plans a retrospective chart review to evaluate the incidence of surgical site infections over the past 5 years. The study will involve collecting patient data, including demographics and outcomes. Which of the following is required before initiating this study?

- A. Obtain individual patient consent
- B. Submit the study for IRB review and approval
- C. No action is needed since it is retrospective
- D. De-identify data and proceed without oversight
- E. Notify patients via public notice

Correct answer is B

Even for retrospective studies using patient data, IRB review and approval are required to ensure ethical standards are met and patients' confidentiality is protected. Depending on the IRB's assessment, the study may qualify for expedited review or a waiver of consent, but the researchers must still seek IRB's approval before proceeding.

▸▸ Question 24

According to HIPAA regulations, when sharing protected health information (PHI) with a third party for quality improvement purposes, a covered entity must first:

- A. Obtain patient authorization for each record shared
- B. De-identify all patient information before sharing
- C. Establish a business associate agreement (BAA)
- D. Notify the Department of Health and Human Services
- E. Encrypt the data and share without additional steps

Correct answer is C

Under HIPAA, when a covered entity shares PHI with a third party (a business associate) for purposes like quality improvement, a BAA must be in place. The BAA ensures that the business associate will appropriately safeguard the PHI.

▸▸ Question 25

Which level of evidence is assigned to a single, well-designed randomized controlled trial (RCT) according to the Agency for Healthcare Research and Quality (AHRQ) system?
- A. Level I
- B. Level II
- C. Level III
- D. Level IV
- E. Level V

Correct answer is A
In the AHRQ system, Level I evidence includes data from well-conducted randomized controlled trials. A single high-quality RCT provides strong evidence due to its design, which minimizes bias and confounding factors.

▸▸ Question 26

A new screening test for a rare neurological disease has a sensitivity of 99% and a specificity of 99%. The disease prevalence is 1 in 10,000. A patient tests positive. What is the most appropriate advice to give this patient?
- A. High likelihood of disease; begin treatment immediately
- B. Low probability of disease; the result is likely a false positive
- C. The test is conclusive; no further testing needed
- D. Repeat the test to confirm results
- E. Ignore the result due to the rarity of the disease

Correct answer is B
In low-prevalence settings, even tests with high sensitivity and specificity can yield a high number of false positives. The positive predictive value is low, meaning a positive result does not strongly indicate disease presence. The patient should be counseled about the low probability and possibly undergo confirmatory testing.

▸▸ Question 27

A neurosurgeon needs to submit billing information for a spinal fusion procedure. Which coding system should be used to specify the surgical procedure performed?
- A. International Classification of Diseases codes
- B. Current Procedural Terminology (CPT) codes
- C. Diagnosis-Related Group codes
- D. National Provider Identifier codes
- E. Healthcare Common Procedure Coding System Level II codes

Correct answer is B
CPT codes are used by physicians to describe and bill for medical, surgical, and diagnostic services. They provide a uniform language for reporting procedures and services.

▸▸ Question 28

A neurosurgery resident participates in a hospital committee focused on reducing postoperative complications through system changes. This activity is an example of which ACGME core competency?
- A. Patient care
- B. Medical knowledge
- C. Systems-based practice
- D. Professionalism
- E. Practice-based learning and improvement

Correct answer is C
Systems-based practice involves understanding and engaging with the healthcare system to improve patient care. Participating in committees to enhance systemic processes reflects this competency.

▸▸ Question 29

In a randomized controlled trial, which aspect is most critical in minimizing the impact of unknown confounding variables?
- A. Blinding of participants and investigators
- B. Random allocation of participants to groups
- C. Stratification of participants
- D. Large sample size
- E. Use of placebo controls

Correct answer is B
Randomization is key to ensuring that confounding variables are evenly distributed between groups, minimizing their impact on the study outcome.

▸▸ Question 30

A neurosurgeon is analyzing data from a study comparing two surgical techniques. He notes that

patients lost to follow-up are disproportionately from one group. This introduces which type of bias?
- A. Selection bias
- B. Information bias
- C. Attrition bias
- D. Observer bias
- E. Recall bias

Correct answer is C
Attrition bias occurs when participants drop out of a study unevenly across groups, potentially affecting the validity of the results.

▸▸ Question 31

A study reports that a new medication reduces the risk of stroke from 4 to 2%. What is the number needed to treat (NNT) to prevent one additional stroke?
- A. 25
- B. 50
- C. 75
- D. 100
- E. 200

Correct answer is B
NNT is calculated as 1 divided by the absolute risk reduction (ARR). ARR = 4% – 2% = 2% (or 0.02). NNT = 1 / 0.02 = 50.

▸▸ Question 32

A neurosurgery resident identifies that postoperative infection rates are higher in their unit compared to national benchmarks. He conducts a literature review and implements evidence-based practices to reduce infections. This demonstrates which ACGME core competency?
- A. Patient care
- B. Practice-based learning and improvement (PBLI)
- C. Systems-based practice
- D. Professionalism
- E. Medical knowledge

Correct answer is B
This competency involves self-directed learning and applying evidence to improve patient outcomes. By identifying an issue, conducting a literature review, and implementing evidence-based interventions, the resident demonstrates mastery of the PBLI **competency at** the level expected by the time of program completion. This highlights an ability to critically evaluate practice, seek knowledge, and integrate improvements to enhance patient care.

▸▸ Question 33

A study compares outcomes before and after a new surgical protocol is implemented. Patients treated before the change serve as controls. This study design is susceptible to which type of bias?
- A. Selection bias
- B. Historical bias
- C. Confirmation bias
- D. Observer bias
- E. Publication bias

Correct answer is B
When comparing groups from different time periods, historical bias can occur due to changes over time unrelated to the intervention, such as improvements in supportive care.

▸▸ Question 34

Which statistical metric assesses how well study findings can be applied to the general population?
- A. Internal validity
- B. External validity
- C. Reliability
- D. Specificity
- E. Sensitivity

Correct answer is B
External validity, or generalizability, refers to the extent to which study results can be applied to populations beyond the study sample.

▸▸ Question 35

A neurosurgeon plans to submit a research proposal involving de-identified patient data. According to the Common Rule, which of the following is true regarding IRB review?
- A. IRB review is not required for de-identified data
- B. Full IRB review is mandatory
- C. Expedited IRB review is required
- D. Informed consent from patients is needed
- E. The study cannot proceed without patient authorization

Correct answer is A

Under the **Common Rule (45 CFR 46)**, research involving **de-identified data** is typically **exempted** from IRB review because it does not involve human subjects as defined by federal regulations. De-identified data means that all **personal identifiers** (e.g., names, medical record numbers, or any information that could potentially re-identify the individual) are removed, making it impossible to trace the data back to specific individuals.

However, researchers should consult their institution's IRB to confirm that their de-identification process aligns with regulatory standards and institutional policies. If there is any question about whether the data are fully de-identified, the IRB may still conduct a limited review to ensure compliance.[18,19,20]

▸▸ Question 36

In designing a multicenter RCT, which strategy best reduces selection bias?

- A. Randomizing participants at each site
- B. Ensuring equal sample sizes at all centers
- C. Blinding data analysts to group assignments
- D. Using strict inclusion and exclusion criteria
- E. Allowing clinicians to choose patient assignments

Correct answer is D

Using strict inclusion and exclusion criteria helps ensure that participants are selected consistently, reducing selection bias.

▸▸ Question 37

A neurosurgery resident observes that patients with a certain genetic marker have different outcomes after surgery. She initiates a study to explore this association. Which type of study design is most appropriate?

- A. Case report
- B. Cross-sectional study
- C. Cohort study
- D. Case–control study
- E. Randomized controlled trial

Correct answer is C

A cohort study follows a group with a shared characteristic over time to observe outcomes, suitable for exploring associations between exposures (genetic markers) and outcomes.

▸▸ Question 38

When reporting study results, which measure is most appropriate to describe the precision of an estimated treatment effect?

- A. *p*-Value
- B. Confidence interval
- C. Standard deviation
- D. Mean difference
- E. Risk ratio

Correct answer is B

A confidence interval provides a range within which the true effect size is expected to lie, indicating the precision of the estimate.

▸▸ Question 39

A neurosurgeon wants to test a new device that requires FDA approval. Before starting the clinical trial, she must ensure compliance with which regulatory body's guidelines?

- A. Institutional Review Board
- B. Department of Health and Human Services
- C. Food and Drug Administration (FDA)
- D. Centers for Medicare and Medicaid Services
- E. Occupational Safety and Health Administration

Correct answer is C

The FDA regulates clinical trials involving new medical devices, ensuring safety and efficacy before approval.[21,22]

▸▸ Question 40

A neurosurgical study aims to determine if a new intervention is superior to the standard treatment. The null hypothesis states there is no difference between treatments. If the study incorrectly concludes that the new intervention is better when it is not, this is an example of:

- A. Type I error
- B. Type II error
- C. Beta error
- D. Statistical power
- E. Confounding variable

Correct answer is A

A Type I error occurs when the null hypothesis is incorrectly rejected, concluding that a difference exists when it does not.

References

[1] Rosenthal JW, Bakillah E, Acker RC, et al. Pilot study of provider adherence to language services for surgical patients with limited English proficiency. Am J Surg 2025;247: 116473

[2] Jain S, Chanmin Z, Havasy J, et al. Stepping up informed consent: navigating foot and ankle orthopedics. Foot Ankle Spec 2025:19386400251336807

[3] Ahmed S, Reichert Z, Santillanes G, et al. Civil monetary penalties from violations of the emergency medical treatment and labor act for patients arriving or leaving with law enforcement. West J Emerg Med 2025;26(3):712–719

[4] Terp S, Wang B, Burner E, et al. Civil monetary penalties resulting from Violations of the Emergency Medical Treatment and Labor Act (EMTALA) involving psychiatric emergencies, 2002 to 2018. Acad Emerg Med 2019;26 (5):470–478

[5] Weaver MD, Sullivan JP, Landrigan CP, Barger LK. Systematic review of the impact of physician work schedules on patient safety with meta-analyses of mortality risk. Jt Comm J Qual Patient Saf 2023;49(11):634–647

[6] Weaver MD, Landrigan CP, Sullivan JP, et al. National improvements in resident physician-reported patient safety after limiting first-year resident physicians' extended duration work shifts. BMJ Qual Saf 2022;32(2):81–89

[7] Awan M, Zagales I, McKenney M, et al. ACGME 2011 duty hours restrictions and their effects on surgical residency training and patients outcomes: a systematic review. J Surg Educ 2021;78(6):e35–e46

[8] Schwartz LP, Hursh SR, Boyle L, et al. Fatigue in surgical residents: an analysis of duty-hours and the effect of hypothetical naps on predicted performance. Am J Surg. 2020;221(5):866–871

[9] Cheng S, Duan W, Zhou W. From symbolism to substance: evaluating state disclosure laws and the case for federal oversight. Front Health Serv 2025;5:1666949

[10] Cronin C, Drmanovic A, Hammadeh Z, et al. Trends in research payments from industry to dermatologists. Cureus 2025;17(10):e94824

[11] CMS Open Payments Program. Accessed May 6, 2025 at: https://www.cms.gov/openpayments/program-participants/reporting-entities/data-collection

[12] Huang LL, Yang JH, Hong WW, et al. Tracing missing surgical specimens: a quality improvement strategy for adverse events based on root cause analysis. Risk Manag Healthc Policy 2025;18:2139–2150

[13] Mohamed A, Fuad U, Hagroo A, Elasad A. Best practices for surgical safety in orthopaedics: a comprehensive review of checklist implementation. Cureus 2025;17(8):e89476

[14] Ong J, Hansemann BK, Lee PP, Weizer JS. Safety outcomes following implementation of a systematic cataract surgery protocol at a tertiary referral eye center. J Patient Saf 2025;21(7):460–466

[15] Ries SA, Zolfaghari EJ, Higaki A, et al. Gender disparities in cardiothoracic surgical conference scholarly interactions: A prime opportunity for change in culture. JTCVS Open 2025;24:521–526

[16] Alshamrani KM, Basalamah EK, AlQahtani GM, et al. Saudi radiology trainees' insights on safety and professionalism in the workplace. Peer J 2025;13:e19257

[17] Wasserstein RL, Lazar NA. The ASA's statement on p-values: context, process, and purpose. Am Stat 2016;70(2):129–133

[18] Indrayan A. P values, power, and medical significance for credible results. J Postgrad Med 2025;71(2):91–94

[19] Miola AC, Espósito ACC, Miot HA. Techniques for randomization and allocation for clinical trials. J Vasc Bras 2025;23: e20240046

[20] Bhowmik B, Siddiquee T, Munir SB, et al. Faith-based lifestyle intervention for diabetes prevention among adults in Bangladesh: a cluster randomized clinical trial. JAMA Netw Open 2025;8(10):e2538101

[21] Almarie B, Pacheco-Barrios K, Gianlorenco AC, et al. Clinical trial design in FDA submissions for neuromodulation devices, 1960–2023: a systematic review and meta-analysis. Expert Rev Med Devices 2025;22(9):1027–1050

[22] Hendrickson BA, McShea C, Hammad TA, et al. Publicly available clinical trial safety data: review and a call for standardization and improved reporting practices. Pharmaceut Med 2025

Index

Note: Page numbers set **bold** or *italic* indicate headings or figures, respectively.

A

B

C

T

U

V

W

X